Primary Mental Health Care in a New Era

Primary Mental Health Care in a New Era

Editors

Athanassios Tselebis
Argyro Pachi

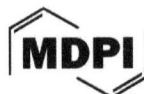

Basel • Beijing • Wuhan • Barcelona • Belgrade • Novi Sad • Cluj • Manchester

Editors
Athanassios Tselebis
"Sotiria" General Hospital of
Chest Diseases
Athens, Greece

Argyro Pachi
"Sotiria" General Hospital of
Chest Diseases
Athens, Greece

Editorial Office
MDPI
St. Alban-Anlage 66
4052 Basel, Switzerland

This is a reprint of articles from the Special Issue published online in the open access journal *Healthcare* (ISSN 2227-9032) (available at: https://www.mdpi.com/journal/healthcare/special_issues/Primary_Era).

For citation purposes, cite each article independently as indicated on the article page online and as indicated below:

Lastname, A.A.; Lastname, B.B. Article Title. *Journal Name* **Year**, *Volume Number*, Page Range.

ISBN 978-3-0365-9651-8 (Hbk)
ISBN 978-3-0365-9650-1 (PDF)
doi.org/10.3390/books978-3-0365-9650-1

© 2023 by the authors. Articles in this book are Open Access and distributed under the Creative Commons Attribution (CC BY) license. The book as a whole is distributed by MDPI under the terms and conditions of the Creative Commons Attribution-NonCommercial-NoDerivs (CC BY-NC-ND) license.

Contents

About the Editors vii

Preface ix

Athanasios Tselebis and Argyro Pachi
Primary Mental Health Care in a New Era
Reprinted from: *Healthcare* **2022**, *10*, 2025, doi:10.3390/healthcare10102025 1

Argyro Pachi, Christos Sikaras, Ioannis Ilias, Aspasia Panagiotou, Sofia Zyga, Maria Tsironi, et al.
Burnout, Depression and Sense of Coherence in Nurses during the Pandemic Crisis
Reprinted from: *Healthcare* **2022**, *10*, 134, doi:10.3390/healthcare10010134 5

Christos Sikaras, Sofia Zyga, Maria Tsironi, Athanasios Tselebis, Argyro Pachi, Ioannis Ilias and Aspasia Panagiotou
The Mediating Role of Depression and of State Anxiety on the Relationship between Trait Anxiety and Fatigue in Nurses during the Pandemic Crisis
Reprinted from: *Healthcare* **2023**, *11*, 367, doi:10.3390/healthcare11030367 17

Patrick R. Krill, Hannah M. Thomas, Meaghyn R. Kramer, Nikki Degeneffe and Justin J. Anker
Stressed, Lonely, and Overcommitted: Predictors of Lawyer Suicide Risk
Reprinted from: *Healthcare* **2023**, *11*, 536, doi:10.3390/healthcare11040536 31

Janett V. Chávez Sosa, Flor M. Mego Gonzales, Zoila E. Aliaga Ramirez, Mayela Cajachagua Castro and Salomón Huancahuire-Vega
Depression Associated with Caregiver Quality of Life in Post-COVID-19 Patients in Two Regions of Peru
Reprinted from: *Healthcare* **2022**, *10*, 1219, doi:10.3390/healthcare10071219 47

Argyro Pachi, Athanasios Tselebis, Ioannis Ilias, Effrosyni Tsomaka, Styliani Maria Papageorgiou, Spyros Baras, et al.
Aggression, Alexithymia and Sense of Coherence in a Sample of Schizophrenic Outpatients
Reprinted from: *Healthcare* **2022**, *10*, 1078, doi:10.3390/healthcare10061078 57

Yao-Yu Lin, Wen-Jiuan Yen, Wen-Li Hou, Wei-Chou Liao and Mei-Ling Lin
Mental Health Nurses' Tacit Knowledge of Strategies for Improving Medication Adherence for Schizophrenia: A Qualitative Study
Reprinted from: *Healthcare* **2022**, *10*, 492, doi:10.3390/healthcare10030492 81

Francisco Javier Ruiz-Sánchez, Maria do Rosário Martins, Salete Soares, Carlos Romero-Morales, Daniel López-López, Juan Gómez-Salgado and Ana María Jiménez-Cebrián
Impact of Multiple Sclerosis and Its Association with Depression: An Analytical Case-Control Investigation
Reprinted from: *Healthcare* **2022**, *10*, 2218, doi:10.3390/healthcare10112218 97

Aniel Jessica Leticia Brambila-Tapia, Fabiola Macías-Espinoza, Yesica Arlae Reyes-Domínguez, María Luisa Ramírez-García, Aris Judit Miranda-Lavastida, Blanca Estela Ríos-González, et al.
Association of Depression, Anxiety, Stress and Stress-Coping Strategies with Somatization and Number of Diseases According to Sex in the Mexican General Population
Reprinted from: *Healthcare* **2022**, *10*, 1048, doi:10.3390/healthcare10061048 105

Mohammed Ahmed Aleisa, Naif Saud Abdullah, Amar Abdullah A. Alqahtani, Jaber Ahmed J Aleisa, Mohammed R. Algethami and Najim Z. Alshahrani
Association between Alexithymia and Depression among King Khalid University Medical Students: An Analytical Cross-Sectional Study
Reprinted from: *Healthcare* **2022**, *10*, 1703, doi:10.3390/healthcare10091703 . . . . **115**

Alicia Ponce-Valencia, Diana Jiménez-Rodríguez, Agustín Javier Simonelli-Muñoz, Juana Inés Gallego-Gómez, Gracia Castro-Luna and Paloma Echevarría Pérez
Adaptation of the Highly Sensitive Person Scale (HSP) and Psychometric Properties of Reduced Versions of the Highly Sensitive Person Scale (R-HSP Scale) in Spanish Nursing Students
Reprinted from: *Healthcare* **2022**, *10*, 932, doi:10.3390/healthcare10050932 . . . . **129**

Antonella Gagliano, Carola Costanza, Marzia Bazzoni, Ludovica Falcioni, Micaela Rizzi, Costanza Scaffidi Abbate, et al.
Effectiveness of an Educational Filmmaking Project in Promoting the Psychological Well-Being of Adolescents with Emotive/Behavioural Problems
Reprinted from: *Healthcare* **2023**, *11*, 1695, doi:10.3390/healthcare11121695 . . . . **141**

Júlia Gisbert-Pérez, Manuel Martí-Vilar and Francisco González-Sala
Prospect Theory: A Bibliometric and Systematic Review in the Categories of Psychology in Web of Science
Reprinted from: *Healthcare* **2022**, *10*, 2098, doi:10.3390/healthcare10102098 . . . . **155**

About the Editors

Athanassios Tselebis

Dr. Tselebis Athanassios was born and raised in Thessaloniki. He studied Psychology at the Aristotle University of Thessaloniki. He has a Master's degree in Social and Child Psychiatry from the Medical School of the University of Ioannina and a Doctoral degree (PhD) in Epidemiology from the Medical School of the University of Crete. He has worked for more than 20 years as a Clinical Psychologist at the Psychiatric Department of the General Hospital of Chest Diseases in Athens. He has a substantial educational and research background with numerous publications in national and international peer-reviewed journals.

Argyro Pachi

Dr. Pachi Argyro was born and raised in Athens. She studied at the National and Kapodistrian University of Athens' School of Medicine and holds a Master's degree in the "Mental Health Promotion and Prevention of Psychiatric Disorders" from the National and Kapodistrian University of Athens. She has worked for more than 30 years in primary, secondary, and tertiary psychiatric care. For the last five years, she has been the Director of the Psychiatric Department of the General Hospital of Chest Diseases in Athens. She has a substantial educational and research background with numerous publications in national and international peer-reviewed journals.

Preface

Working as mental health professionals in a General Chest Diseases Hospital, which was exclusively treating patients with COVID-19 during the pandemic, we have witnessed healthcare personnel being emotionally overwhelmed and patients and their relatives under great psychological and physical stress. We also experienced tremendous pressure while trying to evaluate their psychological distress under unprecedented circumstances in times of health crisis and organize more targeted and effective support interventions. Our aim was to gather information on the current psychosocial and mental health needs of the community population, globally, during the COVID-19 pandemic. The motivation was to communicate a paradigm shift to better address the multiple challenges in Primary Mental Health Care. The pluralistic content and the diverse approaches of the included research articles make the published contributions valuable from a research and clinical point of view, for health professionals, trainees, and the broader reader audience. We would like to thank all contributing authors and all included participants for their commitment and support.

Athanassios Tselebis and Argyro Pachi
Editors

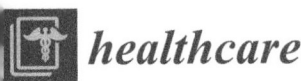

Editorial

Primary Mental Health Care in a New Era

Athanasios Tselebis * and Argyro Pachi

Psychiatric Department, "Sotiria" General Hospital of Chest Diseases, 11527 Athens, Greece
* Correspondence: atselebis@yahoo.gr; Tel.: +30-210-776-3186

Clinical experience and scientific studies highlight the pivotal role that primary health care services have and should have as a gateway to the health care system and as a first point of contact for patients with mental disorders, particularly—but not exclusively—for patients with a disorder in the spectrum of common mental disorders [1,2]. The role of primary mental health care is early diagnosis and intervention, assessment, treatment planning, referral, monitoring, and prevention at the individual and community level [3]. The principles underlying primary mental health care are accessibility; integrated, coordinated, and continuous care with efficiency; reduction in disparities and improvement in well-being for all; and respect for human rights [4]. A variety of cost-effective mental health delivery models for primary care are available, such as collaborative care [5] and various integrated care models [6].

The population's mental health has deteriorated during the COVID-19 pandemic with the high prevalence of psychological distress forewarning increased rates of mental health disorders [7]. Additionally, the pandemic inadvertently induced global economic recession while at the same time widening pre-pandemic health, social, and economic inequalities [8]. As a consequence, vulnerable populations have been disproportionately afflicted in the COVID-19 era [9]. People suffering from a mental health disorder or disability [10,11], those who are educationally or economically disadvantaged, racial and ethnic minorities, refugees, migrants [12], the homeless, minors, and the elderly are among those adversely affected. Additionally, nontraditional cases are seeking psychosocial counselling, including employed parents as well as school and university students. The effects of the pandemic on diverse populations require the implementation of targeted approaches to mental health care delivery. Scheduling studies without delay by following a pragmatic approach to research, considering current views and experiences and concentrating on providing insightful and practical information in order to prioritize mental health needs among vulnerable populations and effectively allocate resources, is imperative.

Primary mental health care providers are dealing first and foremost with the mental health consequences induced by the pandemic [13]. Managing increasing demand in general practice, primary care professionals have promptly applied digital mental health services to expand the reach and accessibility of mental health care. Digital interventions, such as online platforms, are extensively being used to provide help and support to people with mental health needs [14]. Teleconsultations via telephone or videoconference replaced, as an effective alternative, in-person medical counseling, providing cost-effective interventions remotely while providing immediate access to health care [15,16]. During the changing context of the pandemic, alternative methods of communication were adopted to approach individuals who did not actively access medical care. Screening for and contacting susceptible individuals, organizing and engaging government-provided community services, and monitoring enlisted populations to ensure equitable access to mental health care are of outmost importance. In the planning and organization of health care, involving health care professionals from physicians to community health workers required strengthening personnel, enhancing family practitioners' mental health training, and expanding public psychological services, including through digital modalities, to alleviate emotional

Citation: Tselebis, A.; Pachi, A. Primary Mental Health Care in a New Era. *Healthcare* **2022**, *10*, 2025. https://doi.org/10.3390/healthcare10102025

Received: 29 September 2022
Accepted: 11 October 2022
Published: 14 October 2022

Publisher's Note: MDPI stays neutral with regard to jurisdictional claims in published maps and institutional affiliations.

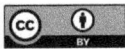

Copyright: © 2022 by the authors. Licensee MDPI, Basel, Switzerland. This article is an open access article distributed under the terms and conditions of the Creative Commons Attribution (CC BY) license (https://creativecommons.org/licenses/by/4.0/).

distress and overcome adversities. Concerns were raised for individuals recovering from the SARS-CoV-2 virus and their caregivers [17], health care staff working on the front lines [18], and socially diverse populations markedly affected by varying degrees of lockdown protocols, such as frail geriatric individuals, people dismissed from employment, working mothers, and youth. It remains unknown whether the implemented programs can keep up with the increasing demands arising during the pandemic.

Enduring challenges emerge when attempting to integrate mental health care within the primary health care system in today's environment. Several issues originated during the pandemic, while others pre-existed and were aggravated [19]. A survey conducted by the World Health Organization disclosed that the vast majority (93%) of 130 countries suspended outpatient and community mental health services [20]. Meanwhile, ministerial recommendations insisted on enhanced cooperation and teamwork between primary and community mental health services with secondary specialized mental health care, emphasizing the need for community services' contribution in quality health interventions, and underscoring mental health care in primary and community-based settings. Few recent articles have investigated how best to overcome these barriers in the post-COVID-19 era [21]. Addressing emerging barriers and challenges to treating common mental health conditions and interventions to enhance the primary care of mental health disorders, aiming to review how mental health needs might be managed in the post-COVID-19 era, is a priority.

By the time this Special Issue was launched, the world was responding to the COVID-19 pandemic and already confronting significant mental health problems. Other diseases with distinct epidemiological profiles along with socioeconomic factors constitute the background wherein pandemics prevail. The syndemic approach in the field of mental diseases captures the individual experiences and the environmental socioeconomic impacts, influencing the direction of clinical practice, policy development, and research priorities and dictating what types of interventions matter [22]. Evidence suggests that implementing community interventions may mitigate the adverse mental health consequences of these environmental risk factors [23]. Promoting the COVID-19 vaccination program, financial support measures to counteract recession and inflation, addressing stigma issues reinforced during the pandemic, building the national response framework for pandemic conditions including plans for mental health services, and the dissemination of computerized transformation and innovation are among adaptive responses in different countries to cope with the mental health repercussions.

Global pandemics, climate change, war, and socioeconomic and energy crises outline a frightful environmental scenario. Contextual issues and the impact of social determinants should primarily be considered when implementing practical strategies and promoting interventions. Nowadays, more than ever, mental health care delivery needs a paradigm shift, for pragmatic applications at the clinical level and for scientific purposes, promoting biopsychosocial integrated mental health care with an emphasis on community-based psychosocial support [24]. Recognition of the central role of environmental context in mental health outcomes and earlier mental health interventions at the community level, rather than only at the individual level, serves as a prerequisite in order to reform mental health research and service delivery [25]. According to this transformational shift, social and psychological needs can be addressed at the community level so that fewer people access hospital clinics with staff that may be overwhelmed in dealing with the structural and social issues contributing to patients' mental health needs.

Unfortunately, the mental health care system has always focused on treating the acute phase of psychiatric disorders, minimizing and questioning the effectiveness of mental health prevention and promotion processes. Specific primary prevention approaches (universal, selective, and indicated), or the "stepped care" approach, mostly remain theoretical formulations either fragmentally applied or somehow absent from practical strategies and interventions. The literature suggests that several risk factors are interrelated and tend to have synergistic effects, such as social risk factors combined with the pandemic-induced stressors [26]. People with mental health disorders or disabilities and people who have already been exposed to multiple risk factors may be less able to cope with their impacts, compared to those who have never been exposed to any risk factors. The cumulative effects of environmental risk factors in genetically vulnerable populations increase the likelihood of developing a mental disorder. Data and research are needed to identify the multiple pathways through which risks contribute to a diversity of adverse outcomes among various populations. In these circumstances, the results of epidemiological studies and interventions aimed at understanding the nature of the disease, especially for multifactorial disorders, and detecting or intervening in environmental, social, and other factors involved in the etiopathogenesis of the disorders, are of outmost importance and have practical application.

Since exposure to environmental stressors is unavoidable, strengthening the protective factors that contribute to psychological resilience serves in adaptive coping. Preventive interventions aim to implement strategies, allocate available resources, and modify environmental factors so that they do not cause stress but benefit people's wellbeing. The determinants that compromise mental health are largely beyond the health sector, making effective initiatives more complex and difficult. This underlines the urgent need for interdisciplinary collaboration, multidisciplinary engagement, and transdisciplinary approaches, in order to develop comprehensive strategies to address needs on a global scale. In addition, mental health promotion and prevention call for governments and policy makers to fully recognize the impact of poverty and social disadvantage on the mental health of the population [27]. Changing our perspective about public mental health care requires skills such as assessing community needs, identifying and prioritizing high-risk groups, and intervening with methods such as counseling, training, and crisis intervention. In this way, by providing people more accessible and effective alternatives in a timely manner, we can prevent emergency mental health issues needing urgent secondary mental health care. Addressing persistent and systemic gaps in the mental health delivery system [28] demands reform and structural changes at the institutional, organizational, and administrative level and a package of feasible, safe, and cost-effective community-based interventions with short- and long-term benefits beyond mental health outcomes (educational, functional, and societal).

Author Contributions: Conceptualization, A.P.; formal analysis, A.T.; investigation, A.P.; resources, A.T.; data curation, A.P.; writing—original draft preparation, A.T.; writing—review and editing, A.P.; visualization, A.T.; supervision, A.T. All authors have read and agreed to the published version of the manuscript.

Funding: This research received no external funding.

Conflicts of Interest: The authors declare no conflict of interest.

References

1. Anonymous. What is primary care mental health?: WHO and Wonca Working Party on Mental Health. *Ment. Health Fam. Med.* **2008**, *5*, 9–13.
2. Kyanko, K.A.; ACurry, L.; EKeene, D.; Sutherland, R.; Naik, K.; Busch, S.H. Does Primary Care Fill the Gap in Access to Specialty Mental Health Care? A Mixed Methods Study. *J. Gen. Intern. Med.* **2022**, *37*, 1641–1647. [CrossRef] [PubMed]
3. Ashcroft, R.; Donnelly, C.; Dancey, M.; Gill, S.; Lam, S.; Kourgiantakis, T.; Adamson, K.; Verrilli, D.; Dolovich, L.; Kirvan, A.; et al. Primary care teams' experiences of delivering mental health care during the COVID-19 pandemic: A qualitative study. *BMC Fam. Pract.* **2021**, *22*, 143. [CrossRef]
4. Gómez-Restrepo, C.; Cepeda, M.; Torrey, W.C.; Suarez-Obando, F.; Uribe-Restrepo, J.M.; Park, S.; Acosta, M.P.J.; Camblor, P.M.; Castro, S.M.; Aguilera-Cruz, J.; et al. Perceived access to general and mental healthcare in primary care in Colombia during COVID-19: A cross-sectional study. *Front. Public Health* **2022**, *10*, 896318. [CrossRef]
5. Moise, N.; Wainberg, M.; Shah, R.N. Primary care and mental health: Where do we go from here? *World J. Psychiatry* **2021**, *11*, 271–276. [CrossRef] [PubMed]
6. Ulupinar, D. The need for integrated primary and behavioral healthcare care in the post-pandemic era. *Asian J. Psychiatry* **2021**, *63*, 102772. [CrossRef] [PubMed]

7. Chennapragada, L.; Sullivan, S.R.; Hamerling-Potts, K.K.; Tran, H.; Szeszko, J.; Wrobleski, J.; Mitchell, E.L.; Walsh, S.; Goodman, M. International PRISMA scoping review to understand mental health interventions for depression in COVID-19 patients. *Psychiatry Res.* **2022**, *316*, 114748. [CrossRef] [PubMed]
8. Gong, Y.; Liu, X.; Zheng, Y.; Mei, H.; Que, J.; Yuan, K.; Yan, W.; Shi, L.; Meng, S.; Bao, Y.; et al. COVID-19 Induced Economic Slowdown and Mental Health Issues. *Front. Psychol.* **2022**, *13*, 777350. [CrossRef] [PubMed]
9. Nam, S.H.; Nam, J.H.; Kwon, C.Y. Comparison of the Mental Health Impact of COVID-19 on Vulnerable and Non-Vulnerable Groups: A Systematic Review and Meta-Analysis of Observational Studies. *Int. J. Environ. Res. Public Health* **2021**, *18*, 10830. [CrossRef]
10. Bahji, A.; Bach, P.; Danilewitz, M.; El-Guebaly, N.; Doty, B.; Thompson, L.; Clarke, D.E.; Ghosh, S.M.; Crockford, D. Strategies to aid self-isolation and quarantine for individuals with severe and persistent mental illness during the COVID-19 pandemic: A systematic review. *Psychiatr. Res. Clin. Pract.* **2021**, *3*, 184–190. [CrossRef] [PubMed]
11. Pachi, A.; Tselebis, A.; Ilias, I.; Tsomaka, E.; Papageorgiou, S.M.; Baras, S.; Kavouria, E.; Giotakis, K. Aggression, Alexithymia and Sense of Coherence in a Sample of Schizophrenic Outpatients. *Healthcare* **2022**, *10*, 1078. [CrossRef] [PubMed]
12. Mengesha, Z.; Alloun, E.; Weber, D.; Smith, M.; Harris, P. "Lived the Pandemic Twice": A Scoping Review of the Unequal Impact of the COVID-19 Pandemic on Asylum Seekers and Undocumented Migrants. *Int. J. Environ. Res. Public Health* **2022**, *19*, 6624. [CrossRef]
13. Rohilla, J.; Tak, P.; Jhanwar, S.; Hasan, S. Primary care physician's approach for mental health impact of COVID-19. *J. Fam. Med. Prim. Care* **2020**, *9*, 3189–3194. [CrossRef] [PubMed]
14. Rauschenberg, C.; Schick, A.; Hirjak, D.; Seidler, A.; Paetzold, I.; Apfelbacher, C.; Riedel-Heller, S.G.; Reininghaus, U. Evidence Synthesis of Digital Interventions to Mitigate the Negative Impact of the COVID-19 Pandemic on Public Mental Health: Rapid Meta-review. *J. Med. Internet Res.* **2021**, *23*, e23365. [CrossRef] [PubMed]
15. Chen, J.A.; Chung, W.J.; Young, S.K.; Tuttle, M.C.; Collins, M.B.; Darghouth, S.L.; Longley, R.; Levy, R.; Razafsha, M.; Kerner, J.C.; et al. COVID-19 and telepsychiatry: Early outpatient experiences and implications for the future. *Gen. Hosp. Psychiatry* **2020**, *66*, 89–95. [CrossRef] [PubMed]
16. Althumairi, A.; AlHabib, A.F.; Alumran, A.; Alakrawi, Z. Healthcare Providers' Satisfaction with Implementation of Telemedicine in Ambulatory Care during COVID-19. *Healthcare* **2022**, *10*, 1169. [CrossRef] [PubMed]
17. Sosa, J.V.C.; Gonzales, F.M.M.; Ramirez, Z.E.A.; Castro, M.C.; Huancahuire-Vega, S. Depression Associated with Caregiver Quality of Life in Post-COVID-19 Patients in Two Regions of Peru. *Healthcare* **2022**, *10*, 1219. [CrossRef]
18. Pachi, A.; Sikaras, C.; Ilias, I.; Panagiotou, A.; Zyga, S.; Tsironi, M.; Baras, S.; Tsitrouli, L.A.; Tselebis, A. Burnout, Depression and Sense of Coherence in Nurses during the Pandemic Crisis. *Healthcare* **2022**, *10*, 134. [CrossRef] [PubMed]
19. Spagnolo, J.; Beauséjour, M.; Fleury, M.J.; Clément, J.F.; Gamache, C.; Sauvé, C.; Couture, L.; Fleet, R.; Knight, S.; Gilbert, C.; et al. Perceptions on barriers, facilitators, and recommendations related to mental health service delivery during the COVID-19 pandemic in Quebec, Canada: A qualitative descriptive study. *BMC Prim. Care* **2022**, *23*, 32. [CrossRef]
20. Henderson, E. WHO Survey: COVID-19 Halted Mental Health Services in 93% of Countries. 2020. Available online: https://www.news-medical.net/news/20201005/WHO-survey-COVID-19-halted-mental-health-services-in-9325-of-countries.aspx (accessed on 5 October 2020).
21. Keyes, B.; McCombe, G.; Broughan, J.; Frawley, T.; Guerandel, A.; Gulati, G.; Kelly, B.D.; Osborne, B.; O'Connor, K.; Cullen, W. Enhancing GP care of mental health disorders post-COVID-19: A scoping review of interventions and outcomes. *Ir. J. Psychol. Med.* **2022**, 1–17. [CrossRef] [PubMed]
22. Di Ciaula, A.; Krawczyk, M.; Filipiak, K.J.; Geier, A.; Bonfrate, L.; Portincasa, P. Noncommunicable diseases, climate change and iniquities: What COVID-19 has taught us about syndemic. *Eur. J. Clin. Investig.* **2021**, *51*, e13682. [CrossRef] [PubMed]
23. McGrath, M.; Duncan, F.; Dotsikas, K.; Baskin, C.; Crosby, L.; Gnani, S.; Hunter, R.M.; Kaner, E.; Kirkbride, J.B.; Lafortune, L.; et al. School for Public Health Research Public Mental Health Programme. Effectiveness of community interventions for protecting and promoting the mental health of working-age adults experiencing financial uncertainty: A systematic review. *J. Epidemiol. Community Health.* **2021**, *75*, 665–673. [CrossRef] [PubMed]
24. Smit, D.; Hill, L.; Walton, I.; Kendall, S.; De Lepeleire, J. European Forum for Primary Care: Position Paper for Primary Care Mental Health: Time for change, now more than ever! *Prim. Health Care Res. Dev.* **2020**, *21*, E56. [CrossRef] [PubMed]
25. Alegría, M.; Zhen-Duan, J.; O'Malley, I.S.; DiMarzio, K. A New Agenda for Optimizing Investments in Community Mental Health and Reducing Disparities. *Am. J. Psychiatry* **2022**, *179*, 402–416. [CrossRef]
26. Boden, M.; Zimmerman, L.; Azevedo, K.J.; Ruzek, J.I.; Gala, S.; Abdel Magid, H.S.; Cohen, N.; Walser, R.; Mahtani, N.D.; Hoggatt, K.J.; et al. Addressing the mental health impact of COVID-19 through population health. *Clin. Psychol. Rev.* **2021**, *85*, 102006. [CrossRef] [PubMed]
27. Compton, M.T.; Shim, R.S. Mental Illness Prevention and Mental Health Promotion: When, Who, and How. *Psychiatr. Serv.* **2020**, *71*, 981–983. [CrossRef] [PubMed]
28. Saif-Ur-Rahman, K.M.; Mamun, R.; Anwar, I. Identifying gaps in primary healthcare policy and governance in low-income and middle-income countries: Protocol for an evidence gap map. *BMJ Open* **2019**, *9*, e024316. [CrossRef] [PubMed]

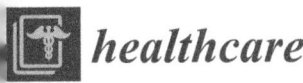 healthcare

Article

Burnout, Depression and Sense of Coherence in Nurses during the Pandemic Crisis

Argyro Pachi [1], Christos Sikaras [2,3], Ioannis Ilias [4], Aspasia Panagiotou [3], Sofia Zyga [3], Maria Tsironi [3], Spyros Baras [1], Lydia Aliki Tsitrouli [1] and Athanasios Tselebis [1,*]

[1] Psychiatric Department, "Sotiria" General Hospital of Chest Diseases, 11527 Athens, Greece; irapah67@otenet.gr (A.P.); spyrosbaras@gmail.com (S.B.); lydiatsitrouli@yahoo.gr (L.A.T.)
[2] Nursing Department, "Sotiria" General Hospital of Chest Diseases, 11527 Athens, Greece; cris.sikaras@gmail.com
[3] Department of Nursing, University of Peloponnese, 22100 Tripoli, Greece; aspasi@uop.gr (A.P.); zygas@uop.gr (S.Z.); tsironi@uop.gr (M.T.)
[4] Department of Endocrinology, "Elena Venizelou" Hospital, 11521 Athens, Greece; iiliasmd@yahoo.com
* Correspondence: atselebis@yahoo.gr; Tel.: +30-210-776-3186

Abstract: During the COVID-19 pandemic, the risk to nurses' mental health has increased rapidly. The aim of the study was to investigate the prevalence of depression and burnout and to evaluate their possible association with the sense of coherence in nursing staff during the pandemic crisis. The Copenhagen Burnout Inventory questionnaire, Beck's Depression Inventory, and the Sense of Coherence questionnaire were completed by 101 male and 559 female nurses. Individual and demographic data were recorded. Regarding depression, 25.5% of respondents exhibited mild depression, 13.5% moderate depression and 7.6% severe depression. In the burnout scale, 47.1% had a pathological value. Female nurses had higher burnout (t test $p < 0.01$, 49.03 vs. 38.74) and depression (t test $p < 0.01$, 11.29 vs. 6.93) scores compared to men and lower levels in the sense of coherence ($p < 0.05$, 59.45 vs. 65.13). Regression evidenced that 43.7% of the variation in the BDI rating was explained by the CBI, while an additional 8.3% was explained by the sense of coherence. Mediation analysis indicated a partial mediation of burnout in the correlation between sense of coherence and depression. The sense of coherence acted as a negative regulator between burnout and depression.

Keywords: depression; sense of coherence; burnout; COVID-19; nurses

1. Introduction

During the COVID-19 pandemic, the risk to nurses' mental health increased rapidly [1–3]. For healthcare workers, the pressure of a professional and social life, along with the occupational hazards associated with exposure to the SARS-CoV-2 virus, lead to increased physical and mental fatigue, as well as to burnout [4–6].

Burnout refers to an occupational syndrome associated with emotional and cognitive changes, including emotional exhaustion, depersonalization or cynicism, and diminished feelings of personal effectiveness resulting from chronic work stress [7]. According to Schaufeli and Greenglass, burnout is defined as "a state of physical, emotional and mental exhaustion resulting from long-term involvement in work situations that are emotionally demanding" [8]. Even before the pandemic, nurses had high levels of burnout; studies have shown that burnout can be diagnosed in more than 35% of nurses [9].

The relationship between depression and burnout is a matter of controversy among researchers [10,11]. There is disagreement whether there is an overlap between burnout and depression. More specifically, researchers have argued that since studies have consistently found average to high correlation between depression and burnout, this may indicate overlap, and that burnout may not be a separate psychological phenomenon but a dimension of depression [12]. Kaschka et al. [13] reported that correlations between burnout and depression often occur, indicating that either there is an overlap between burnout and depression, or that burnout is likely to be a risk factor for developing depression. Regarding the similarity of these two entities at the biological level, in their systematic review, Bakusic et al. [14] found that burnout and depression appear to have a common biological basis. On the other hand, researchers [15,16] argue that an important factor that seems to distinguish burnout from depression is the fact that burnout is work-related, while depression is unconfined and pervasive. More specifically, burnout is related to one's work environment, while depression can occur regardless of environmental conditions (e.g., social or family environment). A recent meta-analysis suggests that although burnout and depression are linked, the magnitude of their relationship is not strong enough to suggest that they are parts of the same construct [17].

Sense of Coherence (SOC) was proposed by Antononsky [18,19] as a construct that expresses the degree to which a person has a diffuse, dynamic but lasting sense that stimuli are internal or external and that stressors are understandable (i.e., predictable, structured and explicable), manageable (i.e., there are resources available to meet the requirements of these stimuli) and meaningful (i.e., the requirements are challenges that are worth committing to and addressing). It has been suggested that a strong SOC helps to manage and deal with stress. This idea is the basis of the "salutogenetic model"; a model that explains how people deal with stressors, such as illness and how people remain reasonably healthy physically and emotionally despite stressors and environmental "insults" [20]. The SOC is often considered to be a stable entity that develops in young adulthood and stabilizes around the age of 30 [20].

From the early 1990s [21] until recently [22], a negative association between depression and SOC is a consistent finding. Studies confirm the effect of SOC on depression in patients with physical illness, such as COPD [23], in multiple sclerosis [24], but also in gynecological cancer [25]. In another study, SOC emerged as a strong predictor of symptoms of adolescent depression [26].

The relationship between SOC and burnout has been much less investigated. A recent study found a negative correlation between them [27], confirming an earlier study [28] with the same results.

There is no study in the literature that examines the role of SOC in the relationship between burnout and depression, although an earlier study [28] simply mentions the existence of correlations between the three variables and concludes that the degree of SOC makes individuals either vulnerable or resistant to both depression and burnout.

The aim of the study was to investigate the prevalence of depression and burnout and to evaluate their possible association with the SOC in nursing staff during the pandemic crisis.

2. Subjects and Methods

2.1. Research Design

This was a descriptive correlational study. Anonymous self-report questionnaires were used to record the data. To ensure and further protect the anonymity of individuals to whom released data refer, the K-anonymity property was applied [29]. The questionnaires were sent to the emails of nurses who had been randomly selected from lists of Greek professional nurses' associations. The first page of the electronic questionnaire clearly stated that the completion and submission of the questionnaire was considered a statement of consent. Participation in the research was voluntary. The sample of the study was the nursing staff of Greek public hospitals who responded to the emails. The study was conducted in the second half of March 2021. This study has been approved from the Clinical Research Ethics Committee of "Sotiria" General Hospital (Number 12253/7-5-20) and from the Ethics Committee of the University of Peloponnese (18 January 2021).

2.2. Study Participants

With a target population of 27,103 nurses, a confidence level of 99%, a margin of error of 5%, and percentage of our sample picking a particular answer = 50% (we used 50%, which is conservative and provides the largest needed sample size for the given level of accuracy), the minimum sample of the study was set at 651 individuals A total of 850 nurses were invited to answer the questionnaires and 660 agreed to participate in the survey.

2.3. Measurement Tools

Demographic and social data from study participants included age, gender, and marital status. Professional information included work experience.

2.4. Copenhagen Burnout Inventory

The Copenhagen Burnout Inventory (CBI) is a tool for measuring personal and occupational burnout, consisting of 19 questions. Answers include "always, often, sometimes, rarely, and never/almost never" or "to a very high degree, to a high degree, somewhat, to a low degree and to a very low degree". The response options are coded in scores of 100, 75, 50, 25, and 0. Possible score range for the burnout scales is 0–100 [29]. Higher scores indicate a higher degree of exhaustion.

The questionnaire includes three subscales:

(I) Personal exhaustion, which assesses the degree of physical and psychological exhaustion the person experiences. It refers to both the physical and psychological exhaustion that accumulates in a person during the day, (e.g.,"How often do you feel physically exhausted?").

(II) Work-related exhaustion, which assesses the degree of physical and psychological exhaustion the individual perceives about work. It describes work-related exhaustion (e.g.,"Is your job emotionally exhausting?").

(III) Patient-related exhaustion, which assesses the degree of physical and psychological exhaustion that is considered by the individual to be related to interaction with patients. It depicts exhaustion as a consequence of interpersonal relationships with patients (e.g.,"Does working with patients absorb your energy?") [30].

For the needs of the study, the Greek adaptation of the questionnaire was used. In reliability analysis, Cronbach's alpha exceeds 0.7 for all subscales indicating a high level of internal consistency [30]. A score higher than 50 was considered as indicative of burnout [31,32].

2.5. Beck's Depression Inventory

Beck's Depression Inventory (BDI) measures the cognitive, emotional, behavioral, and physical manifestations of a person's depression over the past week. It consists of 21 topics which are scored on a scale of 0–3 [33]. The total score is obtained after the sum of the ratings of the 21 topics. The stratification of the severity of depressive symptoms is as follows: 0–9 = without depression, 10–15 = mild depression, 16–23 = moderate depression and ≥ 24 = severe depression. The scale, in its Greek form [22], is a short and reliable tool for measuring depression and has been used by nursing staff in Greece [34]. Internal consistency and reliability are high and retest reliability ranges between 0.48–0.86 for clinical groups and 0.60–0.90 for non-clinical populations. Validity in relation to an external criterion for depression, such as the clinical diagnosis, is considered to be satisfactory [35].

2.6. Sense of Coherence Questionnaire-13

The Sense of Coherence questionnaire (SOC) was developed by Antonovsky to assess how people manage stressful situations and stay well [36]. The SOC-13 scale consists of 13 items, each of which is rated on a Likert scale, ranging from 1 ("very common") to 7 ("very rare or never"). The scale includes three dimensions: comprehensibility (five items, measuring the person's perception of the internal and external elements of its environment as structured and predictable); manageability (four items, referring to the person's ability to meet the demands of stressful environment successfully); and meaningfulness (four items, measuring the person's ability to view those demands as worthy challenges, thus referring to its motivation) [37,38]. Scores range from 13 to 91, with the highest scores indicating a stronger SOC. In this study we used the short version of SOC-13, which has been standardized in the Greek population and seems to be a reliable and valid instrument, with a Cronbach alpha of 0.83 [37].

2.7. Statistical Analysis

All variables were evaluated using descriptive statistics and values were expressed as means and standard deviations for continuous variables. The prevalence of fatigue and depression was determined as a percentage. Independent t-tests were performed to evaluate continuous variables by gender. Analysis of variance (ANOVA) with Bonferroni correction was used to check for differences between groups in continuous variables. Pearson Correlation was performed to determine the strength and direction of the relationship between variables. Linear regression models were built to investigate whether related variables were significant predictors of the independent variable. The evaluation of the linear regression hypotheses (linear relationship, independence, homoscedasticity and normality) was carried out by visual inspection of the variables, residual diagrams and quantile-quantile (QQ) plots. Statistical significance was set at $p < 0.05$ (two-tailed) and analyses were performed using IBM SPSS Statistics 23 (IBM SPSS Statistics for Windows, Version 23.0, IBM Corp, Armonk, NY, USA). Mediation and moderation analyses were conducted using the Hayes SPSS Process Macro. Average scores for the research parameters were compared versus the results obtained in our previous studies in the pre-COVID-19 era [28,35]. IBM SPSS AMOS 23 Graphics was utilized to construct Figure 1.

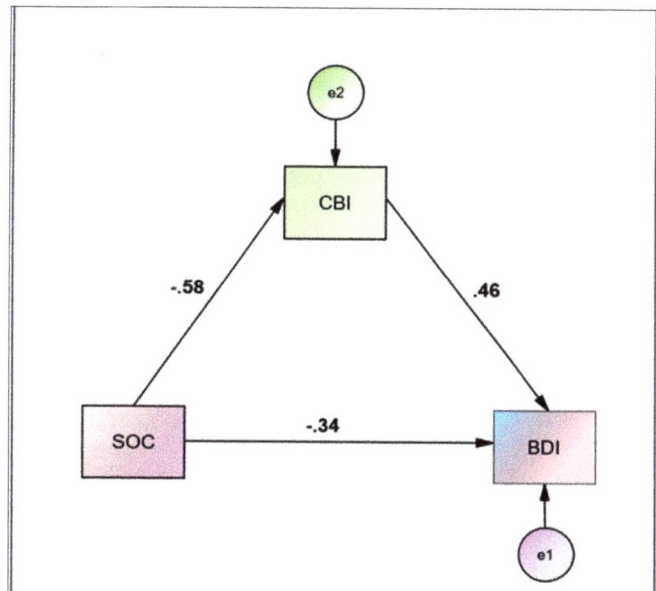

Figure 1. Mediation analysis of Copenhagen Burnout Inventory (CBI) on Sense of Coherence questionnaire (SOC)—Beck's Depression Inventory (BDI) relationship.

3. Results

A total of 101 men (15.3%) and 559 women (84.7%) nurses participated in the study; 375 nurses reported being married (56.8%), 211 (32.0%) unmarried, and 74 (11.2%) divorced. The sample evidenced no difference in marital status (ANOVA $p > 0.05$). Female nurses had higher burnout values (t test $p < 0.01$, 49.03 vs. 38.74) and depression (t test $p < 0.01$, 11.29 vs. 6.93), but also lower SOC values compared to men (t test $p < 0.05$, 59.45 vs. 65.13,

Table 1). Gender differences were statistically significant in both the burnout subscales and the SOC (Table 1).

Regarding depression, 25.5% showed mild depression, 13.5% moderate depression and 7.6% severe depression. On the fatigue scale, 47.1% scored above cutoff. The mean depression score, compared to previous studies [35], was statistically higher in both women (11.29 vs. 8.5 sample t-test $p < 0.01$) and in men (6.93 vs. 4.6 sample t-test $p < 0.01$). The average SOC was statistically lower compared to previous studies [28] in Greek nurses (60.33 vs. 63.6 sample t-test $p < 0.01$).

Table 1. General characteristics of nursing staff and SOC/CBI scores with regards to gender.

P	D.S.	Age	W.E. (in Years)	BDI	Sense of Coherence Questionnaire (SOC)				Copenhagen Burnout Inventory (CBI)			
					Total	A	B	C	Total	Personal Burnout	Work Related Burnout	Patient Related Burnout
Men N = 101	Mean	44.59 *	19.07	6.93 **	65.13 **	24.64 **	18.50 **	21.98 *	38.74 **	38.65 **	42.99 **	33.87 *
	SD	9.42	9.98	5.45	14.01	6.08	5.05	4.76	18.72	18.89	21.77	22.13
Women N = 559	Mean	42.13 *	17.50	11.29 **	59.45 **	21.86 **	16.58 **	20.95 *	49.03 **	52.22 **	54.67 **	39.27 *
	SD	9.89	10.75	8.16	12.94	5.88	4.85	4.39	18.36	19.05	21.67	22.98
Total N = 660	Mean	42.51	17.74	10.62	60.33	22.29	16.88	21.11	47.46	50.14	52.88	38.49
	SD	9.85	10.64	7.95	7.95	5.99	4.93	4.44	18.77	19.63	22.07	22.92

Notes: * independent t-test $p < 0.05$; ** independent t-test $p < 0.01$. Abbreviations: P, Participants; D.S., Descriptive Statistics; W.E., Work Experience; BDI, Beck's Depression Inventory; A, Comprehensibility; B, Manageability; C, Meaningfulness.

Significant negative correlations were evidenced among scores on the SOC scale ($p < 0.01$) with both CBI as well as with BDI scales. However, a positive correlation ($p < 0.01$) was indicated between CBI and BDI (Table 2).

Table 2. Correlations among age, work experience (in years), CBI, SOC, and BDI.

Pearson Correlation N = 660		AGE	Work Experience (in Years)	Sense of Coherence (SOC)	Beck Depression Inventory (BDI)
Work Experience (in Years)	r	0.922 **			
	p	0.001			
Sense of Coherence (SOC)	r	0.114 **	0.075		
	p	0.001	0.054		
Beck Depression Inventory (BDI)	r	0.025	0.038	−0.628 **	
	p	0.518	0.329	0.001	
Copenhagen Burnout Inventory (CBI)	r	0.045	0.094 *	−0.602 **	0.663 **
	p	0.244	0.016	0.001	0.001

Notes: * $p < 0.05$ or ** $p < 0.01$.

A stepwise multiple regression analysis was performed to identify the best predictors for BDI. We defined depression as a dependent variable and as independent variables: work experience, age, burnout and sense of coherence. We tested this model for the absence of multicollinearity. This regression showed that 43.7% of the variation in the BDI score can be explained by the CBI, while an additional 8.3% is explained by SOC; the other variables did not explain the variance in BDI (Table 3).

Table 3. Stepwise multiple regression (only statistically significant variables are included).

Dependent Variable: Beck Depression Inventory (BDI)	R Square	R Square Change	Beta	t	p
Copenhagen Burnout Inventory (CBI)	0.437	0.437	0.661	22.55	0.01 *
Sense of Coherence (SOC)	0.721	0.083	−0.361	−10.66	0.01 *

Notes: Beta = standardized regression coefficient; correlations are statistically significant at the * $p < 0.01$ level.

Bootstrapping was performed with the Hayes SPSS Process Macro to examine whether burnout mediated the relationship between SOC and depressive symptoms: based on 5000 bootstrap samples, a significant indirect relationship between SOC and depressive symptoms was mediated by burnout (Table 4, Figure 1). The outcome variable for the analysis was BDI. The predictor variable for the analysis was SOC. The mediator variable for the analysis was CBI. The indirect effect of CBI on BDI was found to be statistically significant [B= −0.1597, 95% C.I. (−0.1899, −0.1308), $p < 0.05$]. The model explains 42.5% of the variance in the outcome variable. Standardized coefficients for the variables are depicted in Figure 1.

Table 4. Mediation analysis of Copenhagen Burnout Inventory (CBI) on Sense of Coherence (SOC)–Beck Depression Inventory (BDI) relationship.

Variable	b	SE	t	p	95% Confidence Interval	
					LLCI	ULCI
SOC → CBI	−0.8515	0.0442	−19.2810	0.001	−0.9382	−0.7648
SOC → BDI	−0.3759	0.0182	−20.6734	0.001	−0.4115	−0.3402
SOC → CBI → BDI	0.1875	0.0143	13.0854	0.001	0.1594	0.2157
Effects						
Direct	−0.2162	0.0203	−10.6601	0.001	−0.2560	−0.1764
Indirect *	−0.1597	0.0149			−0.1899	−0.1308
Total	−0.3759	0.0182	−20.6734	0.001	−0.4115	−0.3402

* Based on 5000 bootstrap samples.

Finally, the moderation role of SOC in the relationship between CBI and BDI was assessed. A simple moderation analysis was performed using the PROCESS method (with CBI as the predictor variable, BDI as the outcome variable and SOC as the moderator variable) (Table 5). The interaction between CBI and SOC was found to be statistically significant [B = −0.0051, 95% CI (−0.0065, −0.0036) $p < 0.05$]. The effect of CBI on BDI showed corresponding results.

Table 5. Moderation analysis: SOC as a negative moderator of the relationship between CBI and BDI.

Outcome Variable: Beck Depression Inventory (BDI)	b	SE	t	p
Constant	−0.6021 [−6.0401, 4.8359]	2.7694	−0.2174	0.8280
Copenhagen Burnout Inventory (CBI)	0.4945 [0.4037, 0.5853]	0.0463	10.6909	0.001
Sense of coherence (SOC)	0.0246 [−0.0535, 0.1026]	0.0398	0.617	0.5371
Interaction (CBI × SOC)	−0.0051 [−0.0065, −0.0036]	0.0007	−6.9555	0.001

At low moderation (SOC = 47.00) the conditional effect was 0.2564 [95% CI (0.2230, 0.2898), $p < 0.05$]. At middle moderation (SOC = 61.00) the conditional effect was 0.1855

[95% CI (0.1583, 0.2127), $p < 0.05$]. At high moderation (SOC = 74) the conditional effect was 0.1196 [95% CI (0.0864, 0.1529), $p < 0.05$] (Figure 2). These results identify SOC as a negative moderator of the relationship between CBI and BDI.

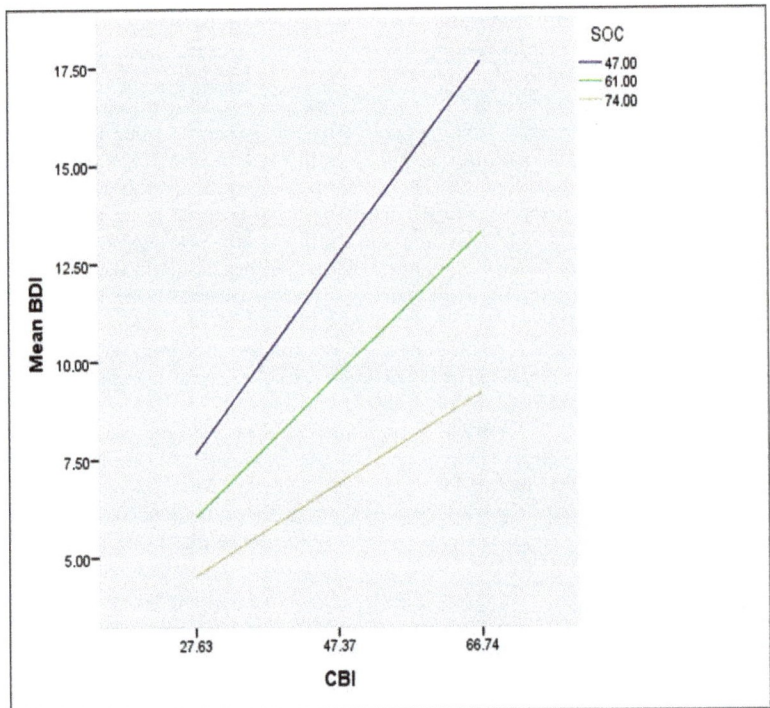

Figure 2. The moderation effect of SOC, between CBI and BDI relationship, at low (47) middle (61) and high (74) degree of SOC.

4. Discussion

A second mental health pandemic is likely to coexist with the COVID pandemic. Nursing staff appear to be particularly vulnerable to the pressure created by the pandemic situation; especially the female population who exhibited higher values of burnout and depression but also lower values of coherence. Scientific studies indicate stronger SOC scores among males compared with females [38,39], but also suggest the dynamic impact of age on SOC [38]. In our sample the female population is significantly younger than males, possibly explaining, in part, the difference in SOC scores, assuming age serves as a confounding variable. Furthermore, research argue that men and women are differentially affected by stressors and make different use of their coping resources [40].These findings are consistent with reviews and meta-analyses indicating that female nurses are more vulnerable to adverse mental health effects; facts that should be taken into consideration in further research on stress, coping, and health [4,41,42].

High rates of burnout and depression in health care workers are a consistent finding in studies worldwide even before COVID-19 [28,43,44]; the pandemic crisis has highlighted the problem. The increase in burnout may be due to the high pressure exerted on hospitals by the pandemic [4]. At the time of the study, cases and admissions to Greek hospitals were on the rise, while work leave for healthcare staff had been suspended for the preceding five months.

In the given period the mental health of the healthcare personnel is especially important for the society as a whole. Firstly, because it has a decisive effect on the quality of health services as mentioned in several studies [45] and, secondly, because it can affect the relationship of public trust in the healthcare system; a factor particularly important in ending the pandemic.

The association between burnout and depression was confirmed in the present study. This correlation (r = 0.66), although being strong, cannot justify an overlap of burnout and depression. The interpretation of the variation of depression from burnout at 43.7% leaves the issue open. Mediation analysis identified burnout as a contributing factor to depression. We would, therefore, prefer to adopt the suggestion given by the World Health Organization, which recognizes burnout as a separate entity, both in International Classification of Diseases (ICD)-10 and ICD-11, giving the code Z 73.0, i.e., as a factor that affects health but not as a separate disease. It is of interest to point out that only one European country has recognized burnout as an occupational disease [46].

The results of the study identify SOC as the negative moderator of the relationship between CBI and BDI. Recent studies highlight the role of SOC in mental health during the pandemic. In particular, a study conducted in eight countries found that a weak SOC was associated with an increased likelihood of "potential depression or anxiety disorder" [47]. A similar result was found in adult samples from Italy [48], and also from Germany [49]. The authors of the latter work explicitly recommended interventions aimed at strengthening the SOC in vulnerable individuals.

Alternatively, interventions have been suggested that use cognitive-behavioral techniques to help people find ways to overcome negative thought patterns and change the way they respond to things that make them feel anxious or upset. Such interventions may include self-help management techniques (e.g., online cognitive behavioral therapy—CBT) [50].

In conclusion, we would like to point out that psychological interventions cannot and should not conceal the real shortcomings of a health system. The theoretical basis of the SOC is to explain why despite the great pressure exerted on them, there were nurses who did not experience burnout and/or depression. The health system is responsible for alleviating the imposed pressure by providing staff with appropriate working conditions, such as adequate supplies and equipment (e.g., PPE), an appropriate patient–nurse ratio, and a work schedule that ensures sufficient rest.

Finally, we will reiterate the message from the World Health Organization for health workers, warning that managing mental health and psychosocial well-being during this pandemic is as important as managing physical health.

The current research was carried out during the COVID-19 pandemic. Therefore, to follow pandemic instructions, data were collected with the online method instead. This meant that nurses without internet access could not participate. Subsequently, the collected data do not represent such groups' considerations and influences the study's generalizability. Additionally, the self-reported data were subject to common method biases. Moreover, owing to the periodical rotation of the nursing personnel, contextual factors relating to the unit where the nurses worked were not included in data collection. Finally, the study was cross-sectional. Therefore, causality between the study's variables cannot be determined.

5. Conclusions

We evidenced high rates of depression and burnout in nursing staff. Mediation analysis highlighted burnout as a factor influencing depression, while sense of coherence functioned as a negative moderator between burnout and depression. Psychological, as well as administrative, interventions are necessary to be implemented immediately to address the problem.

Author Contributions: Conceptualization, A.P. (Argyro Pachi), A.T., C.S.; methodology, A.T., I.I., A.P. (Argyro Pachi); software, A.T., I.I. and A.P. (Aspasia Panagiotou); validation, A.P. (Argyro Pachi), S.Z., M.T.; formal analysis, A.P. (Argyro Pachi), A.T., I.I.; investigation, C.S., A.T.; resources, A.P. (Argyro Pachi); data curation, A.T., I.I., L.A.T., A.P. (Argyro Pachi), S.B.; writing—original draft preparation, A.T., A.P. (Argyro Pachi); writing—review and editing, A.T., C.S., A.P. (Argyro Pachi); supervision,

A.T., A.P. (Argyro Pachi); project administration, A.T., A.P. (Argyro Pachi). All authors have read and agreed to the published version of the manuscript.

Funding: This research received no external funding.

Institutional Review Board Statement: The study was conducted in accordance with the Declaration of Helsinki, and approved by the Clinical Research Ethics Committee of "Sotiria" General Hospital (Number 12253/7-5-20) and from the Ethics Committee of the University of Peloponnese (18 January 2021).

Informed Consent Statement: Informed consent was obtained from all subjects involved in the study since the first page of the electronic questionnaire clearly stated that the completion and submission of the questionnaire was considered a statement of consent. Participation in the research was voluntary.

Data Availability Statement: The data and the questionnaires of the study are available upon request from the corresponding author.

Acknowledgments: We would like to thank all participants in our study.

Conflicts of Interest: The authors declare no conflict of interest.

References

1. Al Maqbali, M.; Al Sinani, M.; Al-Lenjawi, B. Prevalence of stress, depression, anxiety and sleep disturbance among nurses during the COVID-19 pandemic: A systematic review and meta-analysis. *J. Psychosom. Res.* **2021**, *141*, 110343. [CrossRef]
2. Tselebis, A.; Lekka, D.; Sikaras, C.; Tsomaka, E.; Tassopoulos, A.; Ilias, I.; Bratis, D.; Pachi, A. Insomnia, Perceived Stress, and Family Support among Nursing Staff during the Pandemic Crisis. *Healthcare* **2020**, *8*, 434. [CrossRef]
3. Deng, J.; Zhou, F.; Hou, W.; Silver, Z.; Wong, C.Y.; Chang, O.; Huang, E.; Zuo, Q.K. The prevalence of depression, anxiety, and sleep disturbances in COVID-19 patients: A meta-analysis. *Ann. N. Y. Acad. Sci.* **2021**, *1486*, 90–111. [CrossRef]
4. Sikaras, C.; Ilias, I.; Tselebis, A.; Pachi, A.; Zyga, S.; Tsironi, M.; Gil, A.P.R.; Panagiotou, A. Nursing staff fatigue and burnout during the COVID-19 pandemic in Greece. *AIMS Public Health* **2022**, *9*, 94–105. [CrossRef]
5. Ibrahim, F.; Samsudin, E.Z.; Chen, X.W.; Toha, H.R. The Prevalence and Work-Related Factors of Burnout Among Public Health Workforce During the COVID-19 Pandemic. *J. Occup. Environ. Med.* **2022**, *64*, e20–e27. [CrossRef]
6. Batra, K.; Singh, T.P.; Sharma, M.; Batra, R.; Schvaneveldt, N. Investigating the Psychological Impact of COVID-19 among Healthcare Workers: A Meta-Analysis. *Int. J. Environ. Res. Public Health* **2020**, *17*, 9096. [CrossRef]
7. Arnsten, A.F.T.; Shanafelt, T. Physician distress and burnout: The neurobiological perspective. *Mayo Clin. Proc.* **2021**, *96*, 763–769. [CrossRef]
8. Schaufeli, W.B.; Greenglass, E.R. Introduction to special issue on burnout and health. *Psychol. Health* **2001**, *16*, 501–510. [CrossRef]
9. Janeway, D. The Role of Psychiatry in Treating Burnout Among Nurses During the Covid-19 Pandemic. *J. Radiol. Nurs.* **2020**, *39*, 176–178. [CrossRef]
10. Bianchi, R.; Schonfeld, I.S.; Laurent, E. Burnout-depression overlap: A review. *Clin. Psychol. Rev.* **2015**, *36*, 28–41. [CrossRef]
11. Tavella, G.; Parker, G. Distinguishing burnout from depression: An exploratory qualitative study. *Psychiatry Res.* **2020**, *291*, 113212. [CrossRef]
12. Bianchi, R.; Verkuilen, J.; Brisson, R.; Schonfeld, I.S.; Laurent, E. Burnout and depression: Label-related stigma, help-seeking, and syndrome overlap. *Psychiatry Res.* **2016**, *245*, 91–98. [CrossRef]
13. Kaschka, W.P.; Korczak, D.; Broich, K. Burnout: A fashionable diagnosis. *Dtsch. Arztebl. Int.* **2011**, *108*, 781. [CrossRef]
14. Bakusic, J.; Schaufeli, W.; Claes, S.; Godderis, L. Stress, burnout and depression: A systematic review on DNA methylation mechanisms. *J. Psychosom. Res.* **2017**, *92*, 34–44. [CrossRef]
15. Bakker, A.B.; Schaufeli, W.B.; Demerouti, E.; Janssen, P.P.; Van Der Hulst, R.; Brouwer, J. Using equity theory to examine the difference between burnout and depression. *Anxiety Stress Coping* **2000**, *13*, 247–268. [CrossRef]
16. Iacovides, A.; Fountoulakis, K.; Kaprinis, S.; Kaprinis, G. The relationship between job stress, burnout and clinical depression. *J. Affect. Disord.* **2003**, *75*, 209–221. [CrossRef]
17. Koutsimani, P.; Montgomery, A.; Georganta, K. The Relationship Between Burnout, Depression, and Anxiety: A Systematic Review and Meta-Analysis. *Front. Psychol.* **2019**, *13*, 284. [CrossRef]
18. Antonovsky, A. *Health, Stress and Coping*; Jossey Bass Inc.: San Francisco, CA, USA, 1979.
19. Antonovsky, A. *Unraveling the Mystery of Health. How People Manage Stress and Stay Well*; Jossey Bass Inc.: San Francisco, CA, USA, 1987.
20. Eriksson, M.; Mittelmark, M.B. The Sense of Coherence and Its Measurement. In *The Handbook of Salutogenesis*; Springer International Publishing: Cham, Switzerland, 2016.
21. Carstens, J.A.; Spangenberg, J.J. Major depression: A breakdown in sense of coherence? *Psychol. Rep.* **1997**, *80*, 1211–1220. [CrossRef]

22. Généreux, M.; Schluter, P.J.; Landaverde, E.; Hung, K.K.; Wong, C.S.; Mok, C.P.Y.; Blouin-Genest, G.; O'Sullivan, T.; David, M.D.; Carignan, M.E.; et al. The Evolution in Anxiety and Depression with the Progression of the Pandemic in Adult Populations from Eight Countries and Four Continents. *Int. J. Environ. Res. Public Health* **2021**, *18*, 4845. [CrossRef]
23. Tselebis, A.; Bratis, D.; Pachi, A.; Moussas, G.; Karkanias, A.; Harikiopoulou, M.; Theodorakopoulou, E.; Kosmas, E.; Ilias, I.; Siafakas, N.; et al. Chronic obstructive pulmonary disease: Sense of coherence and family support versus anxiety and depression. *Psychiatrike* **2013**, *24*, 109–116.
24. Grothe, L.; Grothe, M.; Wingert, J.; Schomerus, G.; Speerforck, S. Stigma in Multiple Sclerosis: The Important Role of Sense of Coherence and Its Relation to Quality of Life. *Int. J. Behav. Med.* **2021**, 1–7. [CrossRef]
25. Kim, H.S.; Nho, J.H.; Nam, J.H. A serial multiple mediator model of sense of coherence, coping strategies, depression, and quality of life among gynecologic cancer patients undergoing chemotherapy. *Eur. J. Oncol. Nurs.* **2021**, *54*, 102014. [CrossRef]
26. Malinauskiene, V.; Malinauskas, R. Predictors of Adolescent Depressive Symptoms. *Int. J. Environ. Res. Public Health* **2021**, *18*, 4508. [CrossRef]
27. Stoyanova, K.; Stoyanov, D.S. Sense of Coherence and Burnout in Healthcare Professionals in the COVID-19 Era. *Front. Psychiatry* **2021**, *12*, 709587. [CrossRef]
28. Tselebis, A.; Moulou, A.; Ilias, I. Burnout versus depression and sense of coherence: Study of Greek nursing staff. *Nurs. Health Sci.* **2001**, *3*, 69–71. [CrossRef]
29. Samarati, P.; Sweeney, L. *Protecting Privacy When Disclosing Information: K-Anonymity And Its Enforcement through Generalization and Suppression*; Computer Science Laboratory—SRI International: Menlo Park, CA, USA, 1998.
30. Kristensen, T.S.; Borritz, M.; Villadsen, E.; Christensen, K. The Copenhagen Burnout Inventory: A new tool for the assessment of burnout. *Work Stress* **2005**, *19*, 192–207. [CrossRef]
31. Papaefstathiou, E.; Tsounis, A.; Malliarou, M.; Sarafis, P. Translation and validation of the Copenhagen Burnout Inventory amongst Greek doctors. *Health Psychol. Res.* **2019**, *7*, 7678. [CrossRef]
32. Henriksen, L.; Lukasse, M. Burnout among Norwegian midwives and the contribution of personal and work-related factors: A cross-sectional study. *Sex. Reprod. Health* **2016**, *9*, 42–47. [CrossRef]
33. Beck, A.T.; Ward, C.H.; Mendelson, M.; Mock, J.; Erbauch, J. An inventory for measuring depression. *Arch. Gen. Psychiatry* **1961**, *4*, 561–571. [CrossRef]
34. Donias, S.; Demertzis, I. Validation of the Beck depression inventory. In *Proceedings of the 10th Hellenic Congress of Neurology and Psychiatry, Thessaloniki, Greece, 1983*; Varfis, G., Ed.; University Studio Press: Thessaloniki, Greece, 1983; pp. 486–492. (In Modern Greek)
35. Tselebis, A.; Gournas, G.; Tzitzanidou, G.; Panagiotou, A.; Ilias, I. Anxiety and depression in Greek nursing and medical personnel. *Psychol. Rep.* **2006**, *99*, 93–96. [CrossRef]
36. Antonovsky, A. The Structure and properties of the sense of coherence scale. *Soc. Sci. Med.* **1993**, *36*, 725–733. [CrossRef]
37. Anagnostopoulou, T.; Kioseoglou, G. Sense of Coherence Scale. In *Psychometric Tools in Greece*; Stalikas, A., Triliva, S., Roussi, P., Eds.; EllinikaGrammata S.A.: Athens, Greece, 2002; pp. 291–292. (In Modern Greek)
38. Nilsson, K.W.; Leppert, J.; Simonsson, B.; Starrin, B. Sense of coherence and psychological well-being: Improvement with age. *J. Epidemiol. Community Health* **2009**, *64*, 347–352. [CrossRef]
39. Gómez-Salgado, J.; Domínguez-Salas, S.; Rodríguez-Domínguez, C.; Allande-Cussó, R.; Romero-Martín, M.; Ruiz-Frutos, C. Gender perspective of psychological discomfort during COVID-19 confinement among Spanish adult population: A cross-sectional study. *BMJ Open* **2021**, *11*, e051572. [CrossRef]
40. Carmel, S.; Anson, O.; Levenson, A.; Bonneh, D.Y.; Maoz, B. Life events, sense of coherence and health: Gender differences on the kibbutz. *Soc. Sci. Med.* **1991**, *32*, 1089–1096. [CrossRef]
41. Galanis, P.; Vraka, I.; Fragkou, D.; Bilali, A.; Kaitelidou, D. Nurses' burnout and associated risk factors during the COVID-19 pandemic: A systematic review and meta-analysis. *J.Adv. Nurs.* **2021**, *77*, 3286–3302. [CrossRef]
42. Sriharan, A.; West, K.J.; Almost, J.; Hamza, J.A.A.A. COVID-19-Related Occupational Burnout and Moral Distress among Nurses: A Rapid Scoping Review. *Can. J. Nurs. Leadersh.* **2021**, *34*, 7–19. [CrossRef]
43. Elbarazi, I.; Loney, T.; Yousef, S.; Elias, A. Prevalence of and factors associated with burnout among health care professionals in Arab countries: A systematic review. *BMC Health Serv. Res.* **2017**, *17*, 1–10. [CrossRef]
44. Tselebis, A.; Bratis, D.; Karkanias, A.; Apostolopoulou, E.; Moussas, G.; Gournas, G.; Ilias, I. Associations on dimensions of burnout and family support for a sample of Greek nurses. *Psychol. Rep.* **2008**, *103*, 63. [CrossRef]
45. Abraham, C.M.; Zheng, K.; Norful, A.A.; Ghaffari, A.; Liu, J.; Poghosyan, L. Primary care nurse practitioner burnout and perceptions of quality of care. *Nurs. Forum* **2021**, *56*, 550–559. [CrossRef]
46. Lastovkova, A.; Carder, M.; Rasmussen, H.M.; Sjoberg, L.; De Groene, G.J.; Sauni, R.; Vévoda, J.; Vevodova, S.; Lasfargues, G.; Svartengren, M.; et al. Burnout syndrome as an occupational disease in the European Union: An exploratory study. *Ind. Health* **2018**, *56*, 160–165. [CrossRef]
47. Généreux, M.; Schluter, P.J.; Hung, K.K.; Wong, C.S.; Pui Yin Mok, C.; O'Sullivan, T.; David, M.D.; Carignan, M.E.; Blouin-Genest, G.; Champagne-Poirier, O.; et al. One Virus, Four Continents, Eight Countries: An Interdisciplinary and International Study on the Psychosocial Impacts of the COVID-19 Pandemic among Adults. *Int. J. Environ. Res. Public Health* **2020**, *17*, 8390. [CrossRef] [PubMed]

48. Barni, D.; Danioni, F.; Canzi, E.; Ferrari, L.; Ranieri, S.; Lanz, M.; Iafrate, R.; Regalia, C.; Rosnati, R. Facing the COVID-19 Pandemic: The Role of Sense of Coherence. *Front. Psychol.* **2020**, *11*, 578440. [CrossRef] [PubMed]
49. Schäfer, S.K.; Sopp, M.R.; Schanz, C.G.; Staginnus, M.; Göritz, A.S.; Michael, T. Impact of COVID-19 on Public Mental Health and the Buffering Effect of a Sense of Coherence. *Psychother. Psychosom.* **2020**, *89*, 386–392. [CrossRef]
50. Pollock, A.; Campbell, P.; Cheyne, J.; Cowie, J.; Davis, B.; McCallum, J.; McGill, K.; Elders, A.; Hagen, S.; McClurg, D.; et al. Interventions to support resilience and mental health of frontline health and social care professionals during and after a disease outbreak, epidemic or pandemic: A mixed methods systematic review. *Cochrane Database Syst. Rev.* **2020**, *11*, CD013779. [CrossRef] [PubMed]

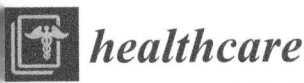

Article

The Mediating Role of Depression and of State Anxiety on the Relationship between Trait Anxiety and Fatigue in Nurses during the Pandemic Crisis

Christos Sikaras [1,2], Sofia Zyga [2], Maria Tsironi [2], Athanasios Tselebis [3,*], Argyro Pachi [3], Ioannis Ilias [4] and Aspasia Panagiotou [2]

1. Nursing Department, "Sotiria" General Hospital of Thoracic Diseases, 11527 Athens, Greece
2. Department of Nursing, University of Peloponnese, 22100 Tripoli, Greece
3. Psychiatric Department, "Sotiria" General Hospital of Chest Diseases, 11527 Athens, Greece
4. Department of Endocrinology, "Elena Venizelou" Hospital, 11521 Athens, Greece
* Correspondence: atselebis@yahoo.gr; Tel.: +30-(210)-776-3186

Abstract: The coronavirus pandemic (COVID-19) is a global health crisis with a particular emotional and physical impact on health professionals, especially nurses. The aim of this study was to investigate the prevalence of anxiety, depression and fatigue and their possible relationships among nurses during the pandemic. The study population consisted of nurses from five tertiary-level public hospitals in Athens who completed the Fatigue Assessment Scale (FAS), Beck Depression Inventory (BDI) and State–Trait Anxiety Inventory (STAI) questionnaires. Gender, age and years of work experience were recorded. The study was conducted from mid-November to mid-December 2021. The sample included 404 nurses (69 males and 335 females) with a mean age of 42.88 years (SD = 10.90) and 17.96 (SD = 12.00) years of work experience. Symptoms of fatigue were noted in 60.4% of participants, while 39.7% had symptoms of depression, 60.1% had abnormal scores on state anxiety and 46.8% on trait anxiety, with females showing higher scores on all scales ($p < 0.05$). High positive correlations ($p < 0.01$) were found between the FAS, BDI, State Anxiety and Trait Anxiety scales. Regression analysis showed that 51.7% of the variance in FAS scores can be explained by trait anxiety, an additional 6.2% by the BDI and 1.2% by state anxiety. Mediation analysis showed that state anxiety and BDI mediate the relationship between trait anxiety and FAS. Finally, BDI was found to exert a moderating role in the relationship between trait anxiety and fatigue. In conclusion, our study showed that nurses continue to experience high rates of anxiety, depression and fatigue. The variation in fatigue appears to be significantly dependent on trait anxiety. Depressive symptomatology and state anxiety exert a parallel positive mediation on the relationship between trait anxiety and fatigue, with depression exhibiting a moderating role in this relationship.

Keywords: depression; anxiety; fatigue; COVID-19; nurses; mediation

Citation: Sikaras, C.; Zyga, S.; Tsironi, M.; Tselebis, A.; Pachi, A.; Ilias, I.; Panagiotou, A. The Mediating Role of Depression and of State Anxiety on the Relationship between Trait Anxiety and Fatigue in Nurses during the Pandemic Crisis. Healthcare 2023, 11, 367. https://doi.org/10.3390/healthcare11030367

Academic Editors: Florin Oprescu and Alyx Taylor

Received: 15 December 2022
Revised: 24 January 2023
Accepted: 26 January 2023
Published: 28 January 2023

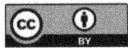

Copyright: © 2023 by the authors. Licensee MDPI, Basel, Switzerland. This article is an open access article distributed under the terms and conditions of the Creative Commons Attribution (CC BY) license (https://creativecommons.org/licenses/by/4.0/).

1. Introduction

The 2019 coronavirus pandemic (COVID-19) has caused a major health crisis worldwide with a huge psychological impact [1–3]. Regarding health professionals, there is consensus across the literature that they are at increased risk of high stress, anxiety, depression, sleep disorders, burnout and post-traumatic stress disorder, with particular emotional and physical impacts [4–8]. In addition, due to the disruption of the balance between their professional and social lives and the occupational risks associated with exposure to the virus, there is an increase in both physical and mental fatigue [9]. Recent studies have shown that nursing staff have higher rates of emotional symptoms compared to other health professionals [10,11]. Work-related fatigue in nurses has been identified as a threat to their health, but it is also associated with negative consequences for safe and quality patient care [12,13]. Work-related fatigue is a complex and multidimensional condition with emotional, physiological, cognitive, mental and sensory components arising as a consequence of excessive work demands and inadequate energy recovery [13]. Moreover, it is positively correlated with levels of anxiety and depression [12]. Anxiety is one of the most common psychiatric disorders in the general population. It consists of a complex cognitive, emotional, physiological and behavioral response related to preparation for anticipated events or circumstances perceived as threatening [14]. Depression is a common mental disorder that presents with a depressed mood, a loss of interest or pleasure, decreased energy, fatigue, feelings of guilt, sleep or appetite disturbances and a lack of concentration [15,16].

Earlier studies had suggested [17,18] that high levels of trait anxiety were a significant risk factor for the development (onset, severity and outcome) of depression. These findings and the high comorbidity between anxiety and depression (up to 60%), but especially the fact that anxiety disorders precede depressive disorders [19], led Sandi and Richter-Levin [20] to hypothesize a "neurocognitive model". According to this model, the neurocognitive style of trait anxiety (neurocognitive maladjustments) plays a central role in the pathological development of depression [20]. More recent studies have argued that high trait anxiety is an important vulnerability phenotype for stress-induced depression [21]. Moreover, studies in breast cancer patients report trait anxiety as an important determinant of both depressive symptoms and fatigue [22,23]. Cognitive theory argues that stressful life events activate some stable underlying dysfunctional maladaptive self-schemata of individuals, which, through automatic cognitive processes, lead to the onset or worsening of depression [24–26]. In summary, trait anxiety makes an individual susceptible to depression [25].

From the above, it is clear that nursing staff are particularly vulnerable to developing physical and psychological problems, especially during the COVID-19 pandemic. It is worth noting that at the time of the study, Greece was experiencing the peak of the fourth wave of the pandemic with the prevalence of the Delta variant, which caused particularly high mortality rates. At that time (mid-November to mid-December 2021), approximately six to seven thousand new cases were being recorded daily, 600–700 patients were hospitalized in intensive care units and 80-100 deaths per day were attributed to COVID-19, with an increasing trend that was difficult to address by the national health system [27], which suffers from a severe shortage of nursing staff [28]. Therefore, the aim of the present study was to study the prevalence of anxiety, depression and fatigue and to investigate the possible relationships among them. By selecting and implementing targeted interventions aimed at enhancing key protective factors, the development of adverse physical and mental conditions can be harnessed.

2. Materials and Methods
2.1. Research Design and Procedure

This was a descriptive correlation study. Data were collected through self-completed questionnaires that were distributed in person to the participants by the researchers. Participation in the study was voluntary. The questionnaire was anonymous, participants had the right to voluntarily withdraw from the study and were aware of the objectives and procedures to be followed.

The study population consisted of a convenience sample of 404 nurses from five large public/academic hospitals in Athens. The above hospitals treated patients with and without COVID-19. The demographics of the study participants included gender and age. Professional information included years of work experience. In the invitation to nurses to participate in the study, an effort was made to make the study sample representative of Greek nurses in terms of gender, years of work and age. The Ethics Committee of the University of Peloponnese approved the study protocol (18699/11-10-2021), as did the Clinical Research Committees of the five hospitals. The study was conducted from mid-November to mid-December 2021.

2.2. Study Participants

With a target population of 27,103 nurses [29] a margin of error of 5%, a confidence level of 95%, and a percentage of the sample selecting a particular response of 50%, the minimum required sample for the study was set at 379. A total of 404 nurses agreed to participate in the study out of 500 nurses who were asked to answer the questionnaires.

2.3. Measures and Instruments

The Fatigue Assessment Scale (FAS) was used to assess fatigue. The FAS consists of 10 questions (e.g., "Fatigue bothers me"). Each question is scored from 1 to 5. Responses include "never, sometimes, often, quite often, always". Total scores range from 10 to 50, with values ≥ 22 indicating fatigue. The FAS questions aim to capture fatigue over the few weeks prior to the questionnaire completion [30]. The reliability and validity of the Greek version of the Fatigue Assessment Scale (FAS) have been tested in a Greek population [21]. The scale has been used in studies of nursing staff in Greece [29]. The internal consistency, as indicated by Cronbach's alpha, was 0.761 [31].

The Beck Depression Inventory (BDI) was used to assess depression. This scale measures the cognitive, emotional, behavioral and physical manifestations of depression in the individual during the week prior to the inventory completion. It consists of 21 items, which are rated on a scale of 0–3 [32]. The items include the following: sadness, pessimism, a feeling of failure, anhedonia, guilt, the expectation of punishment, self-loathing, suicidal ideation, crying, irritability, social withdrawal, indecisiveness, body image, ability to work, insomnia, easy fatigue, anorexia, weight loss, physical preoccupation and loss of libido. The total score is obtained after summing up the scores of the 21 items. The stratification of depressive symptom severity is as follows: 0–9 = no depression, 10–15 = mild depression, 16–23 = moderate depression and ≥ 24 = severe depression. The scale, in its Greek version [33], is a brief and reliable tool for measuring depression and has been applied to nursing staff in Greece [34]. Its internal consistency and reliability are high, and retest reliability ranges from 0.48–0.86 in clinical settings and 0.60–0.90 in the non-clinical population. Validity with respect to an external criterion for depression, such as a clinical diagnosis, is considered satisfactory [33].

The Spielberger State–Trait Anxiety Inventory (STAI-Y Form) was used to assess anxiety. This scale consists of forty items, each of which is scored from 1 to 4. The scale differentiates between anxiety caused by a specific situation (state anxiety) and anxiety that is a more permanent personality trait (trait anxiety). The State Anxiety subscale (STAI Form Y-1) consists of 20 items that assess how the respondent is feeling "right now". In responding to the State Anxiety subscale, individuals select the response that best describes the intensity of their feelings. Answers include "Not at all, somewhat, moderately and a lot". The Trait Anxiety subscale (STAI Form Y-2) consists of 20 items that assess how the respondent feels "in general". In the Trait Anxiety subscale, individuals rate the frequency of their feelings. Answers include "almost never, sometimes, often and almost always". Scores for each subscale can vary from a minimum of 20 to a maximum of 80. Higher scores indicate more anxiety [35]. The scale, in its Greek form, is a short and reliable tool for measuring anxiety. Its internal consistency (Cronbach's alpha) was 0.93 for the State Anxiety subscale and 0.92 for the Trait Anxiety subscale. It is considered to have high internal consistency, reliability and validity [36,37].

2.4. Data Analysis

All variables were evaluated using descriptive statistics, and values were expressed as means and standard deviations for continuous variables. The prevalence of fatigue, anxiety and depression was determined as a percentage. Independent t-tests were conducted to assess continuous variables according to gender. Pearson's correlation was performed to determine the strength and direction of the relationship between variables. Linear regression models were constructed to investigate whether the associated variables were significant predictors of the independent variable. The linear regression hypotheses (linear relationship, independence, homoscedasticity and normality) were assessed by visual inspection of the variables, residual plots and quantile–quantile (QQ) plots. Statistical significance was set at $p < 0.05$ (two-tailed) and analyses were performed using IBM SPSS Statistics 23 (IBM SPSS Statistics for Windows, Version 23.0, IBM Corp, Armonk, NY, USA). Mediation and moderation analyses were performed using the Hayes SPSS Process Macro Models 4 and 5.

3. Results

The sample consisted of 404 nurses (69 men and 335 women) with a mean age of 42.88 years (SD = 10.90) and 17.96 (SD = 12.00) years of experience as nurses (Table 1). In terms of gender (x^2), years of work and age (sample t-test), the sample showed no statistically significant difference ($p > 0.05$) compared to representative samples of the country's nursing workforce from other studies [29].

Table 1. General characteristics of nursing staff and fatigue/anxiety/depression scores with regards to gender.

Participants	Descriptive Statistics	Age	Work Experience (in Years)	Fatigue Assessment Scale	State Anxiety Inventory	Trait Anxiety Inventory	Beck Depression Inventory
Male N = 69	Mean	41.16	15.60	21.25 **	35.47 **	36.32 **	7.06 *
	SD	11.37	11.67	7.43	12.14	11.35	7.15
Female N = 335	Mean	43.23	18.45	24.66 **	40.18 **	40.30 **	9.33 *
	SD	10.79	12.02	7.20	11.59	10.52	7.48
Total N = 404	Mean	42.88	17.96	24.08	39.38	39.62	8.94
	SD	10.90	12.00	7.35	11.80	10.76	7.46

Notes: * independent t-test $p < 0.05$; ** independent t-test $p < 0.01$.

Descriptive statistics of the scales are presented in Table 1. Female nurses showed higher means in all scales compared to the male population (Table 1).

The percentage of nurses who showed fatigue (FAS $\geq$ 22) was 60.4%. The mean fatigue (FAS: 24.08) was statistically lower (sample t-test $p < 0.01$) compared to the mean fatigue (FAS: mean = 25.61, SD = 7.37, N = 701) experienced by nurses in the previous pandemic wave [29]. However, by calculating Hedges' g between the previous measurement and the present measurement, we found a small effect size (g = 0.208).

Regarding depression, 39.7% of the participants had symptoms of depression, (22.4% mild symptoms, 13.7% moderate and 3.6% severe). The mean depressive symptomatology (BDI: 8.94) was shown to be statistically lower (sample t-test $p < 0.01$) compared to the mean depressive symptomatology (BDI: mean = 10.62, SD = 7.65, N = 660) experienced by nurses in a previous phase of the pandemic [34]. By calculating Hedges' g in this instance, we also found a small effect size (g = 0.222).

A total of 60.1% of the participants were found to have abnormal scores in state anxiety and 46.8% in trait anxiety. High positive correlations ($p < 0.01$, Table 2) were found between the fatigue, depression, state anxiety and trait anxiety scales. Age showed a negative correlation with trait anxiety ($p < 0.05$) and a positive correlation ($p < 0.01$) with years of work (Table 2).

Table 2. Correlations among age, work experience (in years), fatigue, anxiety and depression.

Pearson Correlation N = 404		AGE	Work Experience (in Years)	Fatigue Assessment Scale	State Anxiety Inventory	Trait Anxiety Inventory
Work Experience (in Years)	r	0.885 **				
	p	0.001				
Fatigue Assessment Scale	r	−0.096	−0.082			
	p	0.055	0.104			
Spielberger State Anxiety Inventory	r	−0.056	−0.06	0.635 **		
	p	0.258	0.232	0.001		
Spielberger Trait Anxiety Inventory	r	−0.101 *	−0.094	0.715 **	0.789 **	
	p	0.043	0.064	0.001	0.001	
Beck Depression Inventory	r	0.003	0.001	0.707 **	0.603 **	0.750 **
	p	0.951	0.991	0.001	0.001	0.001

* Correlation is significant at the 0.05 level (two-tailed). ** Correlation is significant at the 0.01 level (two-tailed).

A stepwise multiple regression analysis was performed to identify the best predictors of fatigue. With fatigue as the dependent variable, gender, age, years of work, depression, Spielberger Trait Anxiety and Spielberger State Anxiety were given as independent variables. This regression showed that 51.7% of the variance in the Fatigue Assessment Scale score could be explained through the Spielberger Trait Anxiety Inventory, an additional 6.2% was explained through the Beck Depression Inventory and 1.2% through the Spielberger State Anxiety Inventory (Table 3). The other variables did not explain the variance in the Fatigue Assessment Scale.

Table 3. Stepwise multiple regression (only statistically significant variables are included).

Dependent Variable: Fatigue Assessment Scale	R Square	R Square Change	Beta	t	p	Durbin-Watson
Spielberger Trait Anxiety Inventory	0.517	0.517	0.297	4.68	0.01 *	
Beck Depression Inventory	0.577	0.062	0.373	7.58	0.01 *	1.945
Spielberger State Anxiety Inventory	0.591	0.012	0.180	3.43	0.01 *	

Notes: Beta = standardized regression coefficient; correlations are statistically significant at the * $p < 0.01$ level.

With the Hayes SPSS Process Macro (Model 4 with parallel mediators Beck Depression Inventory and Spielberger State Anxiety) bootstrapping was performed in order to first examine whether depression mediates the relationship between trait anxiety and fatigue and, secondly, in the same way, whether state anxiety mediates the relationship between trait anxiety and fatigue.

Based on 5000 bootstrap samples, a significant indirect relationship between trait anxiety and fatigue was found to be mediated by depressive symptomatology (Table 4, Figure 1).

Table 4. Mediation analysis of Beck Depression Inventory (BDI) and Spielberger State Anxiety Inventory (SSAI) on Spielberger Trait Anxiety Inventory (STAI)–Fatigue Assessment Scale (FAS) relationship *.

Variable		b	SE	t	p	95% Confidence Interval	
						LLCI	ULCI
STAI → BDI		0.5256	0.0233	22.5438	0.001	0.4798	0.5715
STAI → SSAI		0.8575	0.0347	24.7243	0.001	0.7993	0.9257
STAI → BDI → FAS		0.3744	0.0484	7.7436	0.001	0.2794	0.4695
STAI → SSAI → FAS		0.1107	0.0325	3.4066	0.001	0.0468	0.1747
STAI → FAS		0.4803	0.0242	19.8655	0.001	0.4237	0.5278
Effects							
Direct		0.1885	0.0433	4.3516	0.001	0.1033	0.2736
Indirect **	Total	0.2918	0.0399			0.2158	0.3689
	BDI	0.1968	0.0311			0.1368	0.2587
	SSAI	0.095	0.0262			0.0446	0.1471
Total (STAI → FAS)		0.4803	0.0242	19.8655	0.001	0.4327	0.5278

* Gender, work experience and age were included in the analysis as covariates variables. They are not shown in the table as they did not give significant statistical results ($p > 0.05$). ** Based on 5000 bootstrap samples.

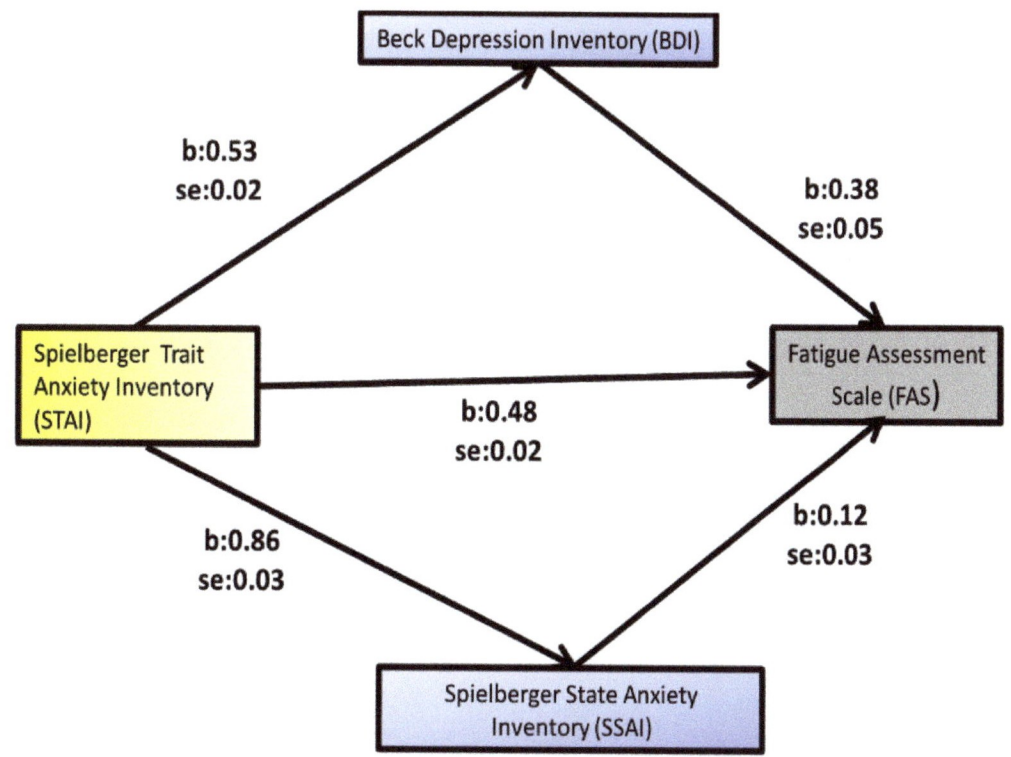

Figure 1. Mediation analysis of Beck Depression Inventory and Spielberger State Anxiety Inventory on Spielberger Trait Anxiety Inventory–Fatigue Assessment Scale relationship (Model 4 with multiple mediators).

The mediator variable for the analysis was the Beck Depression Inventory score. The outcome variable for the analysis was the Fatigue Assessment Scale score. The predictor variable for the analysis was the Trait Anxiety Inventory with the variables gender, work experience and age as covariates. The indirect effect of BDI on fatigue was found to be statistically significant [B = 0.1968, 95% CI (0.1368, 0.2587), $p < 0.05$] (Table 4, Figure 1). The mediation proportion of the model for depression was 41%.

In the same analysis, we used Spielberger State Anxiety as a mediator variable; as an outcome variable, the Fatigue Assessment Scale; as a predictor variable, the Spielberger Trait Anxiety Inventory; and the variables gender, work experience and age as covariates. The indirect effect of Spielberger State Anxiety on fatigue was found to be statistically significant [B = 0.0950, 95% CI (0.0446, 0.1471), $p < 0.05$] (Table 4, Figure 1). The mediation proportion of the model for state anxiety was 20%.

Finally, we examined the moderating role of both the Spielberger State Anxiety and depression in the Spielberger Trait Anxiety–fatigue relationship. Spielberger State Anxiety did not show a moderating role.

In contrast, depression emerged as a positive moderator. Specifically, moderation analysis was performed using the PROCESS method model 5 (with the Spielberger Trait Anxiety Inventory as the predictor variable, the Fatigue Assessment Scale as the outcome variable and the Beck Depression Inventory as the moderator variable). Depression showed a statistically significant moderating role in the Spielberger Trait Anxiety Inventory and Fatigue Assessment Scale relationship ($p < 0.01$, Table 5).

Table 5. Moderation analysis: Beck Depression Inventory (BDI) as a moderator of the relationship between Spielberger Trait Anxiety Inventory (STAI) and Fatigue Assessment Scale (FAS) with Spielberger State Anxiety as a mediator *.

Outcome Variable: Fatigue Assessment Scale (FAS)	b	SE	t	p
Constant	7.3902 [3.1924, 11.5880]	2.1351	3.4614	0.01
Spielberger Trait Anxiety Inventory (STAI)	0.2498 [0.1563, 0.3432]	0.0475	5.2561	0.01
Beck Depression Inventory (BDI)	0.7079 [0.4694, 0.9465]	0.1213	5.834	0.01
Interaction(STAI × BDI)	−0.0070 [−0.0116, −0.0024]	0.0023	−2.9908	0.01

* Gender, work experience and age were included in the analysis as covariate variables. They are not shown in the table as they did not give significant statistical results ($p > 0.05$).

At low moderation (BDI = 1) the conditional effect was 0.2428 [95% CI (0.1512, 0.3343), $p < 0.05$]. At medium moderation (BDI = 8) the conditional effect was 0.1939 [95% CI (0.1096, 0.2783), $p < 0.05$]. At high moderation (BDI = 16) the conditional effect was 0.1381 [95% CI (0.0475, 0.2287), $p < 0.05$] (Figure 2).

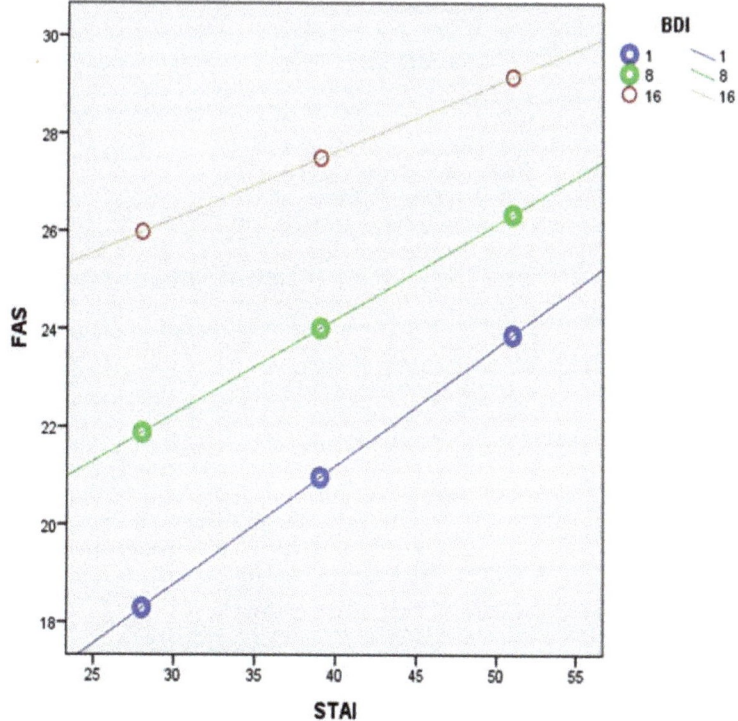

Figure 2. Beck Depression Inventory (BDI) as a moderator of the relationship between Spielberger Trait Anxiety Inventory (STAI) and Fatigue Assessment Scale (FAS), at low (1), middle (8) and high (16) degrees of BDI.

4. Discussion

Alongside the COVID-19 pandemic, an emerging health problem is very likely to co-exist. This problem is pandemic fatigue (PF), which, according to the World Health Organization (WHO), is defined as the physical and mental fatigue that can occur during a pandemic as a consequence of changes in a person's usual activities due to the various measures implemented to reduce the transmission of the virus [38].

Nurses are particularly vulnerable to developing mental and psychological problems, such as higher rates of anxiety, depression, fatigue, mental distress, emotional exhaustion and post-traumatic stress disorder during the peak of the pandemic, potentially increasing the risk of developing PF [39].

Consistent with the above, the results of the present study showed a high prevalence of fatigue, situational and structural anxiety and depression (60.4%, 60.1%, 46.8% and 39.7%, respectively). Our results also showed that Greek nurses had among the highest rates of fatigue [9,12,39], anxiety and depression compared to the findings of studies in other countries [6,10,11].

These findings are probably due, among other reasons, to the fact that Greece, during the period of this study, was experiencing the worst phase of the pandemic [27] in terms of the number of hospitalized patients and mortality, and the resilience of the national health system due to the pandemic was put to test. In addition, it is worth noting that Greece has the lowest ratio of nurses per 1000 inhabitants among European Union countries [28], a finding that partly justifies these findings. Literature data support the positive role of adequate nurse staffing in reducing fatigue, stress and physical and mental exhaustion due to better workload management [39] and subsequent perceived control over work [40].

On the other hand, the resolution of serious problems—such as the provision of personal protective equipment that occurred in the first year of the pandemic [29], the familiarization of nurses with the disease, the increase in information and knowledge about it, and, above all, the complete and universal vaccination of the health care workers' population—are factors that may have been beneficial and may account for the reduction in depression and fatigue compared to the first year of the pandemic. It should be stressed here that this reduction, although statistically significant, does not appear to be clinically important, but it is a finding that may make us more optimistic for the future.

It is known that the prevalence of anxiety and depression is almost twice as high in women as in men [41–45], and studies report that this ratio begins to equalize in the general population with increasing age [46]. In nursing staff, a consistent finding is that the female population has higher rates of anxiety and depression than male nurses [37]. The negative correlation of age with anxiety in the study population confirms the decrease in symptoms of anxiety brought about with increasing age. This negative correlation is well-known among Greek nurses [37]. Studies have tried to explain the increased presence of depressive and anxiety symptomatology by proposing both hormonal factors [46] and social factors [47]. It is possible that both social and instrumental factors are responsible for the presence of increased fatigue in female nurses compared to male nurses.

Statistically significant correlations were found among all the scales considered. Anxiety (state–trait), depression and chronic fatigue were positively correlated with each other. Numerous studies confirm the association between anxiety, depression and fatigue in both nurses [48] and patients with chronic diseases [49]. The findings of this study support a model where trait anxiety accounts for a large proportion of the variance in fatigue.

Furthermore, depressive symptomatology and state anxiety are aggravatingly mediated by depressive symptomatology. This dual mediation works in a parallel fashion, although the mediation effect of depression is twice that of state anxiety. Depressive symptoms are important in this population as they act as a moderator in the relationship between trait anxiety and fatigue. This effect was observed at high, medium and low levels of depression. According to a study by Polikandrioti et al., both anxiety and depression can affect fatigue levels in different ways [50]. People with anxiety are more vulnerable to panic, fear and other high-stress reactions that sequentially increase fatigue levels. In addition, individuals with depression lack motivation or energy to perform either physical or mental tasks and often experience changes in sleep patterns, which in turn increase fatigue levels [50]. However, the association between fatigue and anxiety or depression appears to be a vicious cycle, as a reduction in one can dramatically reduce the risk of developing the other [49], while the presence of one can dramatically increase the risk of developing the other [50].

Ultimately, the nature, as well as the direction, of causality between these variables remains uncertain. While depression appears to be the stronger mediator of the effect of trait anxiety on fatigue, the relationship between the two mediators remains unclear. In future research, it will be useful to use the four-way decomposition method for greater clarity. In addition, our study was synchronic and could not determine with certainty the cause-and-effect relationship beyond the creation of a model. Despite the recent increase in research interest in this area, more longitudinal and/or intervention studies that could further enrich our understanding of the anxiety–fatigue–depression relationship are desirable.

The prevalence of anxiety, depression and fatigue seems to be very high among nurses in Greek hospitals. To reduce the psychological impact of the COVID-19 pandemic on nurses, a number of studies and meta-analyses highlight the positive role of organizational support [51], interventions focused on enhancing resilience [52], appropriate nurse-to-patient ratios [39], proper work time management [53], appropriate remuneration [54], developing fatigue risk management systems (FRMS) [53,55] enhancing a sense of coherence [34] and strengthening family support [56,57]. On the other hand, the use of anxiolytic and antidepressant drugs seems to have increased in the community [58,59] without it being clear what is happening among health professionals. A limitation of the study is that it did not examine the above factors as possible confounding variables.

We have to note that the role of night work was not examined. Nurses working in rotating shifts or at night are exposed to sleep disturbances due to abnormal melatonin secretion at night and circadian rhythm disturbance [60,61]. Nurses are at a high risk of fatigue due to stressful work environments with heavy workloads and non-standard work schedules [62]. Stress and emotional distress are known to predict sleep quality, and all of these factors have been shown to predict fatigue severity [63].

Considering the higher prevalence of insomnia in female nurses compared to other health professionals [64,65] and the fact that they constitute the vast majority of nursing staff, it is proposed to strengthen health protection in this most vulnerable category through prevention and intervention programs oriented towards their psychosocial support [65].

Finally, it is important to mention the willingness of nurses to participate in this research. It is common for Greek nurses to show high rates of acceptance to participate in studies with questionnaires, even in studies conducted online [29]. Nevertheless, the motivation of nurses' acceptance in studies with questionnaires has not been adequately investigated, although it is particularly important as it may influence the prevalence rates of the variables.

5. Conclusions

In the second year of the pandemic, nursing staff continue to experience high rates of anxiety, depression and fatigue. These findings are probably due, among other reasons, to the fact that Greece, during the period of this study, was experiencing the worst phase of the pandemic. The variation in fatigue appears to be significantly dependent on trait anxiety. Depressive symptomatology and state anxiety exert parallel positive mediation on the trait anxiety and fatigue relationship. In this relationship, depression has a moderating role at low, medium and high values. Despite the recent increase in research interest in this area, more longitudinal and/or intervention studies that could further enrich our understanding of the anxiety–fatigue–depression relationship are desirable. Finally, it is proposed to strengthen health protection in this most vulnerable category through prevention and intervention programs oriented toward nurses' psychosocial support.

Author Contributions: Conceptualization, C.S. and A.T.; methodology, C.S., A.T. and A.P. (Aspasia Panagiotou); software, C.S., I.I. and A.P. (Aspasia Panagiotou); validation, A.P. (Argyro Pachi), S.Z. and M.T.; formal analysis, C.S., A.T. and I.I.; investigation, C.S. and A.T.; resources, A.P. (Argyro Pachi); data curation, A.T., I.I. and S.Z.; writing—original draft preparation, C.S. and I.I.; writing—review and editing, A.T., C.S. and A.P. (Argyro Pachi); supervision, A.T. and A.P. (Aspasia Panagiotou); project administration, C.S. and A.T. All authors have read and agreed to the published version of the manuscript.

Funding: This research received no external funding.

Institutional Review Board Statement: The study was conducted in accordance with the Declaration of Helsinki and approved by the Ethics Committee of the University of Peloponnese (18699/11-10-2021).

Informed Consent Statement: Informed consent was obtained from all subjects participating in the study on the first page of the questionnaire. Participation in the research was voluntary.

Data Availability Statement: The data and the questionnaires of the study are available upon request from the corresponding author.

Acknowledgments: We would like to thank all the nurses who participated in our study.

Conflicts of Interest: The authors declare no conflict of interest.

References

1. Mukhtar, S. Psychological health during the coronavirus disease 2019 pandemic outbreak. *Int. J. Soc. Psychiatry* **2020**, *66*, 512–516. [CrossRef] [PubMed]
2. Dubey, S.; Biswas, P.; Ghosh, R.; Chatterjee, S.; Dubey, M.J.; Chatterjee, S.; Lahiri, D.; Lavie, C.J. Psychosocial impact of COVID-19. *Diabetes Metab Syndr.* **2020**, *14*, 779–788. [CrossRef]
3. Tselebis, A.; Pachi, A. Primary Mental Health Care in a New Era. *Healthcare* **2022**, *10*, 2025. [CrossRef] [PubMed]
4. El-Hage, W.; Hingray, C.; Lemogne, C.; Yrondi, A.; Brunault, P.; Bienvenu, T.; Etain, B.; Paquet, C.; Gohier, B.; Bennabi, D.; et al. Health professionals facing the coronavirus disease 2019 (COVID-19) pandemic: What are the mental health risks? *Encephale* **2020**, *46*, S73–S80. [CrossRef]
5. Tselebis, A.; Lekka, D.; Sikaras, C.; Tsomaka, E.; Tassopoulos, A.; Ilias, I.; Bratis, D.; Pachi, A. Insomnia, Perceived Stress, and Family Support among Nursing Staff during the Pandemic Crisis. *Healthcare* **2020**, *8*, 434. [CrossRef] [PubMed]
6. Batra, K.; Singh, T.; Sharma, M.; Batra, R.; Schvaneveldt, N. Investigating the Psychological Impact of COVID-19 among Healthcare Workers: A Meta-Analysis. *Int. J. Environ. Res. Public Health* **2020**, *17*, 9096. [CrossRef]
7. Muller, A.E.; Hafstad, E.V.; Himmels, J.P.W.; Smedslund, G.; Flottorp, S.; Stensland, S.Ø.; Stroobants, S.; Van De Velde, S.; Vist, G.E. The mental health impact of the covid-19 pandemic on healthcare workers, and interventions to help them: A rapid systematic review. *Psychiatr. Res.* **2020**, *293*, 113441. [CrossRef]
8. Lai, J.; Ma, S.; Wang, Y.; Cai, Z.; Hu, J.; Wei, N.; Wu, J.; Du, H.; Chen, T.; Li, R.; et al. Factors associated with mental health outcomes among health care workers exposed to coronavirus disease 2019. *JAMA Netw. Open* **2020**, *3*, e203976. [CrossRef]
9. Sasangohar, F.; Jones, S.L.; Masud, F.N.; Vahidy, F.S.; Kash, B.A. Provider Burnout and Fatigue During the COVID-19 Pandemic: Lessons Learned from a High-Volume Intensive Care Unit. *Obstet. Anesthesia Dig.* **2020**, *131*, 106–111. [CrossRef]
10. Pappa, S.; Ntella, V.; Giannakas, T.; Giannakoulis, V.G.; Papoutsi, E.; Katsaounou, P. Prevalence of depression, anxiety, and insomnia among healthcare workers during the COVID-19 pandemic: A systematic review and meta-analysis. *Brain Behav. Immun.* **2020**, *88*, 901–907. [CrossRef]
11. Marvaldi, M.; Mallet, J.; Dubertret, C.; Moro, M.R.; Guessoum, S.B. Anxiety, depression, trauma- related, and sleep disorders among healthcare workers during the COVID-19 pandemic: A systematic review and meta-analysis. *Neurosci. Biobehav. Rev.* **2021**, *126*, 252–264. [CrossRef]
12. Zhan, Y.-X.; Zhao, S.-Y.; Yuan, J.; Liu, H.; Liu, Y.-F.; Gui, L.-L.; Zheng, H.; Zhou, Y.-M.; Qiu, L.-H.; Chen, J.-H.; et al. Prevalence and Influencing Factors on Fatigue of First-line Nurses Combating with COVID-19 in China: A Descriptive Cross-Sectional Study. *Curr. Med. Sci.* **2020**, *40*, 625–635. [CrossRef]
13. Graham, K.C.; Cvach, M. Monitor Alarm Fatigue: Standardizing Use of Physiological Monitors and Decreasing Nuisance Alarms. *Am. J. Crit. Care* **2010**, *19*, 28–34. [CrossRef] [PubMed]
14. Chand, S.P.; Marwaha, R. Anxiety. In *StatPearls*; StatPearls Publishing: Treasure Island, FL, USA, 2022.
15. Kessing, L.V.; Bukh, J.D.; Bock, C.; Vinberg, M.; Gether, U. Does bereavement-related first episode depression differ from other kinds of first depressions? *Soc. Psychiatry Psychiatr. Epidemiol.* **2009**, *45*, 801–808. [CrossRef]
16. Chand, S.P.; Arif, H. Depression. In *StatPearls*; StatPearls Publishing: Treasure Island, FL, USA, 2022.
17. Kendler, K.S.; Kuhn, J.; Prescott, C.A. The Interrelationship of Neuroticism, Sex, and Stressful Life Events in the Prediction of Episodes of Major Depression. *Am. J. Psychiatry* **2004**, *161*, 631–636. [CrossRef]
18. Hettema, J.M. What is the genetic relationship between anxiety and depression? *Am. J. Med. Genet. Part C: Semin. Med. Genet.* **2008**, *148C*, 140–146. [CrossRef]
19. Bittner, A.; Goodwin, R.D.; Wittchen, H.-U.; Beesdo, K.; Höfler, M.; Lieb, R. What characteristics of primary anxiety disorders predict subsequent major depressive disorder? *J. Clin. Psychiatry* **2004**, *65*, 618–626. [CrossRef]
20. Sandi, C.; Richter-Levin, G. From high anxiety trait to depression: A neurocognitive hypothesis. *Trends Neurosci.* **2009**, *32*, 312–320. [CrossRef]
21. Weger, M.; Sandi, C. High anxiety trait: A vulnerable phenotype for stress-induced depression. *Neurosci. Biobehav. Rev.* **2018**, *87*, 27–37. [CrossRef]
22. Lockefeer, J.P.M.; De Vries, J. What is the relationship between trait anxiety and depressive symptoms, fatigue, and low sleep quality following breast cancer surgery? *Psycho-Oncology* **2012**, *22*, 1127–1133. [CrossRef]
23. De Vries, J.; Van Der Steeg, A.F.; Roukema, J.A. Trait anxiety determines depressive symptoms and fatigue in women with an abnormality in the breast. *Br. J. Health Psychol.* **2009**, *14*, 143–157. [CrossRef] [PubMed]
24. Clark, D.A.; Beck, A.T. Cognitive theory and therapy of anxiety and depression: Convergence with neurobiological findings. *Trends Cogn. Sci.* **2010**, *14*, 418–424. [CrossRef] [PubMed]
25. Wang, T.; Li, M.; Xu, S.; Liu, B.; Wu, T.; Lu, F.; Xie, J.; Peng, L.; Wang, J. Relations between trait anxiety and depression: A mediated moderation model. *J. Affect. Disord.* **2019**, *244*, 217–222. [CrossRef]
26. Mor, N.; Haran, D. Cognitive-behavioral therapy for depression. *Isr. J. Psychiatry Relat. Sci.* **2009**, *46*, 269–273. [PubMed]
27. COVID-19 Coronavirus Pandemic. Available online: https://www.worldometers.info/coronavirus/country/greece/ (accessed on 22 March 2022).
28. Health at a Glance: Europe 2020 State of Health in the EU Cycle. Available online: https://ec.europa.eu/health/system/files/2020-12/2020_healthatglance_rep_en_0.pdf (accessed on 22 March 2022).

29. Sikaras, C.; Ilias, I.; Tselebis, A.; Pachi, A.; Zyga, S.; Tsironi, M.; Gil, A.P.R.; Panagiotou, A. Nursing staff fatigue and burnout during the COVID-19 pandemic in Greece. *AIMS Public Health* **2021**, *9*, 94–105. [CrossRef]
30. De Vries, J.; Michielsen, H.; Van Heck, G.L.; Drent, M. Measuring fatigue in sarcoidosis: The Fatigue Assessment Scale (FAS). *Br. J. Health Psychol.* **2004**, *9*, 279–291. [CrossRef]
31. Alikari, V.; Fradelos, E.; Sachlas, A.; Panoutsopoulos, G.; Lavdaniti, M.; Palla, P.; Lappa, T.; Giatrakou, S.; Stathoulis, J.; Babatsikou, F.; et al. Reliability and validity of the Greek version of "The Fatigue Assessment Scale". *Arch. Hell. Med.* **2016**, *33*, 231–238.
32. Beck, A.T.; Ward, C.H.; Mendelson, M.; Mock, J.; Erbauch, J. An inventory for measuring depression. *Arch. Gen. Psychiatry* **1961**, *4*, 561–571. [CrossRef]
33. Donias, S.; Demertzis, I. Validation of the Beck depression inventory. In *10th Hellenic Congress of Neurology and Psychiatry*; Varfis, G., Ed.; University Studio Press: Thessaloniki, Greece, 1983; pp. 486–492. (In Greek)
34. Pachi, A.; Sikaras, C.; Ilias, I.; Panagiotou, A.; Zyga, S.; Tsironi, M.; Baras, S.; Tsitrouli, L.A.; Tselebis, A. Burnout, Depression and Sense of Coherence in Nurses during the Pandemic Crisis. *Healthcare* **2022**, *10*, 134. [CrossRef]
35. Spielberger, C.D.; Gorsuch, R.L.; Lushene, P.R.; Vagg, P.R.; Jacobs, G.A. *Manual for the State–Trait Spielberger Anxiety Inventory (Form Y)*; Consulting Psychologists Press: Palo Alto, CA, USA, 1983.
36. Fountoulakis, K.N.; Papadopoulou, M.; Kleanthous, S.; Papadopoulou, A.; Bizeli, V.; Nimatoudis, I.; Iacovides, A.; Kaprinis, G.S. Reliability and psychometric properties of the Greek translation of the State-Trait Anxiety Inventory form Y: Preliminary data. *Ann. Gen. Psychiatry* **2006**, *5*, 2. [CrossRef]
37. Tselebis, A.; Gournas, G.; Tzitzanidou, G.; Panagiotou, A.; Ilias, I. Anxiety and Depression in Greek Nursing and Medical Personnel. *Psychol. Rep.* **2006**, *99*, 93–96. [CrossRef]
38. World Health Organization. Pandemic fatigue: Reinvigorating the Public to Prevent COVID-19. 2020. Available online: https://apps.who.int/iris/bitstream/handle/10665/335820/WHO-EURO-2020-1160-40906-55390-eng.pdf (accessed on 3 April 2022).
39. Labrague, L.J. Pandemic fatigue and clinical nurses' mental health, sleep quality and job contentment during the COVID-19 pandemic: The mediating role of resilience. *J. Nurs. Manag.* **2021**, *29*, 1992–2001. [CrossRef] [PubMed]
40. Johnston, D.W.; Allan, J.L.; Powell, D.J.H.; Jones, M.C.; Farquharson, B.; Bell, C.; Johnston, M. Why does work cause fatigue? A real-time investigation of fatigue, and determinants of fatigue in nurses working 12-hour shifts. *Ann. Behav. Med.* **2018**, *53*, 551–562. [CrossRef] [PubMed]
41. Wittchen, H.-U.; Zhao, S.; Kessler, R.C.; Eaton, W.W. DSM-III-R Generalized Anxiety Disorder in the National Comorbidity Survey. *Arch. Gen. Psychiatry* **1994**, *51*, 355–364. [CrossRef]
42. Leach, L.S.; Christensen, H.; Mackinnon, A.J. Gender differences in the endorsement of symptoms for depression and anxiety: Are gender-biased items responsible? *J. Nerv. Ment. Dis.* **2008**, *196*, 128–135. [CrossRef]
43. Weissman, M.M.; Klerman, G.L. Sex differences and the epidemiology of depression. *Arch. Gen. Psychiatry* **1977**, *34*, 98–111. [CrossRef] [PubMed]
44. Jorm, A. Sex and Age Differences in Depression: A Quantitative Synthesis of Published Research. *Aust. New Zealand J. Psychiatry* **1987**, *21*, 46–53. [CrossRef]
45. Kuehner, C. Gender differences in unipolar depression: An update of epidemiological findings and possible explanations. *Acta Psychiatr. Scand.* **2003**, *108*, 163–174. [CrossRef]
46. Faravelli, C.; Alessandra Scarpato, M.; Castellini, G.; Lo Sauro, C. Gender differences in depression and anxiety: The role of age. *Psychiatry Res.* **2013**, *210*, 1301–1303. [CrossRef]
47. Leach, L.S.; Christensen, H.; Mackinnon, A.J.; Windsor, T.D.; Butterworth, P. Gender differences in depression and anxiety across the adult lifespan: The role of psychosocial mediators. *Soc. Psychiatry Psychiatr. Epidemiol.* **2008**, *43*, 983–998. [CrossRef]
48. Jang, H.J.; Kim, O.; Kim, S.; Kim, M.S.; Choi, J.A.; Kim, B.; Dan, H.; Jung, H. Factors Affecting Physical and Mental Fatigue among Female Hospital Nurses: The Korea Nurses' Health Study. *Healthcare* **2021**, *9*, 201. [CrossRef] [PubMed]
49. Brown, L.F.; Kroenke, K. Cancer-related fatigue and its associations with depression and anxiety: A systematic review. *Psychosomatics* **2009**, *50*, 440–447. [CrossRef]
50. Polikandrioti, M.; Tzirogiannis, K.; Zyga, S.; Koutelekos, I.; Vasilopoulos, G.; Theofilou, P.; Panoutsopoulos, G. Effect of anxiety and depression on the fatigue of patients with a permanent pacemaker. *Arch. Med. Sci. Atheroscler. Dis.* **2018**, *3*, 8–17. [CrossRef]
51. Kim, S.C.; Rankin, L.; Ferguson, J. Nurses' mental health from early COVID-19 pandemic to vaccination. *J. Nurs. Scholarsh.* **2021**, *54*, 485–492. [CrossRef] [PubMed]
52. Heath, C.; Sommerfield, A.; Von Ungern-Sternberg, B.S. Resilience strategies to manage psychological distress among healthcare workers during the COVID-19 pandemic: A narrative review. *Anaesthesia* **2020**, *75*, 1364–1371. [CrossRef] [PubMed]
53. Querstret, D.; O'Brien, K.; Skene, D.J.; Maben, J. Improving fatigue risk management in healthcare: A systematic scoping review of sleep-related/fatigue-management interventions for nurses and midwives. *Int. J. Nurs. Stud.* **2019**, *106*, 103513. [CrossRef]
54. Martin-Anatias, N.; Simpson, N.; Sterling, R.; Trnka, S.; Tunufa'i, L. Community healthcare workers' experiences during and after COVID-19 lockdown: A qualitative study from Aotearoa New Zealand. *Health Soc. Care Community* **2022**, *30*, e2761–e2771.
55. Steege, L.M.; Pinekenstein, B.J.; Rainbow, J.G.; Arsenault Knudsen, É. Addressing Occupational Fatigue in Nurses: Current State of Fatigue Risk Management in Hospitals, Part 1. *J. Nurs. Adm.* **2017**, *47*, 426–433. [CrossRef]
56. Tselebis, A.; Bratis, D.; Karkanias, A.; Apostolopoulou, E.; Gournas, G.; Moussas, G.; Ilias, I. Associations on Dimensions of Burnout and Family Support for a Sample of Greek Nurses. *Psychol. Rep.* **2008**, *103*, 63–66. [CrossRef]

57. Bratis, D.; Tselebis, A.; Sikaras, C.; Moulou, A.; Giotakis, K.; Zoumakis, E.; Ilias, I. Alexithymia and its association with burnout, depression and family support among Greek nursing staff. *Hum. Resour. Heath* **2009**, *7*, 72. [CrossRef]
58. Tiger, M.; Wesselhoeft, R.; Karlsson, P.; Handal, M.; Bliddal, M.; Cesta, C.E.; Skurtveit, S.; Reutfors, J. Utilization of antidepressants, anxiolytics, and hypnotics during the COVID-19 pandemic in Scandinavia. *J. Affect. Disord.* **2023**, *323*, 292–298. [CrossRef] [PubMed]
59. González-López, M.D.C.; Díaz-Calvo, V.; Ruíz-González, C.; Nievas-Soriano, B.J.; Rebollo-Lavado, B.; Parrón-Carreño, T. Consumption of Psychiatric Drugs in Primary Care during the COVID-19 Pandemic. *Int. J. Environ. Res. Public Health* **2022**, *19*, 4782. [CrossRef] [PubMed]
60. Knap, M.; Maciag, D.; Trzeciak-Bereza, E.; Knap, B.; Czop, M.; Krupa, S. Sleep Disturbances and Health Consequences Induced by the Specificity of Nurses' Work. *Int. J. Environ. Res. Public Health* **2022**, *19*, 9802. [CrossRef] [PubMed]
61. Tselebis, A.; Zoumakis, E.; Ilias, I. Dream Recall/Affect and the Hypothalamic–Pituitary–Adrenal Axis. *Clocks Sleep* **2021**, *3*, 403–408. [CrossRef]
62. Cho, H.; Steege, L.M. Nurse Fatigue and Nurse, Patient Safety, and Organizational Outcomes: A Systematic Review. *West. J. Nurs. Res.* **2021**, *43*, 1157–1168. [CrossRef]
63. Thorsteinsson, E.B.; Brown, R.F.; Owens, M.T. Modeling the Effects of Stress, Anxiety, and Depression on Rumination, Sleep, and Fatigue in a Nonclinical Sample. *J. Nerv. Ment. Dis.* **2019**, *207*, 355–359. [CrossRef]
64. Dragioti, E.; Tsartsalis, D.; Mentis, M.; Mantzoukas, S.; Gouva, M. Impact of the COVID-19 pandemic on the mental health of hospital staff: An umbrella review of 44 meta-analyses. *Int. J. Nurs. Stud.* **2022**, *131*, 104272. [CrossRef]
65. Italia, S.; Costa, C.; Briguglio, G.; Mento, C.; Muscatello, M.R.A.; Alibrandi, A.; Filon, F.L.; Spatari, G.; Teodoro, M.; Fenga, C. Quality of Life, Insomnia and Coping Strategies during COVID-19 Pandemic in Hospital Workers. A Cross-Sectional Study. *Int. J. Environ. Res. Public Health* **2021**, *18*, 12466. [CrossRef]

Disclaimer/Publisher's Note: The statements, opinions and data contained in all publications are solely those of the individual author(s) and contributor(s) and not of MDPI and/or the editor(s). MDPI and/or the editor(s) disclaim responsibility for any injury to people or property resulting from any ideas, methods, instructions or products referred to in the content.

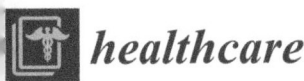

Article

Stressed, Lonely, and Overcommitted: Predictors of Lawyer Suicide Risk

Patrick R. Krill [1], Hannah M. Thomas [2], Meaghyn R. Kramer [2], Nikki Degeneffe [2] and Justin J. Anker [2,*]

[1] Krill Strategies, LLC, Minneapolis, MN 55408, USA
[2] Department of Psychiatry, University of Minnesota, Minneapolis, MN 55454, USA
* Correspondence: anke0022@umn.edu

Abstract: Suicide is a significant public health concern, and lawyers have been shown to have an elevated risk for contemplating it. In this study, we sought to identify predictors of suicidal ideation in a sample consisting of 1962 randomly selected lawyers. Using logistic regression analysis, we found that high levels of work overcommitment, high levels of perceived stress, loneliness as measured by the UCLA loneliness scale, and being male were all significantly associated with an increased risk of suicidal ideation. These results suggest that interventions aimed at reducing work overcommitment, stress, and loneliness, and addressing gender-specific risk factors, may be effective in reducing the risk of suicidal ideation among lawyers. Further research is needed to expand upon these findings and to develop and test interventions specifically tailored to the needs of this population.

Keywords: lawyers; suicidal ideation; occupational stress; loneliness; perceived stress; depression; mental health; work overcommitment

1. Introduction

Lawyers contemplate suicide (suicidal ideation) at an exceedingly high rate. Suicidal ideation, defined as thoughts, ideas, or ruminations about ending one's own life, is the first step to suicide and is predictive of suicide attempts [1,2]. Prior estimates suggest that between 10 and 12 percent of lawyers in the U.S. have contemplated suicide [3–5], compared to 4.2% of adults ≥ 18 years of age in U.S. population [6]. Given the high rates of suicidal ideation among lawyers, it is crucial to identify factors that potentially contribute to their suicide risk.

Lawyers are prone to mental health issues, including anxiety, depression, and substance abuse [3,7], which are strongly linked to suicide risk [8–12]. A nationwide study of ~13,000 lawyers indicated that 28% experienced depression, 19% reported anxiety, 21% had alcohol use problems, and 11% had problems with drug use [3]. Lawyers also experience elevated levels of stress (i.e., perceiving events in one's life or work as unpredictable, uncontrollable, and/or overloaded) [13,14] and loneliness (perceiving one's social needs as not being met) [15–17] which are well-established predictors of suicide risk [18–24]. However, the relative contribution of lawyer mental health, stress, and loneliness to suicide risk has yet to be examined.

Work-related hazards specific to the legal profession may also contribute to suicide risk. For example, lawyers are expected to work long hours, meet tight deadlines, and handle complex legal issues, all while maintaining a high level of professionalism and client satisfaction [5,13,25,26]. This can lead to burnout and feelings of being overwhelmed, which have been linked to increased risk of suicidal ideation [27–35]. Findings from other research, however, demonstrate that the association between job burnout and suicidal ideation disappears after adjusting for depression [36]. This highlights the importance of accounting for psychological distress when seeking to identify workplace predictors of suicidality.

Work-family conflict, or difficulty balancing work and family responsibilities, is a common stressor that can negatively impact mental health [37–40] and there is a growing body of research indicating that work-family conflict is a predictor of suicidal ideation [41,42]. Anker and Krill found that work-family conflict among lawyers was significantly associated with perceived stress and attrition due to burnout in a large sample of lawyers. These findings suggest that work-family conflict may also play a role in suicidal ideation among lawyers.

According to the World Health Organization, men are three times more likely than women to die by suicide even though women tend to experience higher levels of suicidal ideation [43]. Gender differences in suicide risk factors have also been observed across a range of occupational groups [30,44–46]. In relation to lawyers specifically, Anker and Krill (2021) [7] found that women lawyers were more likely to experience moderate to severe levels of work–family conflict, work overcommitment, perceived stress, anxiety, depression, and risky or hazardous levels of alcohol use compared to male lawyers. Owing to their higher prevalence of suicidality risk factors, we hypothesized that women lawyers may be at a higher risk for suicidal ideation than men.

Considering how many lawyers contemplate suicide and the paucity of data examining the relationship between their suicidal ideation and the known risk factors they often experience, further research on the subject is an overdue and essential step in the development of effective suicide prevention strategies tailored to that population. As such, the current study examined the relationship between suicidal ideation, and factors that negatively and disproportionally affect lawyers, including perceived stress, loneliness, work overcommitment, work-family conflict, alcohol use, and prior mental health diagnosis.

2. Materials and Methods

2.1. Participants

Recruitment and Random Selection

The University of Minnesota Institutional Review Board reviewed the study design and protocol. Recruitment was coordinated in collaboration with the California Lawyers Association ("CLA"), a nonprofit, voluntary organization that includes the Sections of the State Bar of California and the California Young Lawyers Association, and the D.C. Bar, the largest unified bar in the United States and an organization which provides an oversight structure to maintain ethical standards and Rules of Professional Conduct. An advertisement was included in newsletters sent by the D.C. Bar and CLA to their respective member lists and posted on their organization's website. The advertisement provided a summary of the study, indicating that the survey was anonymous and that members would be randomly invited to participate in the study via email. Participants were randomly selected from a list of unique de-identified I.D.s supplied by the CLA and D.C. Bar. Each list contained approximately 98,000 IDs (196,000 total IDs). Hence, 40,000 IDs were randomly selected from each list (80,000 total) using the random sample function in the statistical platform R. From that sample, 5292 participants consented to the survey and about 4000 completed the survey. An email notification was sent to randomly selected D.C. Bar and CLA members on behalf of the researchers. Seven days following the email notification, study candidates received an email containing a link to a REDCap (Research Electronic Data Capture) survey. Clicking on the link directed participants to the survey's informed consent page. The study was conducted during the summer of 2020.

2.2. Materials

2.2.1. Descriptive Variables

Demographics and work context. Information regarding age, race, relationship status, and whether respondents had children was collected. Additionally, information on the following work-related variables was collected from participants: the average number of hours worked per week, current position in the legal profession, and whether the current position involved litigation.

2.2.2. Measures

Mental Health Diagnoses. Participants were asked if they ever (lifetime) or currently (past 12 months) had a diagnosis of major depression, anxiety disorder, PTSD, bipolar disorder, alcohol use disorder, substance use disorder, or a non-specified mental health disorder.

Depression. Participants completed the Patient Health Questionnaire-9 (PHQ-9) to assess the prevalence and severity of symptoms of depression [47]. For the PHQ-9, participant depression severity scores were grouped across the following 5 categories: None/Minimal (0–4), Mild (5–9), Moderate (10–14), Moderately Severe (15–19), and Severe (20–27).

Stress. The total score on the Perceived Stress Scale (PSS) was used to assess how unpredictable, uncontrollable, and overloaded respondents found their lives [48]. Scores on the PSS were grouped into Low (0–13), Moderate (14–26), and Severe (27–40) categories for analyses comparing.

Alcohol Use Severity. Scores on the Alcohol Use Disorders Identification Test (AUDIT-C) were used to assess risky drinking (women ≥ 3; men ≥ 4) and high-risk/hazardous drinking (women ≥ 4; men ≥ 5) [49].

Substance Use Severity. Scores on the DAST were used to assess substance use severity and were classified into the following four severity groups: Lifetime abstinence, No problems reported, Low, and Moderate to Severe [50].

Loneliness. Participants completed a 3-item questionnaire adapted from the Revised University of California, Los Angeles (UCLA) Loneliness Scale to assess the prevalence and severity of loneliness [51]. The questionnaire consisted of the following 3 items: "How often do you feel that you lack companionship?", "How often do you feel left out?", and "How often do you feel isolated from others?". Participants responded with "hardly ever or never", "some of the time", and "often". Ratings were summed to produce a loneliness score ranging from 3 to 9, with a higher score indicating greater loneliness. Following methods by Steptoe et al., (2013) [52], participants scores were summed and grouped across 2 categories (Lonely (3–5) and Not Lonely (6–9)).

Work Overcommitment. We used the overcommitment subscale of the Effort–Reward Imbalance (ERI) Questionnaire [53] to assess feelings of being overwhelmed by work demands. Responses on the subscale were on a four-point Likert scale (1 = Strongly Disagree, 2 = Disagree, 3 = Agree, 4 = Strongly Agree).

Work-Family Conflict. The degree to which work interfered with family life was assessed using three items from the Work-Family Conflict (WFC) subscale from the short version of the Copenhagen Psychosocial Questionnaire [54]. Participants rated items are 4-point Likert-scale ranging from 1 (no, not at all) to 4 (yes, certainly).

2.2.3. Outcome Variables

Suicidality/Suicidal Ideation. Participants were classified as endorsing suicidality according to item 9 of the PHQ-9, which can accurately identify individuals at-risk for suicide attempts and death [2,55–58]. Moreover, assessing suicidal ideation with the PHQ-9 allowed for a direct comparison to recent reports of the frequency of suicidality in the legal profession [4]. Participants were considered to have endorsed suicidality if they selected "Several days", "More than half the days", or "Nearly every day" to the item "How often have you had thoughts that you would be better off dead, or of hurting yourself". Participants who selected "Never" for this item were classified as not having suicidality.

2.3. Data Analysis

Demographic and mental health severity scores on the PHQ-9 were compared between men and women using chi-square analyses. Logistic regression analyses were performed to identify associations between predictor variables (e.g., Work–Family Conflict, Work Overcommitment,) and the outcome variables (PHQ-9 suicidality) while controlling for covariates (e.g., COVID-19 impact on PHQ-9 items).

Predictors were entered one at a time in a stepwise fashion, and their impact on the model's overall fit was assessed. Those that significantly contributed to the model were entered into the primary study model. A sensitivity analysis was then conducted to examine the impact of COVID-19 on the primary model by entering a variable representing COVID-19 impact on PHQ-9 suicidality (e.g., a single item added at the end of assessments that asked whether problems defined in the PHQ-9 increased, decreased, or stayed the same since COVID-19). P-values for multiple comparisons were corrected using Holm–Bonferroni adjustments.

3. Results

Of the 80,000 members of the CLA and D.C. Bar that were randomly selected and received a study invitation, 5292 consented. The sample was restricted to lawyers who were employed part- or full-time in a legal setting at the time of the survey and who had complete data on the study measures. The final sample consisted of 1962 participants.

3.1. Descriptive Results

3.1.1. Frequency of Suicidal Ideation

Approximately 8.5% (N = 165) of the participants reported thoughts they would be better off dead, or of hurting themselves "Several days", "More than half the days", or "Nearly every day" and were grouped in the suicidal ideation group. The remaining 91.5% (N = 1797) selected "Not at all" for PHQ-9 item 9 and were grouped in the non-suicidal ideation group.

3.1.2. Demographic Variables

Groups were compared on demographic, occupation, and mental health variables prior to model testing. Women comprised approximately 51% (N = 991) of the sample. Table 1 shows the distribution of demographic variables for participants who endorsed PHQ-9 suicidality vs. those who did not ("Not at all"). There were no differences in the proportion of men and women who endorsed suicidality as a function of gender or race. However, with respect to age, lawyers who endorsed (vs. did not endorse) suicidality tended to be younger. For example, a significantly greater proportion of lawyers from the suicidality group (compared to the non-suicidality group) belonged to the two youngest age groups (30 or younger and 31–40) and a lower proportion of suicidality endorsers belonged to the oldest age group (61 or older).

Table 1. Demographics according to endorsement of PHQ-9 suicidal ideation (N = 1962).

	No Suicidal Ideation (N = 1797)		Suicidal Ideation (N = 165)		χ^2, p-Value
	N	%	N	%	
Gender					$\chi^2(1) = 1.064, 0.302$
Female	914	92.2%	77	7.8%	
Male	883	90.9%	88	9.1%	
Age					$\chi^2(4) = 18.81, <0.001$
30 or younger	126 [a]	85.7%	21 [b]	14.3%	
31–40	465 [a]	89.4%	55 [b]	10.6%	
41–50	425 [a]	93.2%	31 [a]	6.8%	
51–60	408 [a]	91.1%	40 [a]	8.9%	
61 or older	373 [a]	95.4%	18 [b]	4.6%	
Race					$\chi^2(6) = 10.04, 0.123$
Asian or Pacific Islander	125	86.8%	19	13.2%	
Black/African American	85	90.4%	9	9.6%	
Caucasian/White	1457	92.3%	122	7.7%	
Latino/Hispanic	62	91.2%	6	8.8%	
Native American	3	100.0%	0	0.0%	
More than one race	40	83.3%	8	16.7%	
Other	16	94.1%	1	5.9%	

Within each row, each superscript letter denotes column proportions that did not differ significantly at the 0.05 level according to Pearson Chi-Square tests.

3.1.3. Work-Related Demographics

Work-related sample demographics are shown in Table 2 for both groups. The total number of hours worked in a week, the participant's law practice setting, and whether the participant's legal position involved litigation did not significantly differ between groups. There was a trend that approached but did not reach significance ($p = 0.051$) with regards to position in the legal profession, such that a greater proportion of lawyers in the most junior level (junior associate) endorsed (vs. did not endorse) suicidality.

Table 2. Work-related demographics of the study sample according to endorsement of PHQ-9 suicidal ideation (N = 1962).

	No Suicidal Ideation (N = 1797)		Suicidal Ideation (N = 165)		χ^2, p-Value
	N	%	N	%	
Hours worked in a typical week					$\chi^2(7) = 9.674, p = 0.208$
Less than 10 h	28	90.3%	3	9.7%	
11 to 20 h	65	98.5%	1	1.5%	
21 to 30 h	82	91.1%	8	8.9%	
31 to 40 h	405	91.6%	37	8.4%	
41 to 50 h	759	92.1%	65	7.9%	
51 to 60 h	348	90.9%	35	9.1%	
61 to 70 h	81	85.3%	14	14.7%	
71 h or more	25	92.6%	2	7.4%	
Position in Legal Profession					$\chi^2(6) = 14.021, p = 0.051$
Managing partner	315	92.6%	25	7.4%	
Senior partner	262	93.9%	17	6.1%	
Junior partner	115	92.0%	10	8.0%	
Of counsel	138	91.4%	13	8.6%	
Senior associate	254	93.0%	19	7.0%	
Junior associate	195	85.9%	32	14.1%	
Other	414	91.9%	41	9.0%	
Law Practice Setting					$\chi^2(7) = 12.200, p = 0.094$
Sole Practitioner—Private Practice	269	93.4%	19	6.6%	
Private Firm	740	90.7%	76	9.3%	
In-house lawyer: government, public interest, or nonprofit	445	92.5%	36	7.5%	
In-house lawyer: corporation or for-profit institution	233	91.7%	21	8.3%	
Judicial chambers (judge/hearing officer/clerk)	3	60.0%	2	40.0%	
Other law practice setting	39	86.7%	6	13.3%	
College or law school	6	85.7%	1	14.3%	
Other setting (not law practice)	15	100.0%	0	0.0%	
Position Involves Litigation (Yes)	1072	59.7%	105	63.6%	$\chi^2(1) = 1.393, p = 0.238$

3.1.4. Mental health Diagnoses and Symptom Severity

There were no significant group differences concerning current drinking status (current drinker, former drinker, or lifetime abstainer). However, regarding substance use status, a significantly greater proportion of endorsers of suicidality identified as a current substance user (data not shown). Table 3 shows the proportions of lawyers in each suicidality group with a past 12-month mental health diagnosis and the proportion within the severity classifications of the PHQ-9, AUDIT-C, DAST, PSS, and the UCLA loneliness scale. Overall, a greater proportion of lawyers who endorsed suicidal ideation had a current mental health condition (Depression, Anxiety, PTSD, Bipolar Disorder, AUD, or other) and were significantly more likely to be in the moderate, moderately severe, or severe range of depression as measured by the PHQ-9. Similar results indicating greater severity among the suicidality vs. the non-suicidality group were reported concerning (1) hazardous drinking (AUDIT-C), (2) substance use severity (DAST), (3) moderate to high stress (PSS), and (4) loneliness (UCLA Loneliness Scale).

Table 3. The prevalence of mental health diagnoses, severity of depression, alcohol use, substance use, and loneliness in the study sample according to endorsement of PHQ-9 suicidal ideation (N = 1962).

	No Suicidal Ideation (N = 1797)		Suicidal Ideation (N = 165)		χ^2, p-Value
	N	%	N	%	
Past 12-Month Mental Health Diagnosis					
Depression					$\chi^2(2) = 132.47, p < 0.001$
current	152 [a]	9.7%	62 [b]	41.6%	
lifetime	321 [a]	20.5%	31 [a]	20.8%	
no history	1096 [a]	69.9%	56 [b]	37.6%	
total	1569		149		
Anxiety Disorder					$\chi^2(2) = 65.033, p < 0.001$
current	226 [a]	14.5%	54 [b]	39.7%	
lifetime	232 [a]	14.9%	26 [a]	19.1%	
no history	1096 [a]	70.5%	56 [b]	41.2%	
total	1554		136		
PTSD					$\chi^2(2) = 58.780, p < 0.001$
current	22 [a]	1.9%	12 [b]	15.8%	
lifetime	54 [a]	4.6%	8 [b]	10.5%	
no history	1096 [a]	93.5%	56 [b]	73.7%	
total	1172		76		
Bipolar Disorder					$\chi^2(2) = 17.852, p < 0.001$
current	3 [a]	0.3%	2 [b]	3.3%	
lifetime	12 [a]	1.1%	2 [a]	3.3%	
no history	1096 [a]	98.6%	56 [b]	93.3%	
total	1111		60		
Alcohol Use Disorder					$\chi^2(2) = 13.739, p < 0.001$
current	8 [a]	0.7%	3 [b]	4.8%	
lifetime	31 [a]	2.7%	4 [a]	6.3%	
no history	1096 [a]	96.3%	56 [b]	88.9%	
total	1135		63		
Substance Use Disorder					$\chi^2(2) = 2.712, p = 0.258$
current	4	0.4%	1	1.7%	
lifetime	11	1.0%	1	1.7%	
no history	1096	98.6%	56	96.6%	
total	1111		58		
Other					$\chi^2(2) = 17.852, p < 0.001$
current	14 [a]	1.2%	5 [b]	7.9%	
lifetime	20 [a]	1.8%	2 [a]	3.2%	
no history	1096 [a]	97.0%	56 [b]	88.9%	
total	1130		63		
PHQ-9-Depression Severity					$\chi^2(4) = 541.079, p < 0.001$
None/Minimal	1011 [a]	57.8%	12 [b]	7.4%	
Mild	517 [a]	29.5%	33 [b]	20.4%	
Moderate	183 [a]	10.5%	51 [b]	31.4%	
Moderately Severe	34 [a]	1.9%	46 [b]	28.4%	
Severe	5 [a]	0.30%	20 [b]	12.3%	
AUDIT-C-Alcohol Use Severity					$\chi^2(2) = 7.881, p < 0.05$
Low risk	892 [a]	49.6%	74 [a]	44.8%	
Risky drinking	389 [a]	21.6%	27 [a]	16.4%	
Hazardous drinking	516 [a]	28.7%	64 [b]	38.8%	

Table 3. Cont.

	No Suicidal Ideation (N = 1797)		Suicidal Ideation (N = 165)		χ^2, p-Value
	N	%	N	%	
DAST-Substance Use Severity					$\chi^2(3) = 24.952, p < 0.001$
Lifetime abstinence	1418 [a]	78.9%	119 [b]	72.1%	
No problems reported	90 [a]	5.0%	6 [a]	3.6%	
Low	251 [a]	14.0%	26 [a]	15.8%	
Moderate to severe	38 [a]	2.1%	14 [b]	8.5%	
PSS—Perceived Stress Scale					$\chi^2(2) = 237.645, p < 0.001$
Low	812 [a]	45.2%	10 [b]	6.1%	
Moderate	897 [a]	49.9%	98 [b]	59.4%	
High	88 [a]	4.9%	57 [b]	34.5%	
UCLA Loneliness Scale					$\chi^2(1) = 110.338, p < 0.001$
Not Lonely	1224 [a]	68.1%	45 [b]	27.3%	
Lonely	573 [a]	31.9%	120 [b]	72.7%	

Each subscript letter denotes a subset of whose column proportions do not differ significantly from each other at the 0.05 level.

Table 4 shows the proportion of participants in each group with responses to survey items assessing whether participants believed their time in the legal profession has been detrimental to their mental health, led to increased alcohol/substance use, or caused them to contemplate leaving the profession due to mental health, burnout, or stress. A significantly greater proportion of lawyers in the suicidality group reported that their time in the legal profession was detrimental to their mental health, caused an increase in their substance/alcohol use, and considered leaving the profession due to mental health problems or burnout.

Table 4. Proportion of participants with and without PHQ-9 suicidal ideation with responses to items reflecting the perceived relationship between personal mental health and time in the legal profession (N = 1962).

	No Suicidal Ideation (N = 1797)		Suicidal Ideation (N = 165)		χ^2, p-Value
	N	%	N	%	
Has your time in the legal profession been detrimental to your mental health?					$\chi^2(2) = 110.436, p < 0.001$
yes	476 [a]	27.1%	106 [b]	66.3%	
no	943 [a]	53.8%	30 [b]	18.8%	
unsure	335 [a]	19.1%	24 [a]	15.0%	
Has your time in the legal profession caused your use of alcohol and/or other drugs to increase?					$\chi^2(2) = 50.771, p < 0.001$
yes	248 [a]	14.1%	55 [b]	34.2%	
no	1385 [a]	78.9%	89 [b]	55.3%	
unsure	122 [a]	7.0%	17 [a]	10.6%	
Are you considering, or have you left the profession due to mental health, burnout or stress?					$\chi^2(2) = 81.932, p < 0.001$
yes	320 [a]	18.2%	74 [b]	46.0%	
no	1352 [a]	77.0%	72 [b]	44.7%	
unsure	83 [a]	4.7%	15 [b]	9.3%	

Each subscript letter denotes a subset of whose column proportions do not differ significantly from each other at the 0.05 level.

3.2. Predictors of Suicidal Ideation

The results of the logistic regression analyses examining predictors of endorsement of suicidal ideation among lawyers are shown in Table 5. The following predictors did not significantly contribute to the model: alcohol and substance use severity, age, and work-family conflict. As a result, these items were removed in the final, simplified model. The final model contained the following predictors: gender, history of a mental health diagnosis, loneliness, perceived stress, and work overcommitment. Results of the model indicated that the odds of having suicidal ideation were 2.2 times higher among lawyers with high work overcommitment and 1.6 times higher among lawyers with an intermediate level of work overcommitment. Lawyers who screened as lonely on the UCLA loneliness scale were 2.8 times more likely to endorse suicidality than lawyers who did not screen as lonely. Gender was also significantly associated with suicidality, with men being 2 times more likely to endorse suicidality compared to women. Lawyers with a history of at least one mental illness diagnosis were 1.8 times more likely to endorse suicidality compared to lawyers with no history of mental illness. Finally, compared to lawyers with low perceived stress, those with high or intermediate stress levels were 22 times more likely and 5.5 times more likely, respectively, to endorse suicidality.

Table 5. Predictors of PHQ-9 suicidal ideation among lawyers (N = 1962).

	OR	95% CI
Gender (ref. female)		
Male	2.005 ***	(1.401–2.870)
Dx History (ref. no Dx history)		
Yes	1.822 ***	(1.26–2.63)
UCLA Loneliness		
Lonely	2.793 ***	(1.90–4.103)
PSS-Perceived Stress Scale (ref. Low)		
Low		
Intermediate	5.475 ***	(2.750–10.90)
High	22.392 ***	(10.30–48.64)
Work Overcommitment (ref. Low)		
Low		
Intermediate	1.585	(.850–2.96)
High	2.207 **	(1.206–4.039)

* significant difference from referent (** $p \leq 0.01$; *** $p \leq 0.001$); OR = odds ratio; CI = confidence interval.

3.3. Sensitivity Analysis

Accounting for COVID-19. It is important to acknowledge that data collection for the study occurred during the COVID-19 pandemic. In an attempt to control the pandemic's collateral burden on the study outcomes, responses to a single item assessing whether participants believed their PHQ-9 depression symptoms changed since the beginning of the pandemic was entered into the model as a covariate ("Thinking back to before the COVID-19 pandemic, do you believe the frequency of these problems has remained the same, decreased, or increased?"). The results of the model indicated that the perceived influence of COVID-19 on PHQ-9 responses was not a significant predictor of suicidality and that the ORs and significance levels of all the predictors noted in Table 5 were maintained (Supplement Table S1).

4. Discussion

Given the disproportionately high rates of lawyers who contemplate suicide, this study was designed to identify risks for suicidal ideation in the legal profession. To the best of our knowledge, this is the first study to report on factors related to suicidal ideation among lawyers randomly selected from a large sample of practicing lawyers. The first, most notable finding was that 8.5% of lawyers in our sample endorsed suicidal ideation as assessed by the PHQ-9, which is twice as high as the rate in in the general working population and closer to the rate among Utah lawyers (11.9%) noted by Thiese et al. (2021) [4]. The high prevalence of suicidal ideation among lawyers warrants further attention and mitigation efforts that address associated risk factors.

In addition to the high overall rate of suicidal ideation among lawyers, our study demonstrated that perceived stress was significantly associated with increased risk for suicidal thoughts. In fact, the odds of contemplating suicide were a remarkable 22 times higher among lawyers with high (vs. low) stress on the PSS. This finding supports prior studies indicating that perceived stress (as assessed by the PSS) predicts suicidal ideation and suicidal behavior in other populations [19,59,60]. However, the highly conspicuous extent to which it relates to lawyer suicide risk specifically would suggest that stress should be a primary target of suicide prevention and mitigation strategies for that population. A twofold strategy whereby stressors in lawyers' lives are reduced, and their stress tolerance is enhanced, would seem to be the most efficacious approach for mitigating the stress-suicidality risk. To date, however, most efforts to reduce stress within the legal profession have tended to target the individual, e.g., through the provision of personal stress management tools and self-care resources. Where employers have attempted to address the more structural and systemic precipitators of stress (i.e., unrealistic time pressures, unclear expectations, workload control, lack of feedback), employees have generally rated their efforts as 'highly ineffective' [5]. Simply put, it would seem the legal profession has been better at alleviating the effects of stress than in throttling the causes.

To be clear, interventions aimed at helping individuals better cope with stress should remain an essential element of any legal employer's efforts to improve lawyer mental health. Evidence-based self-care interventions for coping with perceived stress have been demonstrated to be effective in numerous settings [61–63]. Considering the profound impact of stress on lawyer suicidality, we believe that all options should remain viable for mitigating stress, including the examination and recalibration of organizational or profession-wide attitudes, norms, and cultures relating to work. Placing increased onus for change on the systems and structure of the profession, as opposed to individual lawyers, would seem appropriate due to the reported experiences of lawyers themselves. Specifically, a significantly greater proportion of lawyers who contemplated suicide indicated that working in the legal profession was detrimental to their mental health and contributed to their substance use, and feelings of burnout (See Table 4). Furthermore, such systemic introspection is both needed and timely in the wake of the COVID-19 pandemic. As noted in a recently published report on workplace mental health from the U.S. Surgeon General, organizational leaders, managers, supervisors, and workers alike have an unprecedented opportunity to examine the role of work in our lives and explore ways to better enable thriving in the workplace and beyond.

The importance of individual and organizational solutions for creating more mentally healthy workplaces is well-established in the literature [64], with upstream approaches being proposed as the most effective to prevent suicide and workplaces being ideal contexts to apply such approaches [65]. By seeking to reduce the incidence and impact of perceived stress among their lawyers, legal employers could be going far upstream with the potential for meaningful reductions in suicidal ideation. An obvious but important fact must be noted, namely that stressors outside of work could certainly contribute to lawyer suicidal ideation and therefore escape the reach of an employer's efforts to reduce stress. To speak practically, employers have an outsized role to play after numerous surveys and studies confirm that occupational pressures and fears are exceedingly the leading source of stress for American adults [66].

Social isolation or loneliness is noted as a common experience among lawyers and law students, often related to the demanding and high-stress nature of the legal profession, as well as the competitive and individualistic culture of law firms and law schools [15,16]. In the present study, lawyers experiencing high levels of loneliness were nearly three times as likely to experience suicidal ideation as those experiencing low levels of loneliness. This finding aligns with previous work demonstrating a relationship between loneliness and suicide risk [18,20,22,23]. Importantly, research has also shown that a sense of relatedness, i.e., how you connect, or relate to others, and whether you feel a sense of belonging at work, among lawyers strongly correlates with improved wellbeing [67]. By making collaboration and regular social interactions in the work environment more of a priority, employers may be able to help mitigate some of the loneliness their lawyers experience. Any such efforts will undoubtedly be complicated by remote and hybrid working models that now predominate the legal field, especially as recent reports from the field suggest that many lawyers are reluctant to return to the office [68]. Given the high rates of alcohol misuse among lawyers and the strong connection between workplace permissiveness towards alcohol and the risk of hazardous drinking among lawyers [7], efforts to combat loneliness and isolation should avoid reliance on alcohol-based events as a primary means of increasing socialization and connection.

Turning to gender, the odds of suicidal ideation were two times higher for men than women. This surprising finding stands in contrast to the 'gender paradox of suicidal behavior' demonstrated by other research, whereby it has been shown that women in most Western countries have higher rates of suicidal ideation but lower rates of mortality than men [69,70]. This finding is also notable because women attorneys experienced higher levels of depression, anxiety, and hazardous drinking than men, which would typically suggest a higher level of corresponding suicide risk. However, after controlling for these variables in our final model, it was revealed that men were more likely to experience suicidal ideation. This would suggest that factors not included in our model, and which may not typically be tied to suicidality, are affecting the tendency of male attorneys to experience suicidal ideation. Further research would be needed to determine the specific reasons for the higher rates of suicidal ideation among male lawyers and the apparent inapplicability of the gender paradox of suicidal behavior to the lawyer population.

Relating to work overcommitment, lawyers with high (vs. low) levels of work overcommitment were two times as likely to endorse suicidal ideation, while those with intermediate levels of overcommitment were 1.5 times more likely to report such thoughts. Work overcommitment, as measured by the ERI questionnaire, has been described as an intrinsic or personality-based coping factor which reflects the need for approval, esteem, and control and it has been shown to be significantly associated with cynicism, exhaustion, and greater psychological distress [71]. According to the ERI model proposed by Siegrist and Montano, 2014 [53], overcommitment involves a desire to control one's work environment and an inability to disconnect from work. Evidence of work overcommitment includes thinking about work immediately upon waking, having people tell you that you sacrifice too much for work, and an inability to relax and switch off work, among other things. High levels of overcommitment to work have been shown to play a detrimental role in lawyer mental health [72], but interventions aimed at reducing such work overcommitment face an uphill climb in the legal profession. Being overly dedicated to one's work is generally highly rewarded in law, beginning in law school and continuing throughout many legal work environments where lawyers are often promoted based on their observed level of commitment to their work, their firm, and their clients. At the same time, research has shown that extrinsic validations and rewards (i.e., grades, rankings, honors, and financial rewards) do not predict lawyer wellbeing but instead that these external considerations that often dominate law schools and law practice are of subordinate importance to lawyer happiness when compared to other basic psychological needs, such as autonomy, relatedness to others, and competence [66]. By raising awareness of the notable downsides of being too committed to one's work, encouraging lawyers to set and maintain appropriate boundaries in their lives, and reframing notions of success to prioritize intrinsic over extrinsic rewards, stakeholders in the legal profession may be able to temper or modulate the harmful effects of work overcommitment without asking lawyers to fully abandon the dedication to their work that may have greatly contributed to elements of their prior success and achievements.

Findings from the present study are consistent with previous research linking mental health disorders (e.g., depression, anxiety) to increased risk for suicidal ideation [73,74].

For example, while suicide accounts for about 1.4% of deaths worldwide, it has been estimated that the risk climbs to 5–8% for those with a mental disorder, such as depression, alcoholism, and schizophrenia [75]. It is well established that mental health disorders can disrupt cognitive and emotional functioning, leading to negative thoughts and behaviors, including suicidal ideation [73]. The present study adds to this literature by demonstrating that these factors are also relevant in the specific context of the legal profession because lawyers with a prior mental health diagnosis were nearly twice as likely to demonstrate suicidal ideation.

Another possible explanation of heightened suicidal ideation among lawyers is workplace culture which may promote unhealthy coping mechanisms and discourage seeking help for mental health problems. Previous research has demonstrated a pronounced reluctance on the part of lawyers to disclose or seek help for a mental health disorder, often due to fear of negative career or professional repercussions [3]. This "sink or swim" mentality and stigma surrounding seeking help for mental health problems may create a toxic work environment that contributes to the high rates of suicidal ideation in the legal profession. One strategy to address this issue involves destigmatizing mental health problems and promoting a culture of help-seeking within the legal profession when mental health problems arise.

Previous research indicates work–family conflict, alcohol use (AUDIT-C), and drug use (DAST) are associated with suicide risk. However, they were not associated with contemplating suicide among our sample of lawyers. This could be due to an overlap between these factors and perceived stress or other variables in the model. For example, other research demonstrates that scores on the AUDIT-C and DAST strongly correlate with perceived stress [76]. As such, it is possible that due to the overlap and strong relationship between perceived stress, alcohol use disorder, and substance use disorder, that the predictors of AUDIT-C and DAST scores did not emerge as significant while perceived stress did. It is important to emphasize that several lines of research implicate alcohol and substance use with suicidality, while several other lines of research demonstrate that lawyers engage in hazardous levels of alcohol and substance use at rates much higher than the general population. Although risky drinking was not a significant predictor of suicidality in this study (likely for the reasons cited above), ours and other's past work clearly indicates a strong connection between problem drinking and psychological distress among lawyers. It is therefore possible that problem drinking impacts the risk for suicidal ideation among lawyers indirectly, by contributing to elements of psychological distress (e.g., perceived stress, poor mental health). Considering these findings, more research is needed to examine the specific contribution of risky drinking to suicidality among lawyers and it would be inappropriate to conclude that it does not meaningfully contribute to their suicide risk.

5. Limitations

There are limitations to the present study that should be considered when interpreting the results. First, the cross-sectional design of the study means that causality cannot be inferred. It is possible that suicidal ideation may also be a cause rather than just a consequence of the predictor variables. Longitudinal studies are needed to establish the direction of the relationship between these variables.

Second, the sample of lawyers in the present study was drawn from two jurisdictions only, California and Washington, D.C. Although those jurisdictions have among the largest lawyer populations in the United States and thereby provide for a large and diverse sample, they may not be representative of the legal profession as a whole. Further research would help confirm the generalizability of these findings to other geographic regions.

Third, the present study relied on self-report measures to assess predictor and outcome variables. Self-report measures are susceptible to bias and may not always reflect an individual's true thoughts, feelings, or behaviors. Future research using objective measures (e.g., medical records, performance assessments) may provide a clearer picture of the relationship between these variables, though such research may be difficult or impractical to conduct.

Finally, although AUDIT scores did not predict suicidal ideation in the present study, drinking is still very relevant to the discussion of suicide in this population given the high rates of problem drinking among lawyers [3,7] and the well-established connection between substance misuse and suicide generally [77]. Future research should continue to examine the relationship between alcohol use and suicidal ideation in this population.

6. Conclusions

Efforts are underway within the legal profession to improve mental health, reduce the stigma associated with mental health disorders, and increase the overall wellbeing of lawyers. To support and inform those efforts, an enhanced empirical understanding of the profession's unique mental health risks is essential, including a better understanding of why lawyers are much more likely than the average person to experience suicidal thoughts. This research has begun to answer that question. To summarize, our findings suggest the profile of a lawyer with the highest risk for suicide is a lonely or socially isolated male with a high level of unmanageable stress, who is overly committed to their work, and may have a history of mental health problems. The heightened risk of suicidal ideation extends well beyond this specific profile, however, thereby necessitating a sustained focus on the factors we identified as predictive of that risk. Overall, these findings underscore the need for interventions to address work-related stress and loneliness in the legal profession. This may include providing education, resources, and support for lawyers to better manage their workload, modifying work demands and expectations, and promoting a culture of openness and support within law firms. Additionally, targeting interventions towards male lawyers may be particularly important given their higher risk of suicidal ideation. Further research is needed to continue exploring the dynamics of the relationship between work overcommitment, loneliness, perceived stress, and suicidal ideation in this population.

Supplementary Materials: The following supporting information can be downloaded at: https://www.mdpi.com/article/10.3390/healthcare11040536/s1, Table S1: Predictors of PHQ-9 suicidal ideation among lawyers controlling for perceived influence of COVID-19 on PHQ-9 depression symptoms (N = 1962).

Author Contributions: Conceptualization, J.J.A. and P.R.K.; methodology, J.J.A.; software, J.J.A. and N.D.; validation, J.J.A. and N.D.; formal analysis, J.J.A.; investigation, J.J.A. and P.R.K.; resources, J.J.A. and P.R.K.; data curation, J.J.A. and N.D.; writing—original draft preparation, J.J.A., H.M.T. and P.R.K.; writing—review and editing, J.J.A., P.R.K. and M.R.K.; visualization, J.J.A. and M.R.K.; supervision, J.J.A. and P.R.K.; project administration, J.J.A. and P.R.K.; funding acquisition, J.J.A. All authors have read and agreed to the published version of the manuscript.

Funding: This research was funded by NIAAA, grant number K01AA024805.

Institutional Review Board Statement: The study design and protocol were reviewed by the University of Minnesota Institutional Review Board and deemed exempt from approval. An Exemption Determination was issued on 20 March 2020.

Informed Consent Statement: Informed consent was obtained from all subjects involved in the study.

Data Availability Statement: Data cannot be shared publicly because they involve human research participants and contain potentially sensitive information related to mental health and substance use. Researchers who meet the criteria for access to confidential data may request to access the data by contacting the corresponding author and completing a University of Minnesota Data Use Agreement.

Acknowledgments: The authors would like to thank the California Lawyers Association and D.C. Bar for their essential support of and commitment to this work.

Conflicts of Interest: The authors declare no conflict of interest.

References

1. Klonsky, E.D.; May, A.M.; Saffer, B.Y. Suicide, Suicide Attempts, and Suicidal Ideation. *Annu. Rev. Clin. Psychol.* **2016**, *12*, 307–330. [CrossRef]
2. Simon, G.E.; Rutter, C.M.; Peterson, D.; Oliver, M.; Whiteside, U.; Operskalski, B.; Ludman, E.J. Does Response on the PHQ-9 Depression Questionnaire Predict Subsequent Suicide Attempt or Suicide Death? *Psychiatr. Serv.* **2013**, *64*, 1195–1202. Available online: https://ps-psychiatryonline-org.ezp2.lib.umn.edu/doi/full/10.1176/appi.ps.201200587 (accessed on 1 December 2013). [CrossRef]
3. Krill, P.R.; Johnson, R.; Albert, L. The Prevalence of Substance Use and Other Mental Health Concerns Among American Lawyers. *J. Addict. Med.* **2016**, *101*, 46–52. [CrossRef] [PubMed]
4. Thiese, M.S.; Allen, J.A.; Knudson, M.; Free, K.; Petersen, P. Depressive Symptoms and Suicidal Ideation Among Lawyers and Other Law Professionals. *J. Occup. Environ. Med./Am. Coll. Occup. Environ. Med.* **2021**, *63*, 381–386. [CrossRef]
5. Buchanan, B.; Coyle, J.; Brafford, A.; Campbell, D.; Camson, J.; Gruber, C.; Harrell, T.; Jaffe, D.; Kepler, T.; Krill, P.; et al. The Path to Lawyer Well-Being: Practical Recommendations for Positive Change (The Report of the National Task Force on Lawyer Well-Being), Part II, Recommendations for Law Schools [Internet]. 2017. Available online: https://papers.ssrn.com/abstract=3021218 (accessed on 14 December 2022).
6. Ivey-Stephenson, A.Z.; Crosby, A.E.; Hoenig, J.M.; Gyawali, S.; Park-Lee, E.; Hedden, S.L. Suicidal thoughts and behaviors among adults aged ≥18 years—United States, 2015–2019. *MMWR Surveill. Summ.* **2022**, *71*, 1–19. [CrossRef]
7. Anker, J.J.; Krill, P.R. Stress, drink, leave: An examination of gender-specific risk factors for mental health problems and attrition among licensed attorneys. *PloS ONE* **2021**, *16*, e0250563. [CrossRef]
8. Bjerkeset, O.; Romundstad, P.; Gunnell, D. Gender differences in the association of mixed anxiety and depression with suicide. *Br. J. Psychiatry J. Ment. Sci.* **2008**, *192*, 474–475. [CrossRef]
9. Davidson, C.L.; Wingate LR, R.; Grant DM, M. Interpersonal Suicide Risk and Ideation: The Influence of Depression and Social Anxiety. *J. Soc.* **2011**, *30*, 842–855. [CrossRef]
10. Gonda, X.; Fountoulakis, K.N.; Kaprinis, G.; Rihmer, Z. Prediction and prevention of suicide in patients with unipolar depression and anxiety. *Ann. Gen. Psychiatry* **2007**, *6*, 23. [CrossRef]
11. Kalin, N.H. Anxiety, Depression, and Suicide in Youth. *Am. J. Psychiatry* **2021**, *178*, 275–279. [CrossRef]
12. Placidi, G.P.; Oquendo, M.A.; Malone, K.M.; Brodsky, B.; Ellis, S.P.; Mann, J.J. Anxiety in major depression: Relationship to suicide attempts. *Am. J. Psychiatry* **2000**, *157*, 1614–1618. [CrossRef] [PubMed]
13. Tsai, F.-J.; Huang, W.-L.; Chan, C.-C. Occupational stress and burnout of lawyers. *J. Occup. Health* **2009**, *51*, 443–450. [CrossRef] [PubMed]
14. Koltai, J.; Schieman, S.; Dinovitzer, R. The Status–Health Paradox: Organizational Context, Stress Exposure, and Well-being in the Legal Profession. *J. Health Soc. Behav.* **2018**, *59*, 20–37. [CrossRef] [PubMed]
15. Achor, S.; Kellerman, G.R.; Reece, A.; Robichaux, A. America's Loneliest Workers, According to Research. Harvard Business Review. Available online: https://hbr.org/2018/03/americas-loneliest-workers-according-to-research (accessed on 19 March 2018).
16. Ash, O. The Prevalence and Effects of Loneliness in the General Population, Lawyer Well-being, and a Survey of Law Students. Ph.D. Thesis, IU McKinney School of Law, Indianapolis, Indiana, 2019. [CrossRef]
17. Ash, O.; Huang, P.H. Loneliness in COVID-19, Life, and Law. *Health Matrix* **2022**, *32*, 55. [CrossRef]
18. Batty, G.D.; Kivimäki, M.; Bell, S.; Gale, C.R.; Shipley, M.; Whitley, E.; Gunnell, D. Psychosocial characteristics as potential predictors of suicide in adults: An overview of the evidence with new results from prospective cohort studies. *Transl. Psychiatry* **2018**, *8*, 22. [CrossRef] [PubMed]
19. Bickford, D.; Morin, R.T.; Nelson, J.C.; Mackin, R.S. Determinants of suicide-related ideation in late life depression: Associations with perceived stress. *Clin. Gerontol.* **2020**, *43*, 37–45. [CrossRef]
20. Calati, R.; Ferrari, C.; Brittner, M.; Oasi, O.; Olié, E.; Carvalho, A.F.; Courtet, P. Suicidal thoughts and behaviors and social isolation: A narrative review of the literature. *J. Affect. Disord.* **2019**, *245*, 653–667. [CrossRef]
21. Cole, A.B.; Wingate, L.R.; Tucker, R.P.; Rhoades-Kerswill, S.; O'Keefe, V.M.; Hollingsworth, D.W. The differential impact of brooding and reflection on the relationship between perceived stress and suicide ideation. *Personal. Individ. Differ.* **2015**, *83*, 170–173. [CrossRef]
22. Motillon-Toudic, C.; Walter, M.; Séguin, M.; Carrier, J.-D.; Berrouiguet, S.; Lemey, C. Social isolation and suicide risk: Literature review and perspectives. *Eur. Psychiatry J. Assoc. Eur. Psychiatr.* **2022**, *65*, e65. [CrossRef]
23. Näher, A.-F.; Rummel-Kluge, C.; Hegerl, U. Associations of suicide rates with socioeconomic status and social isolation: Findings from longitudinal register and census data. *Front. Psychiatry* **2019**, *10*, 898. [CrossRef]
24. Trout, D.L. The role of social isolation in suicide. *Suicide Life-Threat. Behav.* **1980**, *10*, 10–23. [CrossRef]
25. Jackson, S.E.; Turner, J.A.; Brief, A.P. Correlates of burnout among public service lawyers. *J. Organ. Behav.* **1987**, *8*, 339–349. [CrossRef]
26. Nickum, M.; Desrumaux, P. Burnout among lawyers: Effects of workload, latitude and mediation via engagement and over-engagement. *Psychiatry Psychol. Law* **2022**, 1–13. [CrossRef]
27. Alexopoulos, E.C.; Kavalidou, K.; Messolora, F. Suicide mortality patterns in Greek work force before and during the economic crisis. *Int. J. Environ. Res. Public Health* **2019**, *16*, 469. [CrossRef]

28. Choi, B. Job strain, long work hours, and suicidal ideation in US workers: A longitudinal study. *Int. Arch. Occup. Environ. Health* **2018**, *91*, 865–875. [CrossRef] [PubMed]
29. Iannelli, R.J.; Finlayson AJ, R.; Brown, K.P.; Neufeld, R.; Gray, R.; Dietrich, M.S.; Martin, P.R. Suicidal behavior among physicians referred for fitness-for-duty evaluation. *Gen. Hosp. Psychiatry* **2014**, *36*, 732–736. [CrossRef] [PubMed]
30. Kim, S.-Y.; Shin, Y.-C.; Oh, K.-S.; Shin, D.-W.; Lim, W.-J.; Cho, S.J.; Jeon, S.-W. Association between work stress and risk of suicidal ideation: A cohort study among Korean employees examining gender and age differences. *Scand. J. Work. Environ. Health* **2020**, *46*, 198–208. [CrossRef] [PubMed]
31. Kõlves, K.; De Leo, D. Suicide in medical doctors and nurses: An analysis of the Queensland Suicide Register. *J. Nerv. Ment. Dis.* **2013**, *201*, 987–990. [CrossRef]
32. Ross, D.V.; Mathieu, D.S.; Wardhani, M.R.; Gullestrup, M.J.; Kõlves, D.K. Suicidal ideation and related factors in construction industry apprentices. *J. Affect. Disord.* **2022**, *297*, 294–300. [CrossRef]
33. Shanafelt, T.D.; Balch, C.M.; Dyrbye, L.; Bechamps, G.; Russell, T.; Satele, D.; Rummans, T.; Swartz, K.; Novotny, P.J.; Sloan, J.; et al. Special report: Suicidal ideation among American surgeons. *Arch. Surg.* **2011**, *146*, 54–62. [CrossRef]
34. Ullmann, D.; Phillips, R.L.; Beeson, W.L.; Dewey, H.G.; Brin, B.N.; Kuzma, J.W.; Mathews, C.P.; Hirst, A.E. Cause-specific mortality among physicians with differing life-styles. *JAMA J. Am. Med. Assoc.* **1991**, *265*, 2352–2359. [CrossRef]
35. van der Heijden, F.; Dillingh, G.; Bakker, A.; Prins, J. Suicidal thoughts among medical residents with burnout. *Arch. Suicide Res. Off. J. Int. Acad. Suicide Res.* **2008**, *12*, 344–346. [CrossRef]
36. Menon, N.K.; Shanafelt, T.D.; Sinsky, C.A.; Linzer, M.; Carlasare, L.; Brady, K.J.S.; Stillman, M.J.; Trockel, M.T. Association of physician burnout with suicidal ideation and medical errors. *JAMA Netw. Open* **2020**, *3*, e2028780. [CrossRef] [PubMed]
37. Kan, D.; Yu, X. Occupational Stress, Work-Family Conflict and Depressive Symptoms among Chinese Bank Employees: The Role of Psychological Capital. *Int. J. Environ. Res. Public Health* **2016**, *13*, 134. [CrossRef] [PubMed]
38. Obidoa, C.; Reeves, D.; Warren, N.; Reisine, S.; Cherniack, M. Depression and work family conflict among corrections officers. *J. Occup. Environ. Med. /Am. Coll. Occup. Environ. Med.* **2011**, *53*, 1294–1301. [CrossRef] [PubMed]
39. Peter, R.; March, S.; du Prel, J.-B. Are status inconsistency, work stress and work-family conflict associated with depressive symptoms? Testing prospective evidence in the lidA study. *Soc. Sci. Med.* **2016**, *151*, 100–109. [CrossRef] [PubMed]
40. Sugawara, N.; Danjo, K.; Furukori, H.; Sato, Y.; Tomita, T.; Fujii, A.; Nakagami, T.; Kitaoka, K.; Yasui-Furukori, N. Work-family conflict as a mediator between occupational stress and psychological health among mental health nurses in Japan. *Neuropsychiatr. Dis. Treat.* **2017**, *13*, 779–784. [CrossRef] [PubMed]
41. Akram, B.; Bibi, B.; Ahmed, M.; Kauser, N. Work-Family Conflict and Suicidal Ideation Among Physicians of Pakistan: The Moderating Role of Perceived Life Satisfaction. Shibboleth Authentication Request. Available online: https://journals-sagepub-com.ezp1.lib.umn.edu/doi/10.1177/0030222820947246 (accessed on 6 August 2020).
42. Lee, H.-E.; Kim, I.; Kim, H.-R.; Kawachi, I. Association of long working hours with accidents and suicide mortality in Korea. *Scand. J. Work. Environ. Health* **2020**, *46*, 480–487. [CrossRef] [PubMed]
43. Garnett, M.F.; Curtin, S.C.; Stone, D.M. Suicide mortality in the United States, 2000–2020. *NCHS Data Brief* **2022**, *433*, 1–8.
44. Duarte, D.; El-Hagrassy, M.M.; Couto TC, E.; Gurgel, W.; Fregni, F.; Correa, H. Male and Female Physician Suicidality: A Systematic Review and Meta-analysis. *JAMA Psychiatry* **2020**, *77*, 587–597. [CrossRef]
45. Milner, A.J.; Spittal, M.S.; Pirkis, J.; LaMontagne, A.D. Does Gender Explain the Relationship Between Occupation and Suicide? Findings from a Meta-Analytic Study. *Community Ment. Health J.* **2016**, *52*, 568–573. [CrossRef] [PubMed]
46. Milner, A.; Witt, K.; Maheen, H.; LaMontagne, A.D. Access to means of suicide, occupation and the risk of suicide: A national study over 12 years of coronial data. *BMC Psychiatry* **2017**, *17*, 125. [CrossRef] [PubMed]
47. Kroenke, K.; Spitzer, R.L.; Williams, J.B. The PHQ-9: Validity of a brief depression severity measure. *J. Gen. Intern. Med.* **2001**, *16*, 606–613. [CrossRef]
48. Cohen, S.; Kamarck, T.; Mermelstein, R. A global measure of perceived stress. *J. Health Soc. Behav.* **1983**, *24*, 385–396. [CrossRef] [PubMed]
49. Bush, K.; Kivlahan, D.R.; McDonell, M.B.; Fihn, S.D.; Bradley, K.A.; for the Ambulatory Care Quality Improvement Project (ACQUIP). The AUDIT Alcohol Consumption Questions (AUDIT-C): An Effective Brief Screening Test for Problem Drinking. *Arch. Intern. Med.* **1998**, *158*, 1789–1795. [CrossRef] [PubMed]
50. Skinner, H.A. The drug abuse screening test. *Addict. Behav.* **1982**, *7*, 363–371. [CrossRef]
51. Hughes, M.E.; Waite, L.J.; Hawkley, L.C.; Cacioppo, J.T. A short scale for measuring loneliness in large surveys: Results from two population-based studies. *Res. Aging* **2004**, *26*, 655–672. [CrossRef]
52. Steptoe, A.; Shankar, A.; Demakakos, P.; Wardle, J. Social isolation, loneliness, and all-cause mortality in older men and women. *Proc. Natl. Acad. Sci. USA* **2013**, *110*, 5797–5801. [CrossRef] [PubMed]
53. Siegrist, J.; Li, J.; Montano, D. *Psychometric Properties of the Effort-Reward Imbalance Questionnaire*; Duesseldorf University: Düsseldorf, Germany, 2014. Available online: https://www.uniklinik-duesseldorf.de/fileadmin/Fuer-Patienten-und-Besucher/Kliniken-Zentren-Institute/Institute/Institut_fuer_Medizinische_Soziologie/Forschung/PsychometricProperties.pdf (accessed on 14 December 2022).
54. Kristensen, T.S.; Hannerz, H.; Høgh, A.; Borg, V. The Copenhagen Psychosocial Questionnaire—A tool for the assessment and improvement of the psychosocial work environment. *Scand. J. Work. Environ. Health* **2005**, *31*, 438–449. [CrossRef] [PubMed]

55. Bauer, A.M.; Chan, Y.-F.; Huang, H.; Vannoy, S.; Unützer, J. Characteristics, management, and depression outcomes of primary care patients who endorse thoughts of death or suicide on the PHQ-9. *J. Gen. Intern. Med.* **2013**, *28*, 363–369. [CrossRef]
56. Kim, S.; Lee, H.-K.; Lee, K. Which PHQ-9 Items Can Effectively Screen for Suicide? Machine Learning Approaches. *Int. J. Environ. Res. Public Health* **2021**, *18*, 3339. [CrossRef]
57. Mackelprang, J.L.; Bombardier, C.H.; Fann, J.R.; Temkin, N.R.; Barber, J.K.; Dikmen, S.S. Rates and predictors of suicidal ideation during the first year after traumatic brain injury. *Am. J. Public Health* **2014**, *104*, e100–e107. [CrossRef]
58. Walker, J.; Hansen, C.H.; Butcher, I.; Sharma, N.; Wall, L.; Murray, G.; Sharpe, M. Thoughts of Death and Suicide Reported by Cancer Patients Who Endorsed the "Suicidal Thoughts" Item of the PHQ-9 During Routine Screening for Depression. *Psychosomatics* **2011**, *52*, 424–427. [CrossRef]
59. Chen, Y.L.; Kuo, P.H. Effects of perceived stress and resilience on suicidal behaviors in early adolescents. *Eur. Child Adolesc. Psychiatry* **2020**, *29*, 861–870.
60. Abdollahi, A.; Hosseinian, S.; Zamanshoar, E.; Beh-Pajooh, A.; Carlbring, P. The moderating effect of hardiness on the relationships between problem-solving skills and perceived stress with suicidal ideation in nursing students. *Studia Psychologica*. **2018**, *60*, 30–41. [CrossRef]
61. Stillwell, S.B.; Vermeesch, A.L.; Scott, J.G. Interventions to Reduce Perceived Stress Among Graduate Students: A Systematic Review With Implications for Evidence-Based Practice. *Worldviews Evid. -Based Nurs.* **2017**, *14*, 507–513. [CrossRef]
62. Maykrantz, S.A.; Nobiling, B.D.; Oxarart, R.A.; Langlinais, L.A.; Houghton, J.D. Coping with the crisis: The effects of psychological capital and coping behaviors on perceived stress. *Int. J. Workplace Health Manag.* **2021**, *14*, 650–665. [CrossRef]
63. Valosek, L.; Link, J.; Mills, P.; Konrad, A.; Rainforth, M.; Nidich, S. Effect of Meditation on Emotional Intelligence and Perceived Stress in the Workplace: A Randomized Controlled Study. *Perm. J.* **2018**, *22*, 17–172. [CrossRef]
64. Petrie, K.; Crawford, J.; Baker, S.T.E.; Dean, K.; Robinson, J.; Veness, B.G.; Randall, J.; McGorry, P.; Christensen, H.; Harvey, S.B. Interventions to reduce symptoms of common mental disorders and suicidal ideation in physicians: A systematic review and meta-analysis. *Lancet Psychiatry* **2019**, *6*, 225–234. [CrossRef]
65. Howard, M.C.; Follmer, K.B.; Smith, M.B.; Tucker, R.P.; Van Zandt, E.C. Work and suicide: An interdisciplinary systematic literature review. *J. Organ. Behav.* **2022**, *43*, 260–285. [CrossRef]
66. Pfeffer, J. *Dying for a Paycheck: How Modern Management Harms Employee Health and Company Performance—And What We Can Do about It*; Harper Business: New York, NY, USA, 2018; ISBN 978-006-280-092-3.
67. Krieger, L.S.; Sheldon, K.M. What Makes Lawyers Happy? A Data-Driven Prescription to Redefine Professional Success. *Georg. Wash. Law Rev.* **2015**, *83*, 554.
68. American Bar Association Survey: Most Lawyers Want Options for Remote Work, Court, and Conferences. Available online: https://www.americanbar.org/news/abanews/aba-news-archives/2022/09/aba-survey-lawyers-remote-work/ (accessed on 14 December 2022).
69. Canetto, S.S.; Sakinofsky, I. The gender paradox in suicide. *Suicide Life-Threat. Behav.* **1998**, *28*, 1–23. [CrossRef]
70. Schrijvers, D.L.; Bollen, J.; Sabbe, B.G.C. The gender paradox in suicidal behavior and its impact on the suicidal process. *J. Affect. Disord.* **2012**, *138*, 19–26. [CrossRef]
71. Violanti, J.M.; Mnatsakanova, A.; Andrew, M.E.; Allison, P.; Gu, J.K.; Fekedulegn, D. Effort–Reward Imbalance and Overcommitment at Work: Associations With Police Burnout. *Police Q.* **2018**, *21*, 440–460. [CrossRef]
72. Bergin, A.J.; Jimmieson, N.L. Explaining psychological distress in the legal profession: The role of overcommitment. *Int. J. Stress Manag.* **2013**, *20*, 134–161. [CrossRef]
73. Brent, D.A.; Perper, J.A.; Goldstein, C.E.; Kolko, D.J.; Allan, M.J.; Allman, C.J.; Zelenak, J.P. Risk factors for adolescent suicide. A comparison of adolescent suicide victims with suicidal inpatients. *Arch. Gen. Psychiatry* **1988**, *45*, 581–588. [CrossRef]
74. Nock, M.K.; Borges, G.; Bromet, E.J.; Cha, C.B.; Kessler, R.C.; Lee, S. Suicide and suicidal behavior. *Epidemiol. Rev.* **2008**, *30*, 133–154. [CrossRef]
75. Brådvik, L.; Mattisson, C.; Bogren, M.; Nettelbladt, P. Mental disorders in suicide and undetermined death in the Lundby Study. The contribution of severe depression and alcohol dependence. *Arch. Suicide Res. Off. J. Int. Acad. Suicide Res.* **2010**, *14*, 266–275. [CrossRef]
76. McCaul, M.E.; Hutton, H.E.; Stephens MA, C.; Xu, X.; Wand, G.S. Anxiety, anxiety sensitivity, and perceived stress as predictors of recent drinking, alcohol craving, and social stress response in heavy drinkers. *Alcohol. Clin. Exp. Res.* **2017**, *41*, 836–845. [CrossRef]
77. Hawton, K.; Fagg, J.; Simkin, S.; O'Connor, S. Substance abuse and deliberate self-harm. *Am. J. Psychiatry* **2002**, *159*, 2033–2041.

Disclaimer/Publisher's Note: The statements, opinions and data contained in all publications are solely those of the individual author(s) and contributor(s) and not of MDPI and/or the editor(s). MDPI and/or the editor(s) disclaim responsibility for any injury to people or property resulting from any ideas, methods, instructions or products referred to in the content.

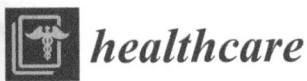

Article

Depression Associated with Caregiver Quality of Life in Post-COVID-19 Patients in Two Regions of Peru

Janett V. Chávez Sosa [1], Flor M. Mego Gonzales [1], Zoila E. Aliaga Ramirez [1], Mayela Cajachagua Castro [1] and Salomón Huancahuire-Vega [2,3,*]

[1] Escuela Profesional de Enfermería, Universidad Peruana Unión (UPeU), Lima 15464, Peru; viki16@upeu.edu.pe (J.V.C.S.); flormego@upeu.edu.pe (F.M.M.G.); estheraliaga@upeu.edu.pe (Z.E.A.R.); mayela@upeu.edu.pe (M.C.C.)
[2] Escuela Profesional de Medicina, Universidad Peruana Unión (UPeU), Lima 15464, Peru
[3] Dirección General de Investigación, Universidad Peruana Unión (UPeU), Lima 15464, Peru
* Correspondence: salomonhuancahuire@upeu.edu.pe; Tel.: +51-997574011

Citation: Chávez Sosa, J.V.; Mego Gonzales, F.M.; Aliaga Ramirez, Z.E.; Cajachagua Castro, M.; Huancahuire-Vega, S. Depression Associated with Caregiver Quality of Life in Post-COVID-19 Patients in Two Regions of Peru. *Healthcare* **2022**, *10*, 1219. https://doi.org/10.3390/healthcare10071219

Academic Editors: Athanassios Tselebis and Argyro Pachi

Received: 16 May 2022
Accepted: 28 June 2022
Published: 29 June 2022

Publisher's Note: MDPI stays neutral with regard to jurisdictional claims in published maps and institutional affiliations.

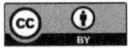

Copyright: © 2022 by the authors. Licensee MDPI, Basel, Switzerland. This article is an open access article distributed under the terms and conditions of the Creative Commons Attribution (CC BY) license (https://creativecommons.org/licenses/by/4.0/).

Abstract: Due to COVID-19, the workload experienced by caregivers has increased markedly which has led them to experience fatigue, anxiety and depression. This study aims to determine the relationship between quality of life and depression in caregivers of post-COVID-19 patients in two regions of Peru. In a cross-sectional analytical study, the sample was non-probabilistic and by snowball, and consisted of 730 caregivers, to whom the questionnaires "Modified Betty Ferell Quality of Life" and the "Beck Depression Inventory" were applied. It was determined that being a male caregiver (OR: 2.119; 95% CI: 1.332–3.369) was associated with a good quality of life. On the other hand, caregivers who had children (OR: 0.391; 95% CI: 0.227–0.675), were vaccinated against COVID-19 (OR: 0.432; 95% CI: 0.250–0.744), were immediate family members (OR: 0.298; 95% CI: 0.117–0.761) and had high depression (OR: 0.189; 95% CI: 0.073–0.490) were associated with poor quality of life. The results of this study allow us to conclude the association between depression and poor quality of life in caregivers of these patients so it is necessary to monitor the mental health of caregivers, and to develop adaptation strategies to pandemic conditions.

Keywords: depression; quality of life; family caregivers; COVID-19

1. Introduction

The growing wave of COVID-19 infections caused a major impact worldwide. This crisis led to a state of emergency that triggered radical preventive measures such as confinement, quarantine and social distancing [1]. The contingency measure taken in response to the pandemic was the limitation of health services at the first level of care and other health facilities, as well as the restriction of outpatient activities, health promotion and risk prevention; this lack of access to the health system, hospitals, appointments, beds and oxygen balloons generated the need for people to assume the role of caregivers and care for their family members with COVID-19 at home. In most cases, caregivers were immediate family members such as father, mother, husband, wife, son, daughter, brother, sister, etc. [2].

A study conducted in the United States indicates that there are about 43.5 million informal caregivers caring for sick or disabled family members; these caregivers are untrained, feel unprepared for this role and experience high levels of stress and depression. Lack of preparation and inadequate development of basic skills for quality caregiving affect the caregiver's emotional well-being, social well-being and finances [3].

At the Latin American level, the workload experienced by caregivers, which includes the parameters of time, difficulty and tasks, is huge and has increased markedly during the pandemic era [4]. According to Ibáñez et al., "the challenges include aspects such as insufficient supply by healthcare personnel, social and socioeconomic determinants of health, disparities, gender-biased burdens and the effect of COVID-19 on families" [5]. Latin American countries face deficiencies in their health systems, which hinder the level of care that the population needs.

Peru has been one of the Latin American countries widely affected by COVID-19, has the highest infection-lethality rate (ILR) due to COVID-19 in the world, and has the fifth highest number of deaths in absolute terms [6]. Even before the pandemic, caregivers of Peruvian patients hospitalized in the medical service were identified as having a poor quality of life [7]. There are different conceptualizations of quality of life related to health. From the nursing point of view, Ferrell et al. describes it as a multidimensional construction that includes well-being or discontent in aspects of life important to the individual, encompassing the interaction of health and psychological, spiritual, socioeconomic and family functioning [8].

Preventive measures taken by the government gave caregivers a new way to manage the prevention of respiratory infections; however, they are not being properly implemented. According to Navarrete et al., the average age of Peruvian caregivers is 33 and 48 years, 95.7% of caregivers in Lima are female, 77.2% of caregivers have not received training on hand washing and 96.7% do not know how to properly manage stress [9].

One of the dimensions of quality of life is spiritual well-being. Spiritual well-being is defined as the satisfaction and experience of a harmonious relationship with oneself/others, nature or a power greater than oneself [10]. Different studies show the importance of spiritual well-being during the COVID-19 pandemic, both for patients with COVID-19 and their caregivers [11,12]. Psychological well-being is another component of quality of life. This is defined by the WHO as the state of complete physical, mental and social well-being, and not merely the absence of disease or illness [13]. There is evidence showing that psychological well-being is positively related to behaviors related to health and spiritual aspects [14].

Another factor affecting quality of life is depression. Depression is a frequently occurring disorder that affects the ability to perform day-to-day tasks effectively and makes it difficult to cope adequately with problems [15]. Therefore, depression is one of the most present and prevalent problems in caregivers because it is directly related to caregiver overload and quality of life; it mainly results from a lack of organization and care by the healthcare system, the absence of a solid support network for the caregiver and insufficient experience in caring for the patient [16]. The Beck Depression Inventory I is one of the most widely used scales in the world to measure the severity of depression symptoms in clinical and non-clinical samples. Based on this scale in its Spanish version, we consider "high depression" scores above 14 [17].

Studies prior to the pandemic found that the frequency of anxiety and depression in primary caregivers of pediatric patients was higher than in the general population [18]. Likewise, in another study, it was found that the quality of life in elderly caregivers was worse compared to younger caregivers due to their frailty, which leads many of them to experience symptoms of depression and a poorer quality of life [19].

There is a variety of research on caregiver quality of life; however, little research has been conducted on the quality of life of caregivers of post-COVID-19 patients. The work performed by the caregiver is of vital importance in the midst of the disease and in the patient's recovery. However, it has a stressful effect on oneself because of the feeling of constant helplessness, the uncertain future and fatigue, which is mainly related to depressive symptomatology and other health conditions in the physical, social, spiritual and occupational areas [20]. As a result, conflicts in the different areas of the caregiver's life generate changes in the family relationship; altering its correct functioning which is expressed through the ability to resolve conflicts, family crises and at the moment of expressing affection and care [21].

Therefore, the study aimed to determine the relationship between quality of life, including physical and psychological well-being, social welfare and spiritual wellness with depression in caregivers of post-COVID-19 patients in two regions of Peru during the second wave of the pandemic.

2. Materials and Methods

The study was a cross-sectional analytical study. The sampling was non-probabilistic and by snowball, and included caregivers of both sexes, over 18 years of age, who were caring for family members or patients diagnosed with COVID-19 and who agreed to participate voluntarily in the study. The sample consisted of 730 caregivers, of whom 366 were from the east of Lima (capital, cost) and 364 from Pucallpa-Ucayali (eastern of Peru, jungle).

For the measurement of quality of life, the modified Betty Ferrell quality of life scale was used, with a reliability of 0.88 by Cronbach's alpha [22]. It has 30 items distributed in four dimensions: physical, psychological, social and spiritual well-being, with a Likert-type response scale. The following classification was used to measure the results of the instrument: 54 to 84 points is equivalent to a poor quality of life and 85 to 115 points as good quality. On the other hand, the depression variable was measured with the Beck Depression Inventory, with a reliability of 0.91 by Cronbach's alpha. This instrument is composed of 21 items, with a Likert-type response scale. The final score ranges from 0 to 13 points equivalent to low depression and from 14 to 35 points as high depression [17].

To collect the data, a letter of request for authorization was first presented to the authorities. For data collection, the survey technique was used, through home visits in the study areas and respecting the biosecurity protocols against COVID-19 imposed by the government. The study has the approval of the Ethics Committee of Peruvian Union University (N° 2021-CE-FCS-UPeU-016) and informed consent was obtained before the application of the questionnaire.

Data analysis was performed using the SPSS v.24 statistical program. For univariate analysis, simple frequency tables were used, and for bivariate analysis, contingency tables and the chi-square test were used. For multivariate analysis, binary logistic regression was used, considering quality of life as the dependent variable: poor (0) and good (1). Similarly, sociodemographic characteristics and depression in caregivers of post-COVID-19 patients were considered as independent variables.

3. Results

Of 730 caregivers, 76.3% were women and 23.7% were men. Likewise, 58.2% were aged 30–59 years, 50.8% were from Lima, 56% were married or cohabiting and 74% had higher education. On the other hand, 83.6% were employed, 46.3% had EsSalud insurance (social security in the country), 84.8% had already been vaccinated against COVID-19, 56.2% had children and 96.4% were direct relatives of the post-COVID-19 patient (Table 1).

Regarding the study variables, 80.1% of the caregivers presented poor quality of life, as did the psychological and spiritual well-being dimensions, with 82.7% and 67.1%, respectively. On the other hand, 86.4% of caregivers had low depression and 13.6% had high depression. The same trend is observed for each of its dimensions (Table 2).

Bivariate analysis showed that sex ($p = 0.000$), age ($p = 0.001$), place of origin ($p = 0.006$), marital status ($p = 0.000$), educational level ($p = 0.017$), type of work ($p = 0.000$), health insurance ($p = 0.009$), COVID-19 vaccination ($p = 0.000$), children ($p = 0.000$), relationship to the patient ($p = 0.044$), and depression were related to caregivers' quality of life (Table 3).

Finally, multivariate analysis found that being a male caregiver (OR: 2.119; 95% CI: 1.332–3.369) was associated with good quality of life. On the other hand, caregivers who had children (OR: 0.391; 95% CI: 0.227–0.675), were vaccinated against COVID-19 (OR: 0.432; 95% CI: 0.250–0.744), were immediate family members (OR: 0.298; 95% CI: 0.117–0.761) and had high depression (OR: 0.189; 95% CI: 0.073–0.490) were associated with poor quality of life (Table 4).

Table 1. General characteristics of caregivers of post-COVID-19 patients.

Variables		n = 730	%
Sex	Male	173	23.7
	Female	557	76.3
Age	Young (18–29 years old)	305	41.8
	Adult (30–59 years)	425	58.2
City	Lima	371	50.8
	Pucallpa-Ucayali	359	49.2
Marital status	Single/Widowed/Divorced	321	44
	Married/Cohabitant	409	56
Level of education	Basic education	190	26
	Higher education	540	74
Type of work	Not working/Retired	120	16.4
	Dependent/Independent	610	83.6
Type of insurance	No insurance	15	2.1
	SIS	286	39.2
	ESSALUD	338	46.3
	PNP/FFAA	11	1.5
	Private	80	11
COVID-19 vaccination	Yes	619	84.8
	No/Not my turn yet	111	15.2
Do you have children?	Yes	410	56.2
	No	320	43.8
Relationship to patient	Immediate family member	704	96.4
	Non-direct relative	26	3.6

Table 2. Descriptive analysis of the study variables.

Variables		n = 730	%
Quality of Life	Good	145	19.9
	Deficient	585	80.1
Physical Well-being	Good	424	58.1
	Deficient	306	41.9
Psychological Well-being	Good	126	17.3
	Deficient	604	82.7
Social Welfare	Good	389	53.3
	Deficient	341	46.7
Spiritual Wellness	Good	240	32.9
	Deficient	490	67.1
Depression	High	99	13.6
	Low	631	86.4
Cognitive Area	High	25	3.4
	Low	705	96.6
Physical Behavioral Area	High	51	7
	Low	679	93
Affective Emotional Area	High	103	14.1
	Low	627	85.9

Table 3. Bivariate analysis according to caregiver quality of life post COVID-19.

Variable		Quality of Life				p-Value
		Good		Deficient		
		n	%	n	%	
Sex	Female	95	65.5	462	79	0.001 *
	Male	50	34.5	123	21	
Age	Young (18–29 years old)	90	62.1	215	36.8	0.000 *
	Adult (30–59 years old)	55	37.9	370	63.2	
City	Lima	59	40.7	312	53.3	0.006 *
	Pucallpa-Ucayali	86	59.3	273	46.7	
Marital status	Single/Widowed/Divorced	92	63.4	229	39.1	0.000 *
	Married/Cohabitant	53	36.6	356	60.9	
Do you have children?	No	100	69	220	37.6	0.000 *
	Yes	45	31	365	62.4	
Studies	Basic education	49	33.8	141	24.1	0.017 *
	Higher education	96	66.2	444	75.9	
Do you have a job?	No	42	29	78	13.3	0.000 *
	Yes	103	71	507	86.7	
Do you have health insurance?	No	7	4.8	8	1.4	0.009 *
	Yes	138	95.2	577	98.6	
Have you been vaccinated against COVID-19?	No	49	33.8	62	10.6	0.000 *
	Yes	96	66.2	523	89.4	
Relationship to patient	Immediate family member	136	93.8	568	97.1	0.044 *
	Non-direct relative	9	6.2	17	2.9	
Depression	High	5	3.4	94	16.1	0.000 *
	Low	140	96.6	491	83.9	

* Statistical significance $p < 0.05$.

Table 4. Multivariate analysis according to the quality of life of the caregiver of post-COVID-19 patients.

Variables		OR	95% CI		p-Value
			LI	LS	
Sex	Male	1	(Reference)		
	Female	2.119	1.332	3.369	0.002 *
Age	Young (18–29 years old)	1	(Reference)		
	Adult (30–59 years)	0.860	0.491	1.507	0.599
City	Lima	1	(Reference)		
	Pucallpa-Ucayali	1.356	0.883	2.084	0.164
Marital status	Single/Widowed/Divorced	1	(Reference)		
	Married/Cohabitant	0.874	0.499	1.530	0.637
Do you have children?	No	1	(Reference)		
	Yes	0.391	0.227	0.675	0.001 *
Studies	Basic education	1	(Reference)		
	Higher education	1.001	0.608	1.647	0.998
Do you have a job?	No	1	(Reference)		
	Yes	0.665	0.383	1.152	0.146
Do you have health insurance?	No	1	(Reference)		
	Yes	0.696	0.214	2.263	0.547
Have you been vaccinated against COVID-19?	No	1	(Reference)		
	Yes	0.432	0.250	0.744	0.002 *
Relationship to patient	Immediate family member	1	(Reference)		
	Non-direct relative	0.298	0.117	0.761	0.011 *
Depression	High	1	(Reference)		
	Low	0.189	0.073	0.490	0.001 *

* Statistical significance $p < 0.05$; LI: lower limit; LS: upper limit.

4. Discussion

In the literature, there are studies that indicate that the quality of life of caregivers is slightly or moderately related to the state of mental, physical and social health. On the other hand, Troschel et al. mentions that the quality of life of caregivers can be significantly reduced if the emotional burden increases [23]. In this work with caregivers of post-COVID-19 patients, it was evidenced that the caregivers presented poor quality of life, especially in the dimensions of psychological and spiritual well-being and it was determined that quality of life is strongly associated with depression, in addition to other factors such as male sex, having children and being a direct relative.

Recent studies have shown lower levels of spiritual well-being than the situation prior to the pandemic, in addition, it has been shown that caregivers of COVID-19 patients express spiritual needs and that they use spiritual coping strategies [24]. During critical health circumstances such as the recent pandemic, many caregivers have questioned the meaning of life and recognized hopelessness, taking refuge in the sacred and using religious practices in search of spiritual well-being [25]. It would be necessary to consider the spiritual aspects of each individual as an important resource in obtaining general well-being.

In relation to the characteristics of the caregivers analyzed in this study, similarities were found with what is described in other investigations [26]. In the study population, the role of caregiver is mainly assumed by women, with 76.3% of the respondents belonging to the female sex. There are also other studies that demonstrate the high prevalence of the female sex as the main caregiver, demonstrated in a study applied to caregivers in China finding that 62.65% of the caregivers were women [27], as well as that of Ito and Tadaka in their work on the Japanese population, where 79.7% of family caregivers were female [28].

This study found that female caregivers had poorer quality of life than male caregivers. The literature indicates that female caregivers are more likely to have higher anxiety and depression and lower social support than male caregivers, which negatively impacts their quality of life [29]. In terms of caregiving approach, male caregivers have a more task-oriented approach to caregiving, while female caregivers use more emotion-oriented coping methods. Additionally, female caregivers tend to report a higher degree of caregiver burden and psychological distress; however, male caregivers may be reluctant to disclose feelings of burden or distress due to traditional views of masculinity that idealize self-sufficiency and stoicism [30].

Next, 56.2% of the caregivers claimed to have children and this was associated with a poor quality of life. In this sense, Pucciarelli, in his study, found that the quality of life of younger family caregivers without children was higher than that of those who had children [31]. The literature indicates that younger mothers perceive a greater burden with each additional child they have than do older mothers [32]. Likewise, each child increases the family burden and this would be related to a poorer quality of life [33].

It was also shown that caregivers who were vaccinated had a poor quality of life. In contrast, a study in the Polish population revealed that fully vaccinated persons had lower levels of anxiety, better quality of life and lower subjective anxiety about being infected with COVID-19 than those awaiting vaccination or those with an incomplete (one dose) vaccination regimen [34]. However, the review of the literature indicates that most of the population presents a local or systemic reaction after the application of the vaccine against COVID-19 and that these reactions could generate work limitation after the application of the second dose, which could affect their quality of life [35,36].

On the other hand, caregivers who were direct relatives of the post-COVID-19 patient presented worse quality of life. Previous studies revealed that family caregivers presented a poor quality of life due to low preparedness for patient care [37]. Likewise, spouses of palliative care partners reported poorer quality of life due to higher levels of unmet support needs [38].

Regarding depression, our study found that 86.4% of caregivers had low depression. Several studies show that caregivers of patients have high percentages of mild to moderate depression [39,40]. In addition, the study found that the higher the level of depression, the poorer the caregiver's quality of life. Similarly, a study of primary caregivers of children with cerebral palsy showed that greater severity of depression is negatively associated with dimensions of quality of life [41]. In the same way, a systematic review revealed that caregivers of patients with Dravet syndrome have high levels of depression and anxiety and that they are associated with fatigue and poor sleep quality, which affected their quality of life [42]. Finally, a study in caregivers of patients with heart failure also showed that depression and anxiety were associated with fatigue and poor sleep quality, which affected their quality of life [43]. These facts indicate that poor mental health, such as the presence of high levels of depression, impairs quality of life conditions. The COVID-19 pandemic has affected the mental health of the population, with several studies showing increased levels of depression [44,45]. Caregivers of post-COVID-19 patients are also included, who in addition to their work as caregivers must face the fear of contagion and the disease. These conditions would be affecting their quality of life, so it is necessary to monitor the mental health of this population group.

The study has some limitations, the main one being that it was carried out in populations of two regions of the country, the capital and the jungle region; it was not carried out in the highlands, so the results cannot be generalized to the entire Peruvian population. In addition, it is a cross-sectional study, so causality cannot be determined. Finally, some factors that could influence the quality of life of caregivers such as caregiver overload and preparation and other mental health conditions such as fear, worry and anxiety were not considered. Despite these limitations, it is necessary to highlight that to our knowledge this is the first report on the quality of life conditions of caregivers of post-COVID-19 patients in the Peruvian population.

5. Conclusions

The recovery process of post-COVID-19 patients depends to a great extent on the work of their caregivers, therefore, their self-care and quality of life should be promoted, including spiritual and psychological well-being. The results of this study allow us to conclude the association between depression and poor quality of life in caregivers of these patients and, in addition, it has been found that having children, having received the vaccine and being a direct relative are associated with a good quality of life. It is necessary to monitor the mental health of caregivers and to develop adaptation strategies to pandemic conditions and, besides, it would be advisable to assign fewer hours of work and greater inclusion in social activities. This will be reflected in better care and recovery of patients post COVID-19.

Author Contributions: Conceptualization, J.V.C.S., M.C.C. and S.H.-V.; methodology, F.M.M.G. and Z.E.A.R.; software, J.V.C.S.; validation, M.C.C. and S.H.-V.; formal analysis, J.V.C.S.; investigation, F.M.M.G. and Z.E.A.R.; data curation, J.V.C.S. and S.H.-V.; writing—original draft preparation, F.M.M.G. and Z.E.A.R.; writing—review and editing, M.C.C. and S.H.-V.; supervision, S.H.-V.; project administration, M.C.C. All authors have read and agreed to the published version of the manuscript.

Funding: This research received no external funding.

Institutional Review Board Statement: The study was conducted according to the guidelines of the Declaration of Helsinki and approved by Peruvian Union University (UPeU) Ethics Committee (2021-CE-FCS-UPeU-016).

Informed Consent Statement: Informed consent was obtained from all subjects involved in the study.

Data Availability Statement: The data presented in this study are available by request to the lead author.

Conflicts of Interest: The authors declare no conflict of interest.

References

1. Tang, J.W.; Caniza, M.A.; Dinn, M.; Dwyer, D.E.; Heraud, J.M.; Jennings, L.C.; Kok, J.; Kwok, K.O.; Li, Y.; Loh, T.P.; et al. An exploration of the political, social, economic and cultural factors affecting how different global regions initially reacted to the COVID-19 pandemic. *Interface Focus* **2022**, *12*, 20210079. [CrossRef] [PubMed]
2. López, H.A.; Álvarez, V.G.; Santibáñez, A.L.V.; Castillo, O.N. Caregiving solutions in Mexican households during COVID-19 lockdown. *SN Soc. Sci.* **2022**, *2*, 49. [CrossRef] [PubMed]

3. Sheth, K.; Lorig, K.; Stewart, A.; Parodi, J.F.; Ritter, P.L. Effects of COVID-19 on Informal Caregivers and the Development and Validation of a Scale in English and Spanish to Measure the Impact of COVID-19 on Caregivers. *J. Appl. Gerontol.* **2021**, *40*, 235–243. [CrossRef] [PubMed]
4. Belji Kangarlou, M.; Fatemi, F.; Paknazar, F.; Dehdashti, A. Occupational Burnout Symptoms and Its Relationship With Workload and Fear of the SARS-CoV-2 Pandemic Among Hospital Nurses. *Front. Public Health* **2022**, *10*, 852629. [CrossRef]
5. Ibáñez, A.; Pina-Escudero, S.D.; Possin, K.L.; Quiroz, Y.T.; Peres, F.A.; Slachevsky, A.; Sosa, A.L.; Brucki, S.M.; Miller, B.L. Dementia caregiving across Latin America and the Caribbean and brain health diplomacy. *Lancet Healthy Longev.* **2021**, *2*, e222–e231. [CrossRef]
6. Sorensen, R.J.; Barber, R.M.; Pigott, D.M.; Carter, A.; Spencer, C.N.; Ostroff, S.M.; Reiner, R.C., Jr.; Abbafati, C.; Adolph, C.; Allorant, A.; et al. Variation in the COVID-19 infection-fatality ratio by age, time, and geography during the pre-vaccine era: A systematic analysis. *Lancet* **2022**, *399*, 1469–1488.
7. Caqueo-Urízar, A.; Alessandrini, M.; Urzúa, A.; Zendjidjian, X.; Boyer, L.; Williams, D.R. Caregiver's quality of life and its positive impact on symptomatology and quality of life of patients with schizophrenia. *Health Qual. Life Outcomes* **2017**, *15*, 76. [CrossRef]
8. Ferrell, B.R.; Dow, K.H.; Grant, M. Measurement of the quality of life in cancer survivors. *Qual. Life Res.* **1995**, *4*, 523–531. [CrossRef]
9. Navarrete-Mejía, P.J.; Parodi, J.F.; Rivera-Encinas, M.T.; Runzer-Colmenares, F.M.; Velasco-Guerrero, J.C.; Sullcahuaman-Valdiglesias, E. Perfil del cuidador de adulto mayor en situación de pandemia por SARS-CoV-2, Lima-Perú. *Rev. Cuerpo Médico Hosp. Nac. Almanzor Aguinaga Asenjo* **2020**, *13*, 26–31. [CrossRef]
10. Sharif Nia, H.; Pahlevan Sharif, S.; Goudarzian, A.H.; Allen, K.A.; Jamali, S.; Heydari Gorji, M.A. The Relationship between Religious Coping and Self-Care Behaviors in Iranian Medical Students. *J. Relig. Health* **2017**, *56*, 2109–2117. [CrossRef]
11. De Diego-Cordero, R.; López-Gómez, L.; Lucchetti, G.; Badanta, B. Spiritual care in critically ill patients during COVID-19 pandemic. *Nurs. Outlook* **2022**, *70*, 64–77. [CrossRef] [PubMed]
12. Bakar, M.; Capano, E.; Patterson, M.; McIntyre, B.; Walsh, C.J. The Role of Palliative Care in Caring for the Families of Patients With COVID-19. *Am. J. Hosp. Palliat. Med.* **2020**, *37*, 866–868. [CrossRef] [PubMed]
13. WHO. Preamble to the Constitution of the World Health Organization as Adopted by the International Health Conference. New York, 19–22 June 1946; Signed on 22 July 1946 by the Representatives of 61 States (Official Records of the World Health Organization 2:100) and Entered into Force on 7 April 1948. 1948. Available online: https://hero.epa.gov/hero/index.cfm/reference/details/reference_id/80385 (accessed on 15 June 2022).
14. Bożek, A.; Nowak, P.F.; Blukacz, M. The Relationship Between Spirituality, Health-Related Behavior, and Psychological Well-Being. *Front. Psychol.* **2020**, *11*, 1997. [CrossRef] [PubMed]
15. Fuhrimann, C.M. Depression: A society's challenge we need to discuss. *Revista Cubana Salud Pública* **2017**, *43*, 136–138.
16. Palacios, E.; Pinzón, D. Sobrecarga, ansiedad y depresión en el cuidador de paciente con enfermedad cerebrovascular. *Repertorio Medicina Cirugía* **2017**, *26*, 118–120. [CrossRef]
17. Valdés, C.; Morales-Reyes, I.; Pérez, J.C.; Medellin, A.; Rojas, G.; Krause, M. Psychometric properties of a spanish version of the Beck depression inventory IA. *Rev. Med. Chil.* **2017**, *145*, 1005–1012. [CrossRef]
18. Aranda-Paniora, F. Depresión y ansiedad en cuidadores primarios en el Instituto Nacional de Salud del Niño. In *Anales de la Facultad de Medicina*; Facultad de Medicina, UNMSM: Lima, Peru, 2017.
19. Melo, L.A.D.; Jesus, I.T.M.D.; Orlandi, F.D.S.; Gomes, G.A.D.O.; Zazzetta, M.S.; Brito, T.R.P.D.; Santos-Orlandi, A.A.D. Frailty, depression, and quality of life: A study with elderly caregivers. *Rev. Bras. Enferm.* **2020**, *73* (Suppl. S3), e20180947. [CrossRef]
20. Laguado-Jaimes, E. Perfil del cuidador del paciente con Enfermedad Renal Crónica: Una revisión de la literatura. *Enfermería Nefrológica* **2019**, *22*, 352–359. [CrossRef]
21. Kimura, H.; Nishio, M.; Kukihara, H.; Koga, K.; Inoue, Y. The role of caregiver burden in the familial functioning, social support, and quality of family life of family caregivers of elders with dementia. *J. Rural. Med.* **2019**, *14*, 156–164. [CrossRef]
22. Parra, L.R.C.; González, G.M.C. Validez y confiabilidad del instrumento de calidad de vida de Betty Ferrell en español, para personas con enfermedad crónica. *Investig. Enfermería Imagen Desarro.* **2016**, *18*, 129–148. [CrossRef]
23. Troschel, F.M.; Ahndorf, F.; Wille, L.M.; Brandt, R.; Jost, J.; Rekowski, S.; Eich, H.T.; Stummer, W.; Wiewrodt, R.; Jetschke, K.; et al. Quality of Life in Brain Tumor Patients and Their Relatives Heavily Depends on Social Support Factors during the COVID-19 Pandemic. *Cancers* **2021**, *13*, 1276. [CrossRef] [PubMed]
24. Coppola, I.; Rania, N.; Parisi, R.; Lagomarsino, F. Spiritual Well-Being and Mental Health During the COVID-19 Pandemic in Italy. *Front. Psychiatry* **2021**, *12*, 626944. [CrossRef] [PubMed]
25. Casaleiro, T.; Caldeira, S.; Cardoso, D.; Apóstolo, J. Spiritual aspects of the family caregivers' experiences when caring for a community-dwelling adult with severe mental illness: A systematic review of qualitative evidence. *J. Psychiatr. Ment. Health Nurs.* **2022**, *29*, 240–273. [CrossRef] [PubMed]
26. Cantillo-Medina, C.P.; Perdomo-Romero, A.Y.; Ramírez-Perdomo, C.A. Habilidad del cuidado, sobrecarga percibida y calidad de vida del cuidador de personas en diálisis. *Enfermería Nefrológica* **2021**, *24*, 184–193. [CrossRef]
27. Huang, Y.; Mao, B.Q.; Ni, P.W.; Wang, Q.; Xie, T.; Hou, L. Investigation of the status and influence factors of caregiver's quality of life on caring for patients with chronic wound during COVID-19 epidemic. *Int. Wound J.* **2021**, *18*, 440–447. [CrossRef]
28. Ito, E.; Tadaka, E. Quality of life among the family caregivers of patients with terminal cancer at home in Japan. *Jpn. J. Nurs. Sci.* **2017**, *14*, 341–352. [CrossRef]

29. Rico-Blázquez, M.; Quesada-Cubo, V.; Polentinos-Castro, E.; Sánchez-Ruano, R.; Rayo-Gómez, M.; del Cura-González, I. Health-related quality of life in caregivers of community-dwelling individuals with disabilities or chronic conditions. A gender-differentiated analysis in a cross-sectional study. *BMC Nurs.* **2022**, *21*, 69. [CrossRef]
30. Robinson, C.A.; Bottorff, J.L.; Pesut, B.; Oliffe, J.L.; Tomlinson, J. The Male Face of Caregiving: A Scoping Review of Men Caring for a Person With Dementia. *Am. J. Mens Health* **2014**, *8*, 409–426. [CrossRef]
31. Pucciarelli, G.; Ausili, D.; Galbussera, A.A.; Rebora, P.; Savini, S.; Simeone, S.; Alvaro, R.; Vellone, E. Quality of life, anxiety, depression and burden among stroke caregivers: A longitudinal, observational multicentre study. *J. Adv. Nurs.* **2018**, *74*, 1875–1887. [CrossRef]
32. Goldsteen, K.; Ross, C.E. The perceived burden of children. *J. Fam. Issues* **1989**, *10*, 504–526. [CrossRef]
33. Çolak, B.; Kahriman, İ. Evaluation of Family Burden and Quality of Life of Parents with Children with Disability. *Am. J. Fam. Ther.* **2022**, *50*, 1–21. [CrossRef]
34. Babicki, M.; Malchrzak, W.; Hans-Wytrychowska, A.; Mastalerz-Migas, A. Impact of Vaccination on the Sense of Security, the Anxiety of COVID-19 and Quality of Life among Polish. A Nationwide Online Survey in Poland. *Vaccines* **2021**, *9*, 1444. [CrossRef] [PubMed]
35. Amodio, E.; Minutolo, G.; Casuccio, A.; Costantino, C.; Graziano, G.; Mazzucco, W.; Pieri, A.; Vitale, F.; Zarcone, M.; Restivo, V. Adverse Reactions to Anti-SARS-CoV-2 Vaccine: A Prospective Cohort Study Based on an Active Surveillance System. *Vaccines* **2022**, *10*, 345. [CrossRef] [PubMed]
36. Arnold, D.T.; Milne, A.; Samms, E.; Stadon, L.; Maskell, N.A.; Hamilton, F.W. Symptoms After COVID-19 Vaccination in Patients With Persistent Symptoms After Acute Infection: A Case Series. *Ann. Intern. Med.* **2021**, *174*, 1334–1336. [CrossRef]
37. Rochmawati, E.; Prawitasari, Y. Perceived caregiving preparedness and quality of life among Indonesian family caregivers of patients with life-limiting illness. *Int. J. Palliat. Nurs.* **2021**, *27*, 293–301. [CrossRef]
38. Norinder, M.; Årestedt, K.; Lind, S.; Axelsson, L.; Grande, G.; Ewing, G.; Holm, M.; Öhlén, J.; Benkel, I.; Alvariza, A. Higher levels of unmet support needs in spouses are associated with poorer quality of life—A descriptive cross-sectional study in the context of palliative home care. *BMC Palliat. Care* **2021**, *20*, 132. [CrossRef]
39. Shukri, M.; Mustofai, M.A.; Md Yasin, M.A.S.; Tuan Hadi, T.S. Burden, quality of life, anxiety, and depressive symptoms among caregivers of hemodialysis patients: The role of social support. *Int. J. Psychiatry Med.* **2020**, *55*, 397–407. [CrossRef]
40. Ayabakan-Cot, D.; Ates, E.; Kurt, B.; Nazlican, E.; Akbala, M. Investigation of depression and quality of life factors in cancer patients' caregivers. *J. Buon.* **2017**, *22*, 524–529.
41. Sonune, S.P.; Gaur, A.K.; Shenoy, A. Prevalence of depression and quality of life in primary caregiver of children with cerebral palsy. *J. Fam. Med. Prim. Care* **2021**, *10*, 4205–4211. [CrossRef]
42. Gonçalves, C.; Martins, S.; Fernandes, L. Dravet syndrome: Effects on informal caregivers' mental health and quality of life—A systematic review. *Epilepsy Behav.* **2021**, *122*, 108206. [CrossRef]
43. Petruzzo, A.; Biagioli, V.; Durante, A.; Gialloreti, L.E.; D'Agostino, F.; Alvaro, R.; Vellone, E. Influence of preparedness on anxiety, depression, and quality of life in caregivers of heart failure patients: Testing a model of path analysis. *Patient Educ. Couns.* **2019**, *102*, 1021–1028. [CrossRef] [PubMed]
44. Olarte-Durand, M.; Roque-Aycachi, J.B.; Rojas-Humpire, R.; Canaza-Apaza, J.F.; Laureano, S.; Rojas-Humpire, A.; Huancahuire-Vega, S. Mood and sleep quality in Peruvian medical students during COVID-19 pandemic. *Rev. Colomb. Psiquiatr.* **2022**, *in press*. [CrossRef]
45. Sáenz, E.D.J.Q.; Salvador-Carrillo, J.F.; Rivera-Lozada, O.; Asalde, C.A.B. Factors related to depression in older adults during the COVID-19 pandemic in two coastal regions of Peru: An analytical cross-sectional study. *F1000Research* **2021**, *10*, 958. [CrossRef]

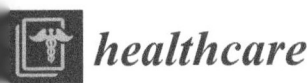

Article

Aggression, Alexithymia and Sense of Coherence in a Sample of Schizophrenic Outpatients

Argyro Pachi [1], Athanasios Tselebis [1,*], Ioannis Ilias [2], Effrosyni Tsomaka [1], Styliani Maria Papageorgiou [1], Spyros Baras [1], Evgenia Kavouria [1] and Konstantinos Giotakis [1]

1. Psychiatric Department, "Sotiria" General Hospital of Chest Diseases, 11527 Athens, Greece; irapah67@otenet.gr (A.P.); tsomaka@gmail.com (E.T.); stellamar4@yahoo.gr (S.M.P.); spyrosbaras@gmail.com (S.B.); e.kavourgia@gmail.com (E.K.); cgiotakis@gmail.com (K.G.)
2. Department of Endocrinology, "Elena Venizelou" Hospital, 11521 Athens, Greece; iiliasmd@yahoo.com
* Correspondence: atselebis@yahoo.gr; Tel.: +30-2107763186

Abstract: Schizophrenia elevates the risk for aggressive behavior, and there is a need to better understand the associated variables predicting aggression for treatment and prevention purposes. The aim of the present study is to determine the relationship between alexithymia, sense of coherence and aggressive behavior in a sample of schizophrenic outpatients. Using a correlational research design, standardized self-report questionnaires assessed aggression (brief aggression questionnaire—BAQ), alexithymia (Toronto Alexithymia Scale—TAS) and sense of coherence (sense of coherence questionnaire—SOC) in a sample of 100 schizophrenic outpatients in clinical remission. Participants reported high levels of aggression and alexithymia along with reduced sense of coherence. Significant negative correlations were evidenced among scores on the SOC scale ($p < 0.001$) with both the TAS as well as with the BAQ scales. However, a positive correlation ($p < 0.001$) was observed between the TAS and BAQ scales. Regression indicated that 27% of the variation in the BAQ rating was explained by the TAS, while an additional 17.8% was explained by the sense of coherence. The difficulty identifying feelings of alexithymia and the comprehensibility and manageability components of sense of coherence significantly predicted anger, hostility and physical aggression. Sense of coherence mediated the relationship between alexithymia and aggression. From the path analysis, comprehensibility emerged as the key factor counterbalancing alexithymic traits and aggressive behaviors, and manageability effectuated higher anger control. The findings hold practical implications for the treatment and rehabilitation of schizophrenic patients.

Keywords: aggression; alexithymia; sense of coherence; schizophrenia; comprehensibility

Citation: Pachi, A.; Tselebis, A.; Ilias, I.; Tsomaka, E.; Papageorgiou, S.M.; Baras, S.; Kavouria, E.; Giotakis, K. Aggression, Alexithymia and Sense of Coherence in a Sample of Schizophrenic Outpatients. *Healthcare* 2022, 10, 1078. https://doi.org/10.3390/healthcare10061078

Academic Editor: David Crompton

Received: 28 April 2022
Accepted: 8 June 2022
Published: 10 June 2022

Publisher's Note: MDPI stays neutral with regard to jurisdictional claims in published maps and institutional affiliations.

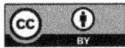

Copyright: © 2022 by the authors. Licensee MDPI, Basel, Switzerland. This article is an open access article distributed under the terms and conditions of the Creative Commons Attribution (CC BY) license (https://creativecommons.org/licenses/by/4.0/).

1. Introduction

Most researchers agree on the presence of an increased risk of aggressive behavior in patients with schizophrenia, but there is considerable heterogeneity in the reported rates of such aggression and uncertainty as to the causes of this heterogeneity [1,2]. Predisposing factors—namely genotype; prenatal and perinatal insults; early adversity as in childhood maltreatment; conduct disorders; comorbid antisocial personality disorder/psychopathy; and precipitating factors, in particular emergence of psychotic symptoms, neurocognitive impairment, substance abuse, nonadherence to treatment and stressful experiences in adult life—can result in risk interactions, increasing the likelihood for the emergence of aggressive behavior [3–5]. In particular, comorbidity with substance abuse increases the incidence of aggressive behavior in patients with schizophrenia with personality traits and social factors probably mediating the relationship between substance abuse and aggressive behavior in these patients [6–9]. Medication nonadherence may also serve as a contributing factor, particularly if it precedes substance abuse [10].

The literature reports differences in brain structure and function associated with aggression in schizophrenia, particularly in areas involved in the formation of psychosis symptoms and affective regulation. The most consistent findings from the structural studies were reduced volumes of the hippocampus and the frontal lobe (i.e., the orbitofrontal and anterior cingulate cortex), and functional studies mainly showed variations in the frontal lobe and amygdala [11,12]. As hypothesized, volume reductions in the hippocampus may predispose individuals with schizophrenia to be less sensitive to social and emotional cues, which might give rise to conflicts and the inability to perceive signals for solutions, leading to conflict escalation [13]. Additionally, functional and neurophysiological studies evidenced an inefficient integration of the information by the dorsal anterior cingulate, between the frontal and limbic regions, in schizophrenia patients with a history of violence during negative emotion processing [14,15]. The anterior cingulate plays a central role in processes that are critical to successful emotion regulation, conflict and performance monitoring, as well as emotional awareness [16,17]. Aberrant dorsal anterior cingulate functional connectivity patterns are consistent with impaired cognitive control over emotions [14]. Aggressive patients display strong reactivity to negative stimuli, which may interfere with response inhibition and lead to impulsive aggression. Relevant research suggested that psychotic symptoms in schizophrenia patients preceded a violent incident only in a small percentage of cases, supporting the idea that behavioral disinhibition and emotional dysregulation are important factors for aggressive behavior in patients with schizophrenia [18].

Aggression in schizophrenia can occur at any time during the disease's course, has significant implications for patient care and treatment and raises the risk of harm. In search for a potential biological signal for early assessing aggressive risk in schizophrenic patients, recent studies identified increased inflammation (CRP levels, leukocyte count and neutrophil to lymphocyte ratio) as a potential biological correlate of aggression [19,20]. The presence of aggressive behavior in schizophrenic patients indicates the severity of the disorder to some degree, and the level of inflammation decreases as the disease goes into remission. The disruptive effect of early-life stress on the immune system is partly involved in brain mechanisms that regulate aggressive behavior in schizophrenia patients, suggesting a link of clinical significance.

A more dynamic feature which has been posited as having an important role in the pathway to aggression is alexithymia [21,22]. Alexithymia is a mental condition characterized by difficulties identifying and describing one's own feelings, externally oriented thinking, and limited imaginative capacity [23]. The majority of research has approached alexithymia as a stable personality trait, thought to be developmental in nature, reflecting a lack in emotion regulation and cognitive processing [24]. Awareness of one's own emotions can prevent us from primitive, uncontrolled emotional responses when facing negative events. Given their inability to identify, manage and express their true emotions, individuals who are alexithymic exhibit high levels of anger and more aggressive behavior. Research indicates that it was primarily the difficulties with identifying feelings aspect of alexithymia that was related to aggression [25]. Brain imaging studies on alexithymia displayed impaired cognitive emotional processing, and—owing to this impairment—alexithymics experience inflexible cognitive regulation. Additionally, they showed weak responses in structures necessary for the representation of emotion used in conscious cognition and stronger responses at levels focused on action [26].

Meta-analyses of functional and structural brain imaging studies have identified the amygdala, the insula, the anterior cingulate cortex and regions of the prefrontal cortex as key correlates of alexithymia in the brain [27–29]. Interestingly, alexithymia is commonly associated with abnormalities of both the anterior cingulate cortex and the insula [30], and impairments in these regions—as suggested—may contribute to aggression, particularly reactive aggression [31]. Contemplating the nature of the alexithymia–aggression relationship, other research evidenced increased right amygdala volume as a common neurobiological denominator for both alexithymia and reactive aggression [31]. Another possible explanation for the association between alexithymia and aggression concerns difficulty labeling emotions. In neuroimaging studies, when labeling emotions, the prefrontal cortex is engaged, while activity in the amygdala is simultaneously reduced, indicating that the cognitive act of labeling emotions dampens the emotional response [32].

Studies have described a variety of deficits in emotion processing in individuals with schizophrenia and identified dysfunction in the domains of emotion expression, emotion experience and emotion recognition [33,34]. Consequently, individuals with schizophrenia who are unable to accurately recognize emotional expressions face problems of adaptability in social life. Inability to decode the social cues projected by others, in which emotions are contained, can lead to misinterpretation of the ambiguous signals received, violation of personal boundaries and possible manifestation of inappropriate or even aggressive behavior. In addition, people with schizophrenia also experience problems in identifying and expressing their own emotions. One of the key areas in which they fall short which is directly related to the expression of their emotional state is that of communication. Although they experience emotions, they often find it difficult to describe and express them in words, sometimes giving the impression that they feel nothing. Emotional dysregulation is closely linked to aggression. Individuals who are unable to express their emotional state experience an uncomfortable, unpleasant and uncontrollable situation that is difficult to tolerate, and thus resort to the use of aggression more easily in order to either communicate this unpleasant experience or to avoid it.

Over recent years, research has indicated that schizophrenia patients are also likely to have reduced empathic ability when interacting with others in everyday life and are less accurate at tracking the positive and negative affective state of another person [35]. These deficits tend to cover every aspect of empathy, from the cognitive to the emotional dimension [36]. Two other concepts closely related to empathy that are compromised in schizophrenia are theory of mind and insight. People with schizophrenia have difficulty processing both their own mental state and those of others, with the result that they are less able to interpret and predict others' behavior. Deficits in the above characteristics can lead to socially dysfunctional and aggressive behaviors. Conversely, understanding another person's emotional and mental state can act as a deterrent to the occurrence of dysfunctional behavior.

Scientific studies support that alexithymia is highly prevalent among schizophrenic patients [37–39]. Whether it is a trait characteristic in deficit patients and a state related to many symptoms, such as flattening of affect, poverty of speech, depression and anxiety in nondeficit patients, or being a separate construct related to dysfunctions in both cognitive and affective processes remains a matter of controversy. Several authors suggested that alexithymia may be a vulnerability factor for the development of schizophrenia and, more specifically, may be an underlying cause of social dysfunction [40,41]. Various core aspects of social cognition have been found to be disrupted in schizophrenia, including emotion recognition [42] and theory of mind [43,44]. Much of the broader social cognitive literature in schizophrenia has focused on the ability to understand the affective states of others, such as via emotion recognition (the ability to decode affective cues) or theory of mind (the ability to understand another's beliefs and desires). In contrast, alexithymia primarily refers to the ability to understand one's own affective experience and therefore seems conceptually closer not only to the construct of emotion regulation, but also to affective empathy (one's emotional response to the cognitive or affective state of another). Neuroimaging studies investigating pathology underlying alexithymia in schizophrenia report gray matter alterations of the left supramarginal gyrus and reduced white matter integrity within the corpus callosum, mostly in the left part of the superior and inferior longitudinal fasciculi, the inferior occipitofrontal fasciculus, the anterior and posterior thalamic radiation and the precuneus white matter [45,46].

Alexithymia has been shown to be associated with both detachment from the self and inadequate differentiation between self and other [47], both of which are included in schizophrenia-spectrum psychopathology. In the same way that the fragmentation of the self may lead to psychotic phenomena, it may also result in impaired ability to differentiate and express one's own emotional experience. Phenomenologically-oriented researchers propose that a disturbance of the basic sense of self is at the clinical core of the schizophrenia spectrum [48]. These abnormal experiences, possibly driven by neurocognitive disturbances, may evolve into first-rank psychotic symptoms [49]. Low baseline levels of basic self-disturbances and further reductions over time independently predict recovery [50]. Significant association between basic self-disturbances and sense of coherence, not mediated by other clinical symptoms, was reported, identifying high levels of basic self-disturbances as independent contributors to poor sense of coherence [51].

Sense of coherence (SOC) was proposed by Antononsky as a construct that expresses the degree to which a person has a diffuse and dynamic, but lasting sense that the internal and external stimuli and stressors in their environment are understandable (i.e., predictable, structured and explicable), manageable (i.e., there are resources available to meet the requirements of these stimuli) and meaningful (i.e., the requirements are challenges that are worth committing to and addressing) [52]. The SOC is often considered to be a stable entity that develops in young adulthood and stabilizes around the age of 30, and as a personality trait it, is more likely to be a predictor of behavior [53,54]. In searching for a relationship between sense of coherence and aggression, a low level of coherence (perceiving stimuli as threatening accompanied by a lack of sufficient internal and external resources to effectively solve problems) may manifest in aggressiveness in the affective and cognitive dimensions (anger, hostility) and also in the instrumental parts of aggressive behavior (verbal, physical aggression) [55].

Sense of coherence and alexithymia exert opposite influences as to the treatment of psychological and physiological disorders, effectuating positive and negative consequences, respectively [56,57]. With reference to relevant evidence, alexithymia may lead to adverse health outcomes as a result of emotion dysregulation and unsuccessful stress and anxiety management, while sense of coherence is regarded as a protective factor that promotes recovery, allowing a person to be resilient in the face of challenges [58,59]. Individuals with a high sense of coherence are likely to perceive stressors as explicable, have confidence in their coping abilities, and feel engaged and motivated to cope with stressors [60]. Inversely, individuals with alexithymia have lower levels of physical functioning, less energy, poorer emotional wellbeing, poorer social functioning and poorer general health [61]. The salutogenesis theory recognizes sense of coherence as a key component of health, whereas alexithymia is presumed to play an important predisposing role in the pathogenesis of diseases. Strengthening the sense of coherence and coping is conducive to recovery [62,63].

According to the salutogenetic approach to the problem of health and disease, higher sense of coherence protects people from the onset of disorders and, if they emerge, aids in accelerating the recovery of health [64,65]. Major mental illnesses, like schizophrenia, are usually expected to run a chronic course with varying trajectories, sometimes in the form of a steady or gradual deterioration and other times with improvements and acute exacerbations with unpredictable effects on outcome. Prognosis varies on a continuum between satisfactory recovery and total disability; although, according to follow-up studies, several schizophrenic patients have a more favorable course outcome [66,67]. Research indicates that people with schizophrenia with a high sense of coherence experienced less severe psychopathological symptoms and a higher overall level of function while also obtaining better results in treatment [68,69].

Over the past decades, evidence of the association between schizophrenia and aggression has accumulated, thereby identifying a multitude of relevant risk factors [70–72]. The presence of alexithymia among patients with schizophrenia has been extensively studied, and heightened levels of alexithymia in a number of different schizophrenia samples have been evidenced [38,41,73,74]. However, studies focused on how alexithymia may give rise to aggression in patients with schizophrenia are scarce [21,75]. The relationship between alexithymia and aggression has also been investigated mostly in community samples, mixed psychiatric and substance dependence inpatients, adolescents, violent offenders and forensic patients [29,76–85]. The association between sense of coherence and aggression has been investigated among juveniles from reformatories, but also among female employees and coronary heart disease patients, as predictors of health-related quality of life [55,86–88]. Sense of coherence in schizophrenia and among delusional patients has been studied in relation to psychopathology and in order to predict remission and risk of relapse [68,89–92]. Finally, the relationship between alexithymia and sense of coherence has been investigated among university students, patients suffering from fibromyalgia and among attention deficit hyperactivity disorder patients [56,58,93].

Schizophrenia-related aggression poses a severe threat to the patient's and society's safety and necessitates the development of interventions with specific or nonspecific anti-aggressive properties. There are various treatment choices apart from pharmacological treatments for addressing aggression in schizophrenia patients. Psychological treatments and other nonpharmacological interventions may be of interest when the etiology of aggression is not a target for pharmacological agents. Elucidating the role of alexithymia on aggression in schizophrenia suggests new modes of treatment which would target these specific underlying impairments. A review examining the effects of psychological interventions on alexithymia concluded that it is partly modifiable with these therapeutic interventions, offering suggestions for future research [94]. Similarly, salutogenic-based approaches offer promising results, strengthening sense of coherence and effectuating positive outcomes in key variables for personal recovery in people with schizophrenia [95,96].

The exploratory purpose of this study was to investigate the possible association between aggression, alexithymia and sense of coherence in a sample of schizophrenic outpatients since there is no study in the literature that simultaneously examines the relationship of these variables. We argue that specific components of sense of coherence, as well as alexithymic traits involving emotional dysregulation, offer insight into schizophrenic outpatients' aggressiveness influencing their self-reported levels of aggression.

The specific aim of this study is to verify whether certain alexithymia and sense of coherence dimensions serve as mediators predicting various aspects of aggression. Differently, considering that sense of coherence is related to the ability to regulate and manage emotions appropriately [87], counterbalancing the limited ability of alexithymic individuals, we aimed to investigate the intervening role of sense of coherence in the relation between alexithymia and aggression. Results would provide a rationale for the development of psychological interventions [75,97] specifically targeted at improving alexithymia and sense of coherence in outpatients with schizophrenia in order to control their aggressive tendencies and cope with their aggressive feelings themselves.

2. Subjects and Methods

2.1. Research Design

In this study, a correlational research design was used. It was conducted with outpatients treated at the Outpatient Psychiatric Department of Sotiria General Hospital between September 2021 and February 2022 after approval from the Clinical Research Ethics Committee of Sotiria General Hospital (Number 24252/27-9-21). According to ethical considerations, participation in the survey was completely voluntary. First, the researchers explained the research objectives and patients were assured that the information would remain confidential. After each participant was informed about the study, they provided written and verbal informed consent. Once recruited, all participants were asked to answer to a semi-structured form designed by research staff to collect demographic data and to fill a battery of self-report questionnaires to assess their self-reported levels of aggression, alexithymia and sense of coherence. At the end, all of the responses were collected anonymously.

2.2. Study Participants

Adopting purposive sampling, the study involved 100 consecutive outpatients with confirmed psychiatric diagnoses of schizophrenia, using the International Classification of Diseases-10 (ICD-10) coding system, who attended the Psychiatry Outpatients Department for maintenance treatment. Eligibility criteria included: (i) aged between 18 and

65 years old; (ii) being in clinical remission in a post-acute phase of illness as defined by no hospitalizations and no changes in psychotropic medication or psychosocial status within 30 days prior to enrollment; (iii) with a history of at least two prior psychiatric hospitalizations (greater diagnostic confidence in confirming schizophrenic disorders), but not more than five hospitalizations (to exclude patients with residual schizophrenia); (iv) coherent verbal contact during the filling of data collection form. Exclusion criteria for participants were psychotic disorders related to clinical medical conditions or substance use; substance addiction and history of substance use in the last six months; uncorrected visual or hearing impairments; neurological disorders or damage to the central nervous system; developmental disability; and signs of intellectual disability, severe cognitive and neuropsychological impairment, personality disorders or schizoid and schizotypal personality traits, other psychiatric comorbidities, namely social anxiety disorder and a record of current substance or alcohol abuse. The majority of participants (68%) were on atypical antipsychotic monotherapy with confirmed antiaggressive properties, while the rest of them were additionally treated with a combination of adjunctive anticonvulsants. A comprehensive health assessment and clinical evaluation of substance abuse were conducted upon study enrollment.

2.3. Minimal Sample Size Calculation

A sample size of 100 was deemed adequate given five independent variables (IVs) to be included in the hierarchical linear regression analysis (N > 50 + 8 m, N = number of Participants and m = number of IVs) [98]. To confirm sample size adequacy, a post hoc power analysis was carried out using G-Power software [99]. The calculation indicated that with a sample size of 100, effect size $f^2 = 0.8116$ (derived from the $R^2 = 0.448$), an alpha of 0.05 and five predictors, an excellent power of 1.00 was identified. The same procedure was followed to verify sample adequacy for the other hierarchical linear regression analyses models built with six predictors. Additionally, a Monte Carlo power analysis for indirect effects was performed through an online application [100]. The results show that a power of 0.95 with a confidence level of 99% is reached with only 60 participants in a simple mediation model. Finally, according to the rule of thumb recommended by Kline [101], an adequate sample size should be 10 times the number of the parameters in path analysis (six parameters were involved in the research path analysis).

2.4. Measurement Tools

Demographic and social data from study participants included age, gender and years of education.

2.5. Brief Aggression Questionnaire

The brief aggression questionnaire (BAQ) is a 12-item self-report measure of aggression. The questionnaire asks participants to rate on a scale from 1 (strongly agree) to 5 (strongly disagree) the degree to which statements describing behaviors and emotions, are characteristic of themselves. The BAQ measures aggression in the domains of physical aggression, verbal aggression, anger, and hostility. The total aggression score was calculated by summing these four factors' scores. Higher scores indicate higher levels of aggression. The questionnaire was translated and back translated, from English to Greek and vice versa, by three bilingual translators and adapted in Greek population [102]. BAQ has been proposed as a valid and reliable instrument (Webster et al., 2014) with adequate temporal stability and convergent validity with other behavioral measures of aggression [103]. Cronbach's alpha in this study was 0.731.

2.6. Sense of Coherence Questionnaire

To measure sense of coherence, we used the short version of a self-rating scale, the sense of coherence questionnaire (SOC-13), developed by Antonovsky [52]. SOC-13 comprises of three components (a) a cognitive component, labeled comprehensibility, representing the ability to understand and integrate internal and external experiences, (b) an instrumental component, labeled manageability, representing the ability to handle challenges and cope with stressful situations and (c) a motivational component, labeled meaningfulness, representing the ability to make sense of experiences and view them as worthy challenges [52,104]. Responses to each question are given using a 7-point Likert scale ranging from 1 ("very common") to 7 ("very rare or never"). Scores range from 13 to 91, with higher numeric values representing a higher degree of SOC. The short version of SOC-13 has been standardized in the Greek population and seems to be a reliable and valid instrument with a Cronbach alpha of 0.83 [104].

2.7. Toronto Alexithymia Scale

The Toronto Alexithymia Scale (TAS-20) is one of the most commonly used self-report measures of alexithymia [105]. It consists of 20 sentences and includes 3 subscales: emotion recognition, which measures the extent to which people report difficulty in identifying their own feelings (DIF); emotion expression, which measures the extent to which people report difficulty in describing feelings to others (DDF); and externally-oriented thinking (EOT), which measures the extent to which people report a tendency to focus on the concrete details of external events rather than of their own inner experience. The sentences are scored using a 5-point Likert scale from 1 (strongly disagree) to 5 (strongly agree) with total scores ranging from 20 to 100. The scale has good reliability and validity in both its original version and in the Greek adaptation [106] that was used in the present study. The distinctive cutoff scores to indicate the degree of alexithymic characteristics were as follows: ≤50 indicated no alexithymia, 51–60 indicated borderline alexithymia, and ≥61 indicated alexithymia [105]. The Cronbach's alpha for the scale in this study was 0.809.

2.8. Statistical Analysis

Descriptive statistics were computed for all variables in the analysis. Independent sample *t*-tests assessed for gender differences. The prevalence of alexithymia was determined as a percentage. The internal consistency reliability of the BAQ, SOC-13 and TAS-20 in our sample was evaluated using Cronbach's alpha coefficient (≥ 0.70). The Shapiro–Wilk test was used to assess the normality of the data. Pearson correlation was performed to determine the strength and direction of the relationship between variables. Hierarchical linear regression analyses were built to investigate whether related variables were significant predictors of aggression while controlling for other covariables. The assumption testing (linear relationship, independence, homoscedasticity and normality) was carried out by visual inspection of the variables, residuals and collinearity statistics and quantile–quantile (QQ) plots, probability–probability (PP) plots and scatterplots. A bootstrap approach was used to test the significance of the indirect effect of alexithymia on aggression through the mediating role of sense of coherence. The SPSS PROCESS Macro (Hayes, 2013) was used to conduct simple mediation analyses, computing 5000 bootstrap resampling with replacement from the original dataset to estimate 95% confidence intervals (CIs) for the indirect effects (CIs that do not include zero indicate a significant indirect effect). For the sake of parsimony, mediation models were run, including TAS-20 and SOC subscales, predicting each of the BAQ subscales. Path analysis was performed in order to concurrently examine the impact of a set of predictor variables (certain TAS-20 and SOC subscales derived from regression and mediation model results) on the BAQ subscales, which were handled as dependent variables and thus identify which are the most important (and significant) paths. This may have implications for the plausibility of our prespecified hypotheses. A structural model with observed variables was tested using a covariance matrix as input and maximum likelihood estimation. Assumptions (linearity, causal closure, unitary variables) were respected. Maximum likelihood estimation (MLE) indices were calculated in order to assess the correspondence of the model with the data: chi-square statistics, root mean square error of approximation (RMSEA) and comparative fit index (CFI). All *p* values were two-tailed, and the statistical significance level was set at $p < 0.05$. SPSS software, version

23, was used for the statistical analysis. SPSS AMOS 23 Graphics enabled the presentation of Figures 1–5.

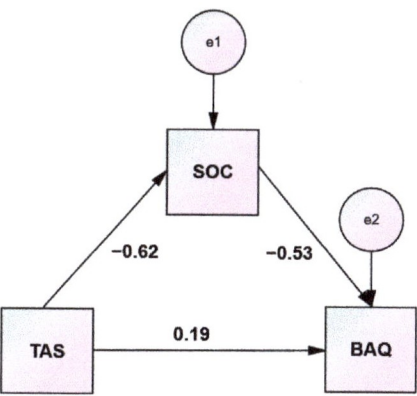

Figure 1. Simple mediation analysis of sense of coherence (SOC) on Toronto alexithymia scale (TAS)–brief aggression questionnaire (BAQ) relationship.

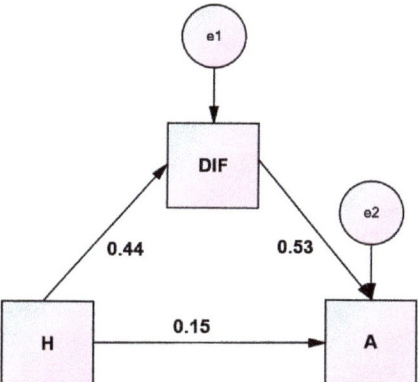

Figure 2. Simple mediation analysis of difficulty identifying feelings (DIF) on hostility (H)–anger (A) relationship.

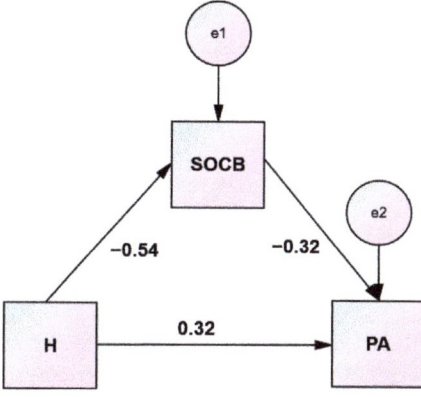

Figure 3. Simple mediation analysis of comprehensibility (SOC B) on hostility (H)–physical aggression (PA) relationship.

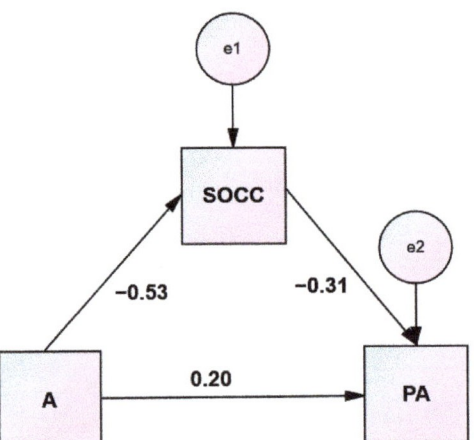

Figure 4. Simple mediation analysis of manageability (SOC C) on anger (A)–physical aggression (PA) relationship.

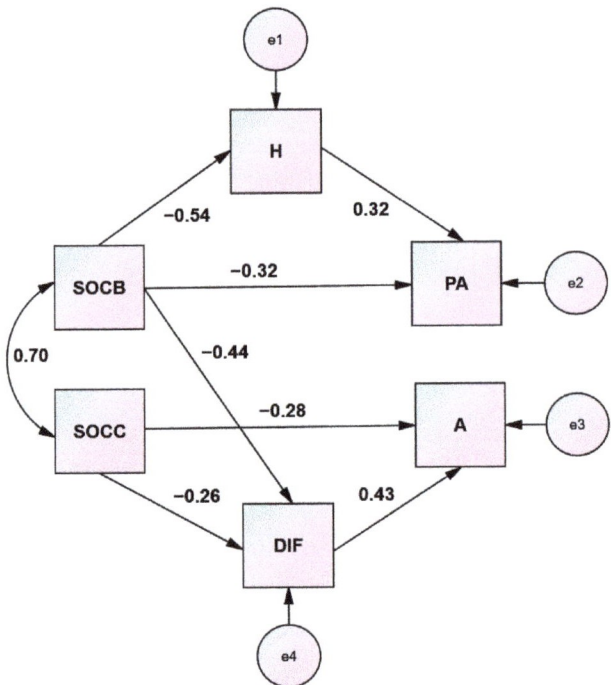

Figure 5. Path model illustrating patterns of effect within a system of research variables. Note: Standardized coefficients are presented.

3. Results

3.1. General Characteristics of Participants and Scores on Outcome Variables

The study included 100 participants (45 men and 55 women). Means and standard deviations for general characteristics of participants and all key variables are presented in Table 1. The mean BAQ score was statistically higher compared to the corresponding score in the Greek general population [107], (30.93 vs. 23.22, sample t-test $p < 0.01$). A total of 22% of schizophrenic participants scored above the cutoff on the TAS scale. The mean TAS score was statistically higher compared to the corresponding score in the general population [61], (49.10 vs. 45.8, sample t-test $p < 0.05$), but comparable to the average score observed among patients with chronic somatic diseases (49.10 vs. 48.2 sample t-test $p > 0.05$) [108]. The average SOC was statistically lower compared to the mean score from the standardization studies [104] in the Greek general population (56.57 vs. 59.85 sample t-test $p < 0.05$). No statistically significant differences were observed between men and women as to the BAQ, TAS, or SOC scores or any of their subscales. Significantly higher BAQ and lower SOC scores were evidenced among alexithymic participants (36.59 ± 8.7 vs. 29.33 ± 7.42, $t = 3.564$, $p = 0.001$ and 45.95 ± 16.33 vs. 59.42 ± 1433, $t = -3.44$, $p = 0.002$, correspondingly).

Table 1. General characteristics of participants and scores on BAQ, TAS, SOC and subscales.

	N	Min	Max	Mean	SD
age	100	21	65	41.71	10.718
education	98	6	18	13.10	3.003
BAQ	100	14	54	30.93	8.247
TAS	100	20	82	49.10	13.369
SOC	99	19	89	56.57	15.697
PA	100	3	15	6.61	3.284
VA	100	4	15	10.06	2.473
H	100	3	15	8.24	3.194
A	100	3	13	6.02	2.655
DIF	100	7	31	16.91	6.741
DDF	100	5	25	13.07	4.965
EOT	100	8	36	19.12	5.524
SOC A	99	4	28	18.82	5.530
SOC B	99	5	35	21.39	7.184
SOC C	99	4	28	16.35	5.877

Abbreviations: P, participants; D.S., descriptive statistics; PA, physical aggression; VA, verbal aggression; H, hostility; A, anger; DIF, difficulty identifying feelings; DDF, difficulty describing feelings; EOT, externally oriented thinking; SOC A; meaningfulness; SOC B, comprehensibility; SOC C, manageability.

3.2. Correlations among Continuous Variables

Significant negative correlations were evidenced among scores on the SOC scale ($p < 0.001$) with both the TAS as well as with BAQ scales. However, a positive correlation ($p < 0.001$) was indicated between TAS and BAQ scales (Table 2).

Results from correlations among subscales of the TAS, BAQ and SOC are presented in Table 3.

Table 2. Correlations among age, education (in years), TAS, BAQ and SOC.

Pearson Correlation N = 100		AGE	Education (in Years)	Sense of Coherence (SOC)	Toronto Alexithymia Scale (TAS)
Education (in years)	r	0.073			
	p	0.478			
Sense of coherence (SOC)	r	−0.021	0.003		
	p	0.838	0.976		
Toronto Alexithymia Scale (TAS)	r	0.044	−0.062	−0.624 **	
	p	0.664	0.545	0.000	
Brief aggression questionnaire (BAQ)	r	0.058	0.057	−0.653 **	0.525 **
	p	0.569	0.575	0.000	0.000

** $p < 0.01$.

Table 3. Correlations among subscales of TAS, BAQ and SOC.

N = 100		DIF	DDF	EOT	TAS	SOC A	SOC B	SOC C	SOC
BAQ	r	0.579 **	0.463 **	0.147	0.525 **	−0.366 **	−0.648 **	−0.608 **	−0.525 **
	p	0.000	0.000	0.144	0.000	0.000	0.000	0.000	0.000
PA	r	0.435 **	0.384 **	0.163	0.429 **	−0.298 **	−0.487 **	−0.419 **	−0.485
	p	0.000	0.000	0.105	0.000	0.003	0.000	0.000	0.000
VA	r	0.140	−0.127	−0.004	0.116	0.068	−0.261 **	−0.310 **	−0.212 *
	p	0.166	0.207	0.967	0.251	0.506	0.009	0.002	0.035
H	r	0.444 **	0.292 **	0.151	0.394 **	−0.328 **	−0.534 **	−0.456 **	−0.531 **
	p	0.000	0.003	0.135	0.000	0.001	0.000	0.000	0.000
A	r	0.595 **	0.495 **	0.078	0.516 **	−0.433 **	−0.517 **	−0.526 **	−0.586 **
	p	0.000	0.000	0.442	0.000	0.000	0.000	0.000	0.000

Abbreviations: PA, physical aggression; VA, verbal aggression; H, hostility; A, anger; DIF, difficulty identifying feelings; DDF, difficulty describing feelings; EOT, externally oriented thinking; SOC A; meaningfulness; SOC B, comprehensibility; SOC C, manageability. * $p < 0.05$ or ** $p < 0.01$.

3.3. Hierarchical Linear Regression Analyses

A three-stage hierarchical linear regression analysis was conducted to evaluate the prediction of BAQ scores from the general characteristics of participants (age, gender and education), TAS scores and SOC scores. For the first block analysis, the predictor variables age, gender (coded as 1 = male, 2 = female) and education were analyzed. The results of the first block revealed the model not to be statistically significant ($p > 0.05$). For the second block analysis, the predictor variable TAS scores were added to the analysis and contributed significantly to the regression model, $F(4, 92) = 8.501$, $p < 0.001$) accounting for 27% of the variation in aggression. Introducing the SOC scores variable at stage three explained an additional 17.8% of variation in aggression and this change in R^2 was significant, $F(5, 91) = 14.757$, $p < 0.001$. Both the TAS scores and SOC scores were significant predictors of aggression. Together, the two independent variables accounted for 44.8% of the variance in aggression. Participants' predicted aggression was equal to 37.84 + 0.108 (TAS) − 0.272 (SOC) (Table 4).

Table 4. Summary of hierarchical regression analysis for variables predicting aggression (BAQ scores).

		Unstandardized Coefficients		Standardized Coefficients				
		B	Std. Error	Beta	t	Sig.	R Square	ΔR^2
Step 1	(constant)	26.906	4.740		5.676	0.000	0.009	0.009
	age	0.053	0.080	0.072	0.660	0.511		
	gender	−0.533	1.771	−0.034	−0.301	0.764		
	education	0.170	0.278	0.065	0.613	0.542		
Step 2	(constant)	11.954	4.850		2.465	0.016	0.270	0.261
	age	0.046	0.069	0.063	0.666	0.507		
	gender	−1.183	1.532	−0.075	−0.772	0.442		
	education	0.273	0.241	0.104	1.135	0.259		
	TAS	0.306	0.053	0.514	5.737	0.000 *		
Step 3	(constant)	37.840	6.391		5.921	0.000	0.448	0.178
	age	0.048	0.060	0.066	0.800	0.426		
	gender	−1.410	1.340	−0.089	−1.052	0.296		
	education	0.235	0.211	0.089	1.117	0.267		
	TAS	0.108	0.059	0.180	1.811	0.073		
	SOC	−0.272	0.050	−0.538	−5.414	0.000 *		

Correlations are statistically significant at the * $p < 0.01$ level. Beta = standardized regression coefficient.

Two-stage hierarchical linear regression analyses were conducted to evaluate the prediction of BAQ and subscales scores from the scores on the TAS and SOC subscales. For the first block analysis, the predictor variables were the scores on TAS subscales. and for the second block analysis, the scores on the SOC subscales were added. In these analyses, DIF, SOC A, SOC B and SOC C predicted the dependent variables (Table 5).

Table 5. Hierarchical regression analyses for variables (TAS and SOC subscales) predicting aggression (BAQ and subscales).

Dependent Variables		Unstandardized Coefficients		Standardized Coefficients				
		B	Std. Error	Beta	t	p	R Square	ΔR^2
	DIF	0.287	0.146	0.232	1.967	0.05 *	33.4	33.4
BAQ	SOC B	−0.415	0.136	−0.363	−3.045	0.003 **	49.9	16.5
	SOC C	−0.349	0.149	−0.250	−2.340	0.021 *		
PA	SOC B	−0.134	0.066	−0.291	−2.041	0.044 *	27.9	7.4
VA	SOC A	0.142	0.044	0.319	2.609	0.011 *	17.1	15.3
	SOC C	−0.118	0.058	−0.281	−2.051	0.043 *		
H	SOC B	−0.174	0.062	−0.392	−2.833	0.006 **	32.5	13.2
A	DIF	0.117	0.050	0.294	2.335	0.022 *	42.7	5.9

Correlations are statistically significant at the * $p < 0.05$ or ** $p < 0.01$ level. Abbreviations: PA, physical aggression; VA, verbal aggression; H, hostility; A, anger; DIF, difficulty identifying feelings; SOC A; meaningfulness; SOC B, comprehensibility; SOC C, manageability. Notes: 1. Results are given for Step 2, when SOC variables are included as independent variables. 2. Only the variables that significantly predicted the dependent variables are shown.

3.4. Simple Mediation Analyses

To clarify the nature of the relationship between alexithymia and aggression and answer one of the research questions, we investigated the underlying mechanism by which alexithymia influences aggression through sense of coherence. The objective was to examine the impact of alexithymia on aggression as mediated by sense of coherence. It was hypothesized that being alexithymic will positively predict aggression. Additionally, it was hypothesized that sense of coherence will mediate this relationship. A simple mediation analysis, using the bootstrap method, was conducted to test these hypotheses. Analyzing the indirect effects, the results reveal that sense of coherence significantly mediated the relationship between alexithymia and aggression [(B 0.2093, 95% C.I. (0.1234, 0.2966), $p < 0.05$, Table 6]. Sense of coherence accounted for 65.55% of total effect. These findings provide some evidence that alexithymic patients are less likely to exhibit aggression provided they have high sense of coherence. Nevertheless, alexithymia still contributes to aggression beyond what is accounted for by sense of coherence. Standardized coefficients for the variables are depicted in Figure 1.

Table 6. Mediation analysis of sense of coherence (SOC) on Toronto alexithymia scale (TAS) – brief aggression questionnaire (BAQ) relationship.

Variable	b	SE	t	p	95% Confidence Interval	
					LLCI	ULCI
TAS → SOC	−0.7367	0.0936	−7.8672	0.000	−0.9225	−0.5508
TAS → BAQ	0.3193	0.0538	5.9358	0.000	0.2125	0.4260
TAS → SOC → BAQ	−0.2841	0.0510	−5.5764	0.000	−0.3853	−0.1830
Effects						
Direct	0.1100	0.0601	1.8285	0.0706	−0.0094	0.2293
Indirect *	0.2093	0.0445			0.1234	0.2966
Total	0.3193	0.0538	5.9358	0.000	0.2125	0.4260

* Based on 5000 bootstrap samples.

A bootstrap approach was used to test the significance of the indirect effect of hostility on anger through the mediating role of difficulty identifying feelings. Results of this mediation analysis are displayed in Table 7 and illustrated in the Figure 2.

Table 7. Mediation analysis of difficulty identifying feelings (DIF) on hostility (H) – anger (A) relationship.

Variable	b	SE	t	p	95% Confidence Interval	
					LLCI	ULCI
H → DIF	0.9366	0.1910	4.9033	0.0000	0.5575	1.3156
H → A	0.3202	0.0775	4.1331	0.0001	0.1665	0.4740
H → DIF → A	0.2080	0.0354	5.8810	0.0000	0.1378	0.2782
Effects						
Direct	0.1255	0.0746	1.6814	0.0959	−0.0226	0.2736
Indirect *	0.1948	0.0493			0.1041	0.2975
Total	0.3202	0.0775	4.1331	0.0001	0.1665	0.4740

* Based on 5000 bootstrap samples. The model explains 60.8% of the variance in the outcome variable.

Results of the mediation analyses to test the significance of the indirect effects of hostility and anger on physical aggression through comprehensibility and manageability are displayed in Tables 8 and 9 and illustrated in Figures 3 and 4.

Table 8. Mediation analysis of comprehensibility (SOC B) on hostility (H)–physical aggression (PA) relationship.

Variable	b	SE	t	p	95% Confidence Interval	
					LLCI	ULCI
H → SOC B	−1.2002	0.1928	−6.2264	0.0000	−1.5828	−0.8176
H → PA	0.5052	0.0913	5.5346	0.0000	0.3241	0.6863
H → SOC B → PA	−0.1446	0.0460	−3.1416	0.0022	−0.2359	−0.0532
Effects						
Direct	0.3317	0.1033	3.2095	0.0018	0.1266	0.5368
Indirect *	0.1735	0.0657			0.0539	0.3085
Total	0.5052	0.0913	5.5346	0.0000	0.3241	0.6863

* Based on 5000 bootstrap samples. The model explains 34.34% of the variance in the outcome variable.

Table 9. Mediation analysis of manageability (SOC C) on anger (A)–physical aggression (PA) relationship.

Variable	b	SE	t	p	95% Confidence Interval	
					LLCI	ULCI
A → SOC C	−1.1650	0.1914	−6.0850	0.0000	−1.5449	−0.7850
A → PA	0.4552	0.1175	3.8728	0.0002	0.2219	0.6884
A → SOC C → PA	−0.1758	0.0600	−2.9278	0.0043	−0.2949	−0.0566
Effects						
Direct	0.2504	0.1331	1.8820	0.0626	−0.0137	0.5145
Indirect *	0.2048	0.0771			0.0594	0.3617
Total	0.4552	0.1175	3.8728	0.0002	0.2219	0.6884

* Based on 5000 bootstrap samples. The model explains 45% of the variance in the outcome variable.

3.5. Path Analysis

Path analysis was used to determine the pathways by which the alexithymia and sense of coherence dimensions interact to influence modes of aggression. From regression and mediation analysis results, it was expected that comprehensibility and manageability would exert their protective effects, counteracting physical aggression and anger both directly and indirectly through hostility and the difficulty identifying feelings dimension of alexithymia. A structural model with observed variables was tested using a covariance matrix as input and maximum likelihood estimation. This type of analysis provides a comprehensive picture of the nature of the associations between the predictor and dependent variables of interest. Comprehensibility and manageability served as predictor variables and physical aggression and anger were treated as the dependent variables. Results suggested that the measures of fit of the model were satisfactory, indicating adequate fit ($p = 0.325$, CMIN/df = 1.156, comparative fit index CFI = 0.995, normed fit index NFI = 0.968, parsimonious normed fit index PNFI = 0.552, incremental fit index IFI = 0.996, Tucker–Lewis index TLI = 0.990 and the root mean square error of approximation RMSEA = 0.040). No modifications were necessary for the model. The nonexistence of an arrow between two variables means that these two variables are not significantly related. Figure 5 presents the set of hypotheses about the relations between the aforementioned variables.

4. Discussion

The present study confirmed high levels of aggression and alexithymia and low levels of sense of coherence among schizophrenic outpatients. Participants with alexithymic characteristics reported higher aggressive tendencies and lower sense of coherence capacities. The observed correlations supported all the main assumptions of the relationships between the study variables. Alexithymia and sense of coherence accounted for 44.8% of the variance in disclosed aggression. The difficulty identifying feelings dimension of alexithymia and the comprehensibility and manageability components of sense of coherence significantly predicted anger, hostility and physical aggression. Sense of coherence mediated the relationship between alexithymia and aggression. The difficulty identifying feelings dimension of alexithymia mediated the relationship between hostility and anger. Comprehensibility mediated the relationship between hostility and physical aggression, and manageability mediated the relationship between anger and physical aggression. From the path analysis, comprehensibility emerged as the key factor counterbalancing alexithymic traits and aggressive behaviors, and manageability effectuated higher anger control. The main hypotheses were supported, indicating that high SOC scores predicted high physical aggression buffering and anger control, both directly and indirectly neutralizing alexithymic traits and hostility.

The presence of hostility in schizophrenic patients is not limited to the acute phase of the disease [109] but persists for a long time after hospitalization [110] and may be a predisposing factor for the emergence of anger and verbal or physical aggression. As opposed to enduring hostility, anger is a temporary but highly intense negative emotional state that usually abates but easily relapses in people who are temperamentally characterized by hostility due to their increased susceptibility to situations of anger [111]. Imaging studies aiming to clarify the neuroanatomical basis of hostility-related dimensions in schizophrenia patients who exhibited high levels of urgency, impulsivity and aggressiveness reported dysfunction of neuronal circuits involving the amygdala, striatum, prefrontal cortex, anterior cingulate cortex, insula and hippocampus [112].

The literature suggests that aggression and alexithymia are related to each other in the mentally ill [21]. Poor emotional awareness [33] and emotion dysregulation [113] are possible implicating mechanisms underlying aggression. By definition, alexithymia is considered to be a disorder of affect regulation [113], and there is evidence that some facets of emotion regulation may be disrupted in schizophrenia [114–116]. A possible etiological sequence is that limited emotional awareness interferes with emotion regulation, effectuating indirect consequences as to emotional response, thereby mediating aggression [117].

Awareness and understanding of emotions are common features of both alexithymia and emotion regulation. Research reports that alexithymics have a variety of emotion regulation difficulties and outline the nature of emotional dysfunction in alexithymia. Nonacceptance of emotional reactions, lack of emotional clarity, difficulties with goal-directed behavior and impulse control, as well as limited access to emotion regulation strategies commonly present in alexithymic individuals [113]. The similarity of content and underlying processes of difficulty in identifying feelings (a dimension of alexithymia) and lack of emotional awareness (a dimension of emotion regulation difficulties) forms a common substrate for both constructs and may be a region of overlap. The observed emotion regulation difficulties in alexithymic individuals appear to be conceptually attributed to a lack of emotional awareness and differentiation [118].

Consistent with results from other studies, it was predominantly the difficulties with identifying feelings (DIF) aspect of alexithymia that was related to aggression [119–121]. Additionally, DIF significantly predicted total BAQ and anger and mediated the relationship between hostility and anger. In other words, the relationship between the cognitive and the affective components of aggression is mediated by the difficulties with identifying feelings dimension of alexithymia. Among those, having difficulty in identifying their feelings of hostile aggression motivated by anger [122] may be considered as a further effort to distract from feelings (or to express feelings in a rather maladaptive way).

Conscious awareness of emotions is acquired when emotional information and experiences are integrated into cognitive processes [123]. Furthermore, it has been argued that many symptoms typical of schizophrenia can be explained by specific cognitive deficits in schizophrenic patients to accurately attribute mental states to themselves or others [124]. Affective theory of mind refers to the ability to comprehend and confront others' affective mental states and differences in "affective" versus "non-affective" theory of mind' tasks have been reported to relate to certain behaviors in schizophrenia, such as violence [125].

The drastic changes in the subjective experiences of schizophrenic patients give rise to stress and bring about everyday challenges. The ability to manage stressful situations, mental resilience and sense of coherence predict and modify the level of psychological wellbeing among patients suffering from mental disorders [69]. The theory of salutogenesis supports the idea that sense of coherence mitigates stress, and results from early studies evidence the protective effects of a salutogenic approach in individuals with serious mental illnesses [126].

The first step when dealing with a stressful situation is to perceive and be knowledgeably aware of its full extent [53]. An individual with higher comprehensibility is more likely to perceive stimuli from the environment as coherent and understandable [127]. Schizophrenic patients usually require support in reassembling their erratic experiences, reflecting upon them and possibly learning something from them. The severity of symptoms and the chronicity of the psychiatric disorder seem to determine their ability to adapt, as does the use of available resources to manage stressors. First-episode psychotic patients in remission appear to be in a more favorable position compared to chronic patients with persistent positive symptoms or in a deficit state [128,129].

In mental health settings where the therapeutic treatment and long-term follow-up of psychiatric patients is sought, the theory of salutogenesis may find practical application through the modification of therapeutic procedures and environmental factors in order to enhance the three components of salutogenesis [130]. The same approach could even be applied in clinical practice in situations involving conflict prevention through communication, emotional regulation, self-management and other de-escalation techniques [131]. The first goal attempted in de-escalation is reducing the patient's level of arousal to enable discussion by gathering the necessary resources through manageability. The patient should be encouraged to communicate openly with staff about their own emotions and to discuss feelings of anger and frustration in order to enhance comprehensibility. Recent evidence supports the effectiveness of integrating milieu therapy in psychiatric acute wards in reducing conflict behaviors among schizophrenia patients [132].

Preventing or managing stress is of paramount importance according to the diathesis–stress model of schizophrenia. Considering that sense of coherence essentially protects against the pressures generated by stressors, should clearly define the purpose of implemented healthcare interventions, in order to avoid negative health outcomes. Since patients with schizophrenia are so vulnerable to the impacts of stressors, the focus of comprehensive psychoeducation should be on reinforcing coping skills by teaching stress reduction techniques and assertiveness training. Additionally, providing schizophrenic patients with education regarding their illness and improving attention along with other cognitive functions would enhance comprehensibility. When facing challenges, equally important for these patients is acknowledging, approaching, and activating or resorting to other available resources, namely family, social and healthcare support.

In summary, it is reasonable to assume that the inability to recognize and describe emotions may, under stressful circumstances, lead to an increased state of unmanageable arousal. Patients with schizophrenia, particularly if they are characterized by temperamental hostility, feel threatened under stressful conditions and tend to react aggressively. Furthermore, in individuals with reduced abilities to regulate emotions with conscious effort or a strong tendency toward impulsivity, the effect is reinforcing. In these cases, the explanation for the apparent aggressive behavior is provided by the indirect effect of alexithymia, which reduces the cognitive and emotional capacities necessary to moderate distressing feelings and inhibit impulsive actions.

Specific therapeutic interventions to improve the ability to identify subjective feelings that target alexithymia and neurocognitive impairments that may make self-reflection difficult could be implemented. Integrative psychotherapy that targets metacognition could assist patients in developing these capacities [133], and cognitive remediation [134] could provide the prerequisites for metacognitively focused psychotherapy to be successful. Additionally, research argues that alexithymic individuals would benefit more from group-based psychological therapy and supportive and educational approaches as opposed to interpretive ones [25]. A recent open-label randomized controlled trial applied an integrated cognitive-based violence intervention program on management of repetitive violence in patients with schizophrenia and evidenced significant improvement of cognitive failure, management of alexithymic features and attribution styles and errors and fostered adequate decision-making styles and emotion regulation capacity. This intervention provided patients a more active role to manage their violent behavior with the involvement of alexithymia [75].

In the last two decades, there has been increasing research interest in the ability of tailored interventions to modify and strengthen the sense of coherence of various target groups [97]. Enhancing comprehensibility for individuals with schizophrenia should be the focus of comprehensive psychoeducation and cognitive remediation. Moreover, aiming to improve prognosis through the implementation of psychosocial rehabilitation interventions requires the identification and reduction of aggravating factors, such as ineffective stress management, as well as the enhancement of protective factors, especially manageability.

Aggressive behavior is a leading public health problem incurring a massive cost on society and, according to epidemiological studies, individuals diagnosed with major mental disorders such as schizophrenia are more likely to be engaged in such behaviors than the general population, with obvious relevance for health care systems. The etiological heterogeneity of aggression and the possible multifactorial contributors to aggressive behaviors, along with the fact that the current treatment approaches and outcomes are so far inferior, justifies the search for new targets for the treatment of aggression in people with schizophrenia [135]. Addressing factors that limit the effectiveness of treatments might decrease the burden of these severe chronic disorders. Given the high observed prevalence of alexithymia and associated negative outcomes, researchers and clinicians examined the feasibility of treating alexithymia [136]. Interventions aiming to increase patients' emotional awareness and their ability to label emotions may promote their successful engagement in cognitive behavioral psychotherapies to regulate unpleasant, angry emotions before they escalate and drive their behavior [137]. There is promising evidence that alexithymia can improve with treatment even after neurological damage [32].

Identified targets for treating aggression in schizophrenia in our study, i.e., alexithymia and sense of coherence, are mostly amenable to psychotherapeutic and psychosocial interventions. Several different psychotherapeutic approaches for schizophrenia have been developed and studied, with cognitive behavior therapy having the strongest evidence base [138]. Providing comprehensive psychological interventions in this clinical population will likely require drawing upon knowledge from several areas of current research and incorporating elements of various psychosocial interventions, such as cognitive remediation, social skills training and psychoeducation [139]. A recent systematic review evidenced the effectiveness of cognitive remediation and social cognitive training in the management of violent and aggressive behaviors in schizophrenia [140]. According to another review, once patients' positive symptoms have stabilized, cognitive behavioral therapy and cognitive remediation are the two psychosocial interventions that have demonstrated positive outcomes for violence in patients with schizophrenia [141].

The presence of contributing factors to aggression, either adverse or protective, namely alexithymia and sense of coherence, acquires importance in light of the possibility of handling their impact on the effectiveness of antiaggressive treatments, particularly in the domain of psychosocial interventions. Testing the efficacy of psychotherapeutic interventions for people with schizophrenia may benefit from an inclusion of aggression as a treatment outcome in clinical trials. Our study proposes alexithymia and sense of coherence as putative targets for addressing aggression in schizophrenia and extends ideas for treatment and research. Future studies should be carried out, especially controlled and follow-up studies, comparing different forms of treatment on more extensive patient populations while considering potential confounding factors and performing objective assessment of aggression, alexithymia and related constructs.

The present study suffers from various limitations. Participants were enrolled from the outpatients department. Subsequently, research findings may not be applied beyond this study population. Additionally, since the data were collected using self-report tools, self-serving bias may be an issue. Specifically, the TAS-20 scale as a measure of alexithymia consists of self-rated agreement statements and presupposes awareness of the deficit to be reported, which raises the concern that emotion recognition deficits that patients do not detect would not be captured by this scale. Moreover, due to social desirability bias, participants might have stated their self-reported levels of aggression in a socially acceptable manner instead of providing answers that are reflective of their genuine aggression level. Finally, the cross-sectional design of the study precluded us from making secure inferences about direction of causality.

5. Conclusions

High rates of aggression and alexithymia, along with low sense of coherence, were observed among schizophrenic outpatients. Alexithymia fueled aggression, and sense of coherence counteracted aggressive tendencies. The difficulty identifying feelings dimension of alexithymia emerged as a liability, and the comprehensibility component of sense of coherence as a protective factor buffering the deleterious consequences towards physical aggression. These results hold practical implications for the treatment and rehabilitation of schizophrenic patients.

Author Contributions: Conceptualization, A.P. and A.T.; methodology, A.T., I.I. and A.P.; software, A.T., I.I. and A.P.; validation, A.P., A.T. and S.B.; formal analysis, A.P., A.T. and E.T.; investigation, A.P., S.M.P. and K.G.; resources, A.P.; data curation, S.M.P., E.T. and A.P.; writing—original draft preparation, A.T., A.P. and E.K.; writing—review and editing, A.T. and A.P.; supervision, A.T. and A.P.; project administration, A.T. and A.P. All authors have read and agreed to the published version of the manuscript.

Funding: This research received no external funding.

Institutional Review Board Statement: The study was conducted in accordance with the Declaration of Helsinki and approved by the Clinical Research Ethics Committee of Sotiria General Hospital (Number 24252/27-9-21).

Informed Consent Statement: Informed consent was obtained from all subjects involved in the study. Participation in the research was voluntary.

Data Availability Statement: The data and the questionnaires of the study are available upon request from the corresponding author.

Acknowledgments: We would like to thank all participants in our study.

Conflicts of Interest: The authors declare no conflict of interest.

References

1. Monahan, J.; Steadman, H.J.; Silver, E.; Appelbaum, P.S.; Robbins, P.C.; Mulvey, E.P.; Roth, L.H.; Grisso, T.; Banks, S.M. *Rethinking Risk Assessment: The MacArthur Study of Mental Disorder and Violence*; Oxford University Press: Oxford, UK, 2001.
2. Hodgins, S. Aggressive Behavior Among Persons with Schizophrenia and Those Who Are Developing Schizophrenia: Attempting to Understand the Limited Evidence on Causality. *Schizophr. Bull.* **2017**, *43*, 1021–1026. [CrossRef] [PubMed]
3. Cho, W.; Shin, W.S.; An, I.; Bang, M.; Cho, D.Y.; Lee, S.H. Biological Aspects of Aggression and Violence in Schizophrenia. *Clin. Psychopharmacol. Neurosci.* **2019**, *17*, 475–486. [CrossRef]
4. Hodgins, S.; Klein, S. New Clinically Relevant Findings about Violence by People with Schizophrenia. *Can. J. Psychiatry* **2017**, *62*, 86–93. [CrossRef]
5. Volavka, J.; Citrome, L. Pathways to aggression in schizophrenia affect results of treatment. *Schizophr. Bull.* **2011**, *37*, 921–929. [CrossRef] [PubMed]
6. Fazel, S.; Langstrom, N.; Hjern, A.; Grann, M.; Lichtenstein, P. Schizophrenia, substance abuse, and violent crime. *JAMA* **2009**, *301*, 2016–2023. [CrossRef] [PubMed]

7. Lamsma, J.; Cahn, W.; Fazel, S.; GROUP and NEDEN Investigators. Use of illicit substances and violent behaviour in psychotic disorders: Two nationwide case-control studies and meta-analyses. *Psychol. Med.* **2020**, *50*, 2028–2033. [CrossRef] [PubMed]
8. Jones, M.T.; Harvey, P.D. Neurocognition and social cognition training as treatments for violence and aggression in people with severe mental illness. *CNS Spectr.* **2019**, *25*, 145–153. [CrossRef]
9. Ndoro, S. Understanding aggressive behaviour in patients with schizophrenia through social cognitive theory: A narrative literature review. *Br. J. Ment. Health Nurs.* **2020**, *9*, 1–10. [CrossRef]
10. Wu, Y.; Kang, R.; Yan, Y.; Gao, K.; Li, Z.; Jiang, J.; Chi, X.; Xia, L. Epidemiology of schizophrenia and risk factors of schizophrenia-associated aggression from 2011 to 2015. *J. Int. Med. Res.* **2018**, *46*, 4039–4049. [CrossRef]
11. Widmayer, S.; Sowislo, J.F.; Jungfer, H.A.; Borgwardt, S.; Lang, U.E.; Stieglitz, R.D.; Huber, C.G. Structural Magnetic Resonance Imaging Correlates of Aggression in Psychosis: A Systematic Review and Effect Size Analysis. *Front. Psychiatry* **2018**, *9*, 217. [CrossRef]
12. Fjellvang, M.; Grøning, L.; Haukvik, U.K. Imaging Violence in Schizophrenia: A Systematic Review and Critical Discussion of the MRI Literature. *Front. Psychiatry* **2018**, *9*, 333. [CrossRef] [PubMed]
13. Yang, Y.; Raine, A.; Han, C.B.; Schug, R.A.; Toga, A.W.; Narr, K.L. Reduced hippocampal and parahippocampal volumes in murderers with schizophrenia. *Psychiatry Res. Neuroimaging* **2010**, *182*, 9–13. [CrossRef] [PubMed]
14. Tikàsz, A.; Potvin, S.; Dugré, J.R.; Fahim, C.; Zaharieva, V.; Lipp, O.; Mendrek, A.; Dumais, A. Violent Behavior Is Associated with Emotion Salience Network Dysconnectivity in Schizophrenia. *Front. Psychiatry* **2020**, *11*, 143. [CrossRef] [PubMed]
15. Krakowski, M.I.; De Sanctis, P.; Foxe, J.J.; Hoptman, M.J.; Nolan, K.; Kamiel, S.; Czobor, P. Disturbances in Response Inhibition and Emotional Processing as Potential Pathways to Violence in Schizophrenia: A High-Density Event-Related Potential Study. *Schizophr. Bull.* **2016**, *42*, 963–974. [CrossRef]
16. Botvinick, M.M.; Cohen, J.D.; Carter, C.S. Conflict monitoring and anterior cingulate cortex: An update. *Trends Cogn. Sci.* **2004**, *8*, 539–546. [CrossRef]
17. McRae, K.; Reiman, E.M.; Fort, C.L.; Chen, K.; Lane, R.D. Association between trait emotional awareness and dorsal anterior cingulate activity during emotion is arousal-dependent. *Neuroimage* **2008**, *41*, 648–655. [CrossRef]
18. Swanson, J.W.; Swartz, M.S.; Van Dorn, R.A.; Elbogen, E.B.; Wagner, H.R.; Rosenheck, R.A.; Stroup, T.S.; McEvoy, J.P.; Lieberman, J.A. A national study of violent behavior in persons with schizophrenia. *Arch. Gen. Psychiatry* **2006**, *63*, 490–499. [CrossRef]
19. Barzilay, R.; Lobel, T.; Krivoy, A.; Shlosberg, D.; Weizman, A.; Katz, N. Elevated C-reactive protein levels in schizophrenia inpatients is associated with aggressive behavior. *Eur. Psychiatry* **2016**, *31*, 8–12. [CrossRef]
20. Tong, Z.; Zhu, J.; Wang, J.J.; Yang, Y.J.; Hu, W. The Neutrophil-Lymphocyte Ratio Is Positively Correlated with Aggression in Schizophrenia. *Biomed. Res. Int.* **2022**, *2022*, 4040974. [CrossRef]
21. Velotti, P.; Garofalo, C.; Petrocchi, C.; Cavallo, F.; Popolo, R.; Dimaggio, G. Alexithymia, emotion dysregulation, impulsivity and aggression: A multiple mediation model. *Psychiatry Res.* **2016**, *237*, 296–303. [CrossRef]
22. De Schutter, M.A.; Kramer, H.J.; Franken, E.J.; Lodewijkx, H.F.; Kleinepier, T. The influence of dysfunctional impulsivity and alexithymia on aggressive behavior of psychiatric patients. *Psychiatry Res.* **2016**, *243*, 128–134. [CrossRef] [PubMed]
23. Messina, A.; Beadle, J.N.; Paradiso, S. Towards a classification of alexithymia: Primary secondary and organic. *J. Psychopathol.* **2014**, *20*, 38–49.
24. Luminet, O.; Nielson, K.A.; Ridout, N. Having no words for feelings: Alexithymia as a fundamental personality dimension at the interface of cognition and emotion. *Cogn. Emot.* **2021**, *35*, 435–448. [CrossRef] [PubMed]
25. Hemming, L.; Haddock, G.; Shaw, J.; Pratt, D. Alexithymia and Its Associations with Depression, Suicidality, and Aggression: An Overview of the Literature. *Front. Psychiatry* **2019**, *10*, 203. [CrossRef]
26. Kano, M.; Fukudo, S. The alexithymic brain: The neural pathways linking alexithymia to physical disorders. *Biopsychosoc. Med.* **2013**, *7*, 1. [CrossRef]
27. Han, D.; Li, M.; Mei, M.; Sun, X. The functional and structural characteristics of the emotion network in alexithymia. *Neuropsychiatr. Dis. Treat.* **2018**, *14*, 991–998. [CrossRef]
28. Goerlich, K.; Aleman, A. Neuroimaging Studies of Alexithymia. In *Alexithymia: Advances in Research, Theory, and Clinical Practice*; Luminet, O., Bagby, R., Taylor, G., Eds.; Cambridge University Press: Cambridge, UK, 2018; pp. 207–249.
29. Ihme, K.; Dannlowski, U.; Lichev, V.; Stuhrmann, A.; Grotegerd, D.; Rosenberg, N.; Kugel, H.; Heindel, W.; Arolt, V.; Kersting, A.; et al. Alexithymia is related to differences in gray matter volume: A voxel-based morphometry study. *Brain Res.* **2013**, *1491*, 60–67. [CrossRef]
30. Goerlich-Dobre, K.S.; Bruce, L.; Martens, S.; Aleman, A.; Hooker, C.I. Distinct associations of insula and cingulate volume with the cognitive and affective dimensions of alexithymia. *Neuropsychologia* **2014**, *53*, 284–292. [CrossRef]
31. Farah, T.; Ling, S.; Raine, A.; Yang, Y.; Schug, R. Alexithymia and reactive aggression: The role of the amygdala. *Psychiatry Res. Neuroimaging* **2018**, *281*, 85–91. [CrossRef]
32. Neumann, D.; Malec, J.F.; Hammond, F.M. The Relations of Self-Reported Aggression to Alexithymia, Depression, and Anxiety After Traumatic Brain Injury. *J. Head Trauma Rehabil.* **2017**, *32*, 205–213. [CrossRef]
33. Baslet, G.; Termini, L.; Herbener, E. Deficits in emotional awareness in schizophrenia and their relationship with other measures of functioning. *J. Nerv. Ment. Dis.* **2009**, *197*, 655–660. [CrossRef] [PubMed]
34. Tremeau, F. A Review of Emotion Deficits in Schizophrenia. *Dialogues Clin. Neurosci.* **2006**, *8*, 59–70. [CrossRef] [PubMed]

35. Lee, J.; Zaki, J.; Harvey, P.O.; Ochsner, K.; Green, M.F. Schizophrenia patients are impaired in empathic accuracy. *Psychol. Med.* **2011**, *41*, 2297–2304. [CrossRef] [PubMed]
36. Varachhia, S.; Ferguson, E.; Doody, G.A. A Meta-Analysis Taxonomizing Empathy in Schizophrenia. *J. Psychiatry Depress. Anxiety* **2018**, *4*, 016. [CrossRef]
37. Stanghellini, G.; Ricca, V. Alexithymia and Schizophrenias. *Psychopathology* **1995**, *28*, 263–272. [CrossRef]
38. Todarello, O.; Porcelli, P.; Grilletti, F.; Bellomo, A. Is alexithymia related to negative symptoms of schizophrenia? *Psychopathology* **2015**, *38*, 310–314. [CrossRef]
39. Van't Wout, M.; Aleman, A.; Bermond, B.; Kahn, R.S. No words for feelings: Alexithymia in schizophrenia patients and first-degree relatives. *Compr. Psychiatry* **2007**, *48*, 27–33. [CrossRef]
40. Van der Meer, L.; van't Wout, M.; Aleman, A. Emotion regulation strategies in patients with schizophrenia. *Psychiatry Res.* **2009**, *170*, 108–113. [CrossRef]
41. Fogley, R.; Warman, D.; Lysaker, P.H. Alexithymia in schizophrenia: Associations with neurocognition and emotional distress. *Psychiatry Res.* **2014**, *218*, 1–6. [CrossRef]
42. Phillips, M.L.; Drevets, W.C.; Rauch, S.L.; Lane, R. Neurobiology of emotion perception: II. Implications for major psychiatric disorders. *Biol. Psychiatry* **2003**, *54*, 515–528. [CrossRef]
43. Bailey, P.E.; Henry, J.D. Separating component processes of theory of mind in schizophrenia. *Br. J. Clin. Psychol.* **2010**, *49*, 43–52. [CrossRef] [PubMed]
44. Brüne, M. "Theory of mind" in schizohrenia: A review of the literature. *Schizophr. Bull.* **2005**, *31*, 21–42. [CrossRef] [PubMed]
45. Kubota, M.; Miyata, J.; Sasamoto, A.; Kawada, R.; Fujimoto, S.; Tanaka, Y.; Sawamoto, N.; Fukuyama, H.; Takahashi, H.; Murai, T. Alexithymia and reduced white matter integrity in schizophrenia: A diffusion tensor imaging study on impaired emotional self-awareness. *Schizophr. Res.* **2012**, *141*, 137–143. [CrossRef] [PubMed]
46. Kubota, M.; Miyata, J.; Hirao, K.; Fujiwara, H.; Kawada, R.; Fujimoto, S.; Tanaka, Y.; Sasamoto, A.; Sawamoto, N.; Fukuyama, H.; et al. Alexithymia and regional gray matter alterations in schizophrenia. *Neurosci. Res.* **2011**, *70*, 206–213. [CrossRef]
47. De Rick, A.; Vanheule, S. The relationship between perceived parenting, adult attachment style and alexithymia in alcoholic inpatients. *Addict. Behav.* **2006**, *31*, 1265–1270. [CrossRef]
48. Parnas, J. Self and schizophrenia: A phenomenological perspective. In *The Self in Neuroscience and Psychiatry*; Kircher, T., David, A., Eds.; Cambridge University Press: Cambridge, UK, 2013; pp. 127–141.
49. Nelson, B.; Whitford, T.J.; Lavoie, S.; Sass, L.A. What are the neurocognitive correlates of basic self-disturbance in schizophrenia? Integrating phenomenology and neurocognition. Part 1 (Source monitoring deficits). *Schizophr. Res.* **2014**, *152*, 12–19. [CrossRef]
50. Svendsen, I.H.; Øie, M.G.; Møller, P.; Nelson, B.; Haug, E.; Melle, I. Basic self-disturbances independently predict recovery in psychotic disorders: A seven year follow-up study. *Schizophr. Res.* **2019**, *212*, 72–78. [CrossRef]
51. Svendsen, I.H.; Øie, M.G.; Møller, P.; Nelson, B.; Melle, I.; Haug, E. Basic self-disturbances are associated with Sense of Coherence in patients with psychotic disorders. *PLoS ONE* **2020**, *15*, e0230956. [CrossRef]
52. Antonovsky, A. The Structure and properties of the sense of coherence scale. *Soc. Sci. Med.* **1993**, *36*, 725–733. [CrossRef]
53. Eriksson, M.; Mittelmark, M. The sense of coherence and its measurement. In *The Handbook of Salutogenesis*; Mittelmark, M.B., Sagy, S., Eriksson, M., Bauer, G.F., Pelikan, J.M., Lindström, B., Espnes, G.A., Eds.; Springer: Berlin/Heidelberg, Germany, 2017; pp. 97–106.
54. Feldt, T.; Leskinen, E.; Kinnunen, U.; Ruoppila, I. The stability of sense of coherence: Comparing two age groups over a 5-year follow-up study. *Pers. Individ. Differ.* **2003**, *35*, 1151–1165. [CrossRef]
55. Gierowski, J.K.; Cyboran, M.; Poranska, A. Relationship between Coherence and Aggression, Taking Into Account Psychological Gender, in Juvenile Girls and Boys. *Probl. Forensic Sci.* **2008**, *74*, 121–149.
56. Allah-Gholilo, K.; Abolghasemi, A.; Dehghan, H.; Imani, H. The Association of Alexithymia and Sense of Coherence with Life Satisfaction in Attention Deficit Hyperactivity Disorder. *Zahedan J. Res. Med. Sci.* **2015**, *17*, e977. [CrossRef]
57. O'Carroll, R.E.; Ayling, R.; O'Reilly, S.M.; North, N.T. Alexithymia and sense of coherence in patients with total spinal cord transection. *Psychosom. Med.* **2003**, *65*, 151–155. [CrossRef] [PubMed]
58. Sancassiani, F.; Preti, A.; Cacace, E.; Ruggiero, V.; Testa, G.; Romano, F.; Carta, M.G. Alexithymia and sense of coherence: Does their impact on fibromyalgia suggest new targets for therapy? *Gen. Hosp. Psychiatry* **2019**, *59*, 78–79. [CrossRef] [PubMed]
59. Banni, S. Alexithymia, Sense of Coherence and Dysregulation of Biorhythms in Fibromyalgia: Implications for Pain Management and Quality of Life. Ph.D. Thesis, Università degli Studi di Cagliari, Cagliari, Italy, 2015.
60. Richardson, C.G.; Ratner, P.A. Sense of coherence as a moderator of the effects of stressful life events on health. *J. Epidemiol. Community Health* **2005**, *59*, 979–984. [CrossRef] [PubMed]
61. Mattila, A.K.; Saarni, S.I.; Salminen, J.K.; Huhtala, H.; Sintonen, H.; Joukamaa, M. Alexithymia and health-related quality of life in a general population. *Psychosomatics* **2009**, *50*, 59–68. [CrossRef]
62. Antonovsky, A. *Unravelling the Mystery of Health: How People Manage Stress and Stay Well*; Jossey-Bass: San Francisco, CA, USA, 1987.
63. Langeland, E.; Wahl, A.K.; Kristoffersen, K.; Hanestad, B.R. Promoting coping: Salutogenesis among people with mental health problems. *Issues Ment. Health Nurs.* **2007**, *28*, 275–295. [CrossRef] [PubMed]
64. Cederblad, M.; Hansson, K. Sense of coherence—A concept influencing health and quality of life in a Swedish psychiatric at-risk group. *Isr. J. Med. Sci.* **1996**, *32*, 194–199. [PubMed]

65. Langeland, E.; Wahl, A.K.; Kristoffersen, K.; Nortvedt, M.; Hanestad, B.R. Sense of coherence predicts change in life satisfaction among home-living residents in the community with mental health problems: A 1-year follow-up study. *Qual. Life Res.* **2007**, *16*, 939–946. [CrossRef] [PubMed]
66. Torgalsbøen, A.K.; Rund, B.R. Lessons learned from three studies of recovery from schizophrenia. *Int. Rev. Psychiatry* **2002**, *14*, 312–317. [CrossRef]
67. Harrow, M.; Grossman, L.; Jobe, T.H.; Herbener, E.S. Do patients with schizophrenia ever show periods of recovery? A 15-years multi-follow-up study. *Schizophr. Bull.* **2005**, *31*, 723–734. [CrossRef]
68. Witkowska-Łuć, B. Schizophrenia and sense of coherence. *Psychiatr. Pol.* **2018**, *52*, 217–226. [CrossRef] [PubMed]
69. Izydorczyk, B.; Sitnik-Warchulska, K.; Kühn-Dymecka, A.; Lizińczyk, S. Resilience, Sense of Coherence, and Coping with Stress as Predictors of Psychological Well-Being in the Course of Schizophrenia. The Study Design. *Int. J. Environ. Res. Public Health* **2019**, *16*, 1266. [CrossRef] [PubMed]
70. Huber, C.G.; Hochstrasser, L.; Meister, K.; Schimmelmann, B.G.; Lambert, M. Evidence for an agitated-aggressive syndrome in early-onset psychosis correlated with antisocial personality disorder, forensic history, and substance use disorder. *Schizophr. Res.* **2016**, *175*, 198–203. [CrossRef] [PubMed]
71. Bobes, J.; Fillat, O.; Arango, C. Violence among schizophrenia out-patients compliant with medication: Prevalence and associated factors. *Acta Psychiatr. Scand.* **2009**, *119*, 218–225. [CrossRef]
72. Caqueo-Urízar, A.; Fond, G.; Urzúa, A.; Boyer, L.; Williams, D.R. Violent behavior and aggression in schizophrenia: Prevalence and risk factors. A multicentric study from three Latin-America countries. *Schizophr. Res.* **2016**, *178*, 23–28. [CrossRef] [PubMed]
73. Stündağ, M.; Gulec, H.; Inanç, L.; Sevinç, E.; Semiz, M. Is alexithymia a separate dimension in schizophrenia? *Anatol. J. Psychiatry* **2020**, *21*, 85663. [CrossRef]
74. Maggini, C.; Raballo, A. Alexithymia and schizophrenic psychopathology. *Acta Biomed.* **2004**, *75*, 40–49. [PubMed]
75. Hsu, M.C.; Ouyang, W.C. Effects of Integrated Violence Intervention on Alexithymia, Cognitive, and Neurocognitive Features of Violence in Schizophrenia: A Randomized Controlled Trial. *Brain Sci.* **2021**, *11*, 837. [CrossRef] [PubMed]
76. Kupferberg, S.L. The relation between alexithymia and aggression in a nonclinical sample. *Diss. Abstr. Int. Sect. B Sci. Eng.* **2002**, *63*, 3011.
77. Sfeir, E.; Geara, C.; Hallit, S.; Obeid, S. Alexithymia, aggressive behavior and depression among Lebanese adolescents: A cross-sectional study. *Child Adolesc. Psychiatry Ment. Health* **2020**, *14*, 32. [CrossRef]
78. Garofalo, C.; Velotti, P.; Zavattini, G.C. Emotion regulation and aggression: The incremental contribution of alexithymia, impulsivity, and emotion dysregulation facets. *Psychol. Violence* **2018**, *8*, 470–483. [CrossRef]
79. Mancinelli, E.; Li, J.-B.; Lis, A.; Salcuni, S. Adolescents' Attachment to Parents and Reactive–Proactive Aggression: The Mediating Role of Alexithymia. *Int. J. Environ. Res. Public Health* **2021**, *18*, 13363. [CrossRef]
80. Manninen, M.; Therman, S.; Suvisaari, J.; Ebeling, H.; Moilanen, I.; Huttunen, M.; Joukamaa, M. Alexithymia is common among adolescents with severe disruptive behavior. *J. Nerv. Ment. Dis.* **2011**, *199*, 506–509. [CrossRef]
81. Konrath, S.; Novin, S.; Li, T. Is the relationship between alexithymia and aggression context-dependent? Impact of group membership and belief similarity. *Pers. Individ. Differ.* **2012**, *53*, 329–334. [CrossRef]
82. Dehghani, F.; Falahi, P. Does impulsivity mediate the relationship between alexithymia and aggression? *J. Fundam. Ment. Health* **2021**, *23*, 57–62.
83. Hemming, L.; Shaw, J.; Haddock, G.; Carter, L.A.; Pratt, D. A Cross-Sectional Study Investigating the Relationship between Alexithymia and Suicide, Violence, and Dual Harm in Male Prisoners. *Front. Psychiatry* **2021**, *12*, 670863. [CrossRef]
84. Parry, C.L. The Nature of the Association between Male Violent Offending and Alexithymia. Ph.D. Thesis, Edith Cowan University, Joondalup, WA, Australia, 2012. Available online: https://ro.ecu.edu.au/theses/483 (accessed on 7 February 2022).
85. Evren, C.; Cinar, O.; Evren, B.; Umut, G.; Can, Y.; Bozkurt, M. Relationship between Alexithymia and Aggression in a Sample of Men with Substance Dependence. *Klin. Psikofarmakol. Bülteni Bull. Clin. Psychopharmacol.* **2015**, *25*, 233–242. [CrossRef]
86. Kivimäki, M.; Elovainio, M.; Vahtera, J.; Nurmi, J.E.; Feldt, T.; Keltikangas-Järvinen, L.; Pentti, J. Sense of coherence as a mediator between hostility and health: Seven-year prospective study on female employees. *J. Psychosom. Res.* **2002**, *52*, 239–247. [CrossRef]
87. Silarova, B.; Nagyova, I.; Rosenberger, J.; van Dijk, J.P.; Reijneveld, S.A. Sense of coherence as a mediator between hostility and health-related quality of life among coronary heart disease patients. *Heart Lung.* **2016**, *45*, 126–131. [CrossRef] [PubMed]
88. Julkunen, J.; Ahlström, R. Hostility, anger, and sense of coherence as predictors of health-related quality of life. Results of an ASCOT substudy. *J. Psychosom. Res.* **2006**, *61*, 33–39. [CrossRef] [PubMed]
89. Bengtsson-Tops, A.; Brunt, D.; Rask, M. The structure of Antonovsky's sense of coherence in patients with schizophrenia and its relationship to psychopathology. *Scand. J. Caring Sci.* **2005**, *19*, 280–287. [CrossRef]
90. Gassmann, W.; Christ, O.; Lampert, J.; Berger, H. The influence of Antonovsky's sense of coherence (SOC) and psychoeducational family intervention (PEFI) on schizophrenic outpatients' perceived quality of life: A longitudinal field study. *BMC Psychiatry* **2013**, *13*, 10. [CrossRef] [PubMed]
91. Bengtsson-Tops, A.; Hansson, L. The validity of Antonovsky's Sense of Coherence measure in a sample of schizophrenic patients living in the community. *J. Adv. Nurs.* **2001**, *33*, 432–438. [CrossRef] [PubMed]
92. Bergstein, M.; Weizman, A.; Solomon, Z. Sense of coherence among delusional patients: Prediction of remission and risk of relapse. *Compr. Psychiatry.* **2008**, *49*, 288–296. [CrossRef]

93. Yıldız, B. Investigation the mediator role of sense of coherence in the relationship between self differentiation and alexitymia in university students. *Turk. Psychol. Couns. Guid. J.* **2020**, *10*, 603–616.
94. Cameron, K.; Ogrodniczuk, J.; Hadjipavlou, G. Changes in alexithymia following psychological intervention: A review. *Harv. Rev. Psychiatry* **2014**, *22*, 162–178. [CrossRef]
95. Aci, O.S.; Kutlu, F.Y. The effect of salutogenic approach-based interviews on sense of coherence and resilience in people with schizophrenia: A randomized controlled trial. *Perspect. Psychiatr. Care* **2021**, 1–9. [CrossRef]
96. Veltro, F.; Latte, G.; Pontarelli, I.; Pontarelli, C.; Nicchiniello, I.; Zappone, L. Long term outcome study of a salutogenic psychoeducational recovery oriented intervention (Inte.G.R.O.) in severe mental illness patients. *BMC Psychiatry* **2022**, *22*, 240. [CrossRef]
97. Langeland, E.; Vaandrager, L.; Nilsen, A.B.V.; Schraner, M.; Meier Magistretti, C. Effectiveness of Interventions to Enhance the Sense of Coherence in the Life Course. In *The Handbook of Salutogenesis*; Mittelmark, M.B., Sagy, S., Eriksson, M., Bauer, G.F., Pelikan, J.M., Lindström, B., Espnes, G.A., Eds.; Springer: Berlin/Heidelberg, Germany, 2022.
98. Tabachnick, B.G.; Fidell, L.S. *Using Multivariate Statistics*, 5th ed.; Pearson Education, Inc.: Boston, MA, USA, 2007.
99. Faul, F.; Erdfelder, E.; Lang, A.-G.; Buchner, A. Statistical power analyses using G*Power 3.1: Tests for correlation and regression analyses. *Behav. Res. Methods* **2009**, *41*, 1149. [CrossRef]
100. Schoemann, A.M.; Boulton, A.J.; Short, S.D. Determining Power and Sample Size for Simple and Complex Mediation Models. *Soc. Psychol. Pers. Sci.* **2017**, *8*, 379–386. [CrossRef]
101. Kline, R.B. *Methodology in the Social Sciences. Principles and Practice of Structural Equationmodeling*; Guilford Press: New York, NY, USA, 1998.
102. Pachi, A.; Giotakis, K.; Fanouraki, E.; Vouraki, G.; Bratis, D.; Tselebis, A. Adaptation of the Brief Aggression Questionnaire (BAQ) in Greek population. *Encephalos* **2021**, *58*, 6–23.
103. Webster, G.D.; DeWall, C.N.; Pond, R.S., Jr.; Deckman, T.; Jonason, P.K.; Le, B.M.; Nichols, L.A.; Orozco Schember, T.; Crysel, L.C.; Crosier, B.S.; et al. The Brief Aggression Questionnaire: Psychometric and Behavioral Evidence for an Efficient Measure of Trait Aggression. *Aggress. Behav.* **2014**, *40*, 120–139. [CrossRef] [PubMed]
104. Anagnostopoulou, T.; Kioseoglou, G. Sense of Coherence Scale. In *Psychometric Tools in Greece*; Stalikas, A., Triliva, S., Roussi, P., Eds.; Ellinika Grammata: Athens, Grece, 2002; pp. 291–292, (In Modern Greek).
105. Bagby, R.M.; Parker, J.D.; Taylor, G.J. The Twenty-Item Toronto Alexithymia Scale—I. Item selection and cross-validation of the factor structure. *J. Psychosom. Res.* **1994**, *38*, 23–32. [CrossRef]
106. Anagnostopoulou, T.; Kioseoglou, G. Toronto Alexithymia Scale. In *Psychometric Tools in Greece*; Stalikas, A., Triliva, S., Roussi, P., Eds.; Ellinika Grammata: Athens, Grece, 2002; pp. 100–101. (In Modern Greek)
107. Tselebis, A.; Bratis, D.; Roubi, A.; Anagnostopoulou, M.; Giotakis, K.; Pachi, A. Anger management during the COVID-19 lockdown: The role of resilience and family support. *Encephalos* **2022**, *59*, 1–10.
108. Tselebis, A.; Kosmas, E.; Bratis, D.; Moussas, G.; Karkanias, A.; Ilias, I.; Siafakas, N.; Vgontzas, A.; Tzanakis, N. Prevalence of alexithymia and its association with anxiety and depression in a sample of Greek chronic obstructive pulmonary disease (COPD) outpatients. *Ann. Gen. Psychiatry* **2010**, *9*, 16. [CrossRef] [PubMed]
109. Raja, M.; Azzoni, A. Hostility and violence of acute psychiatric inpatients. *Clin. Pract. Epidemiol. Ment. Health* **2005**, *1*, 11. [CrossRef]
110. Ochoa, S.; Suarez, D.; Novick, D.; Arranz, B.; Roca, M.; Baño, V.; Haro, J.M. Factors predicting hostility in outpatients with schizophrenia: 36-month results from the SOHO study. *J. Nerv. Ment. Dis.* **2013**, *201*, 464–470. [CrossRef]
111. Smith, T.W. Concepts and methods in the study of anger, hostility, and health. In *Anger, Hostility and the Heart*; Siegman, A.W., Smith, T.W., Eds.; Lawrence Erlbaum: Hillsdale, NJ, USA, 1994; pp. 23–42.
112. Perlini, C.; Bellani, M.; Besteher, B.; Nenadić, I.; Brambilla, P. The neural basis of hostility-related dimensions in schizophrenia. *Epidemiol. Psychiatr. Sci.* **2018**, *27*, 546–551. [CrossRef]
113. Pandey, R.; Saxena, P.; Dubey, A. Emotion regulation difficulties in alexithymia and mental health. *Eur. J. Psychol.* **2011**, *7*, 604–623. [CrossRef]
114. Taylor, G.J.; Bagby, R.M.; Parker, J.D.A. *Disorders of Affect Regulation: Alexithymia in Medical and Psychiatric Illness*; Cambridge University Press: Cambridge, UK, 1997.
115. Henry, J.D.; Green, M.J.; De Lucia, A.; Restuccia, C.; McDonald, S.; O'Donnell, M. Emotion dysregulation in schizophrenia: Reduced amplification of emotional expression is associated with emotional blunting. *Schizophr. Res.* **2007**, *95*, 197–204. [CrossRef]
116. Henry, J.D.; Rendell, P.G.; Green, M.J.; McDonald, S.; O'Donnell, M. Emotion regulation in schizophrenia: Affective, social and clinical correlates of suppression and reappraisal. *J. Abnorm. Psychol.* **2008**, *117*, 473–478. [CrossRef] [PubMed]
117. Jenkins, A.L.; McCloskey, M.S.; Kulper, D.; Berman, M.E.; Coccaro, E.F. Selfharm behavior among individuals with intermittent explosive disorder and personality disorders. *J. Psychiatr. Res.* **2014**, *60*, 125–131. [CrossRef] [PubMed]
118. Gratz, K.L.; Roemer, L. Multidimensional assessment of emotion regulation and dysregulation: Development, factor structure, and initial validation of the difficulties in emotion regulation scale. *J. Psychopathol. Behav. Assess.* **2004**, *26*, 41–54. [CrossRef]
119. Hornsveld, R.H.J.; Kraaimaat, W. Alexithymia in Dutch violent forensic psychiatric outpatients. *Psychol. Crime Law* **2012**, *18*, 833–846. [CrossRef]
120. Ates, M.A.; Algul, A.; Gulsun, M.; Gecici, O.; Ozdemir, B.; Basoglu, C. The relationship between alexithymia, aggression and psychopathy in young adult males with antisocial personality disorder. *Noropsikiyatri Ars. Neuropsychiatry* **2009**, *46*, 135–139.

121. Teten, A.L.; Miller, L.A.; Bailey, S.D.; Dunn, N.J.; Kent, T.A. Empathic deficits and alexithymia in trauma-related impulsive aggression. *Behav. Sci. Law* **2008**, *26*, 823–832. [CrossRef]
122. Spielberger, C.D.; Reheiser, E.C.; Sydeman, S.J. Measuring the experience, expression, and control of anger. *Issues Compr. Pediatr. Nurs.* **1995**, *18*, 207–232. [CrossRef]
123. Damasio, A.R. *Descartes Error: Emotion, Reason and the Human Brain*; G P Putnam's Sons: New York, NY, USA, 1994.
124. Frith, C.D. *The Cognitive Neuropsychology of Schizophrenia*; Lawrence Erlbaum: Hove, UK, 1992.
125. Abu-Akel, A.; Abushua'leh, K. "Theory of mind" in violent and nonviolent patients with paranoid schizophrenia. *Schizophr. Res.* **2004**, *69*, 45–53. [CrossRef]
126. Landsverk, S.S.; Kane, C.F. Antonovsky's sense of coherence: Theoretical basis of psychoeducation in schizophrenia. *Issues Ment. Health Nurs.* **1998**, *19*, 419–431.
127. Antonovsky, A. The salutogenic model as a theory to guide health promotion. *Health Promot. Int.* **1996**, *11*, 11–18. [CrossRef]
128. Torgalsbøen, A.K.; Fu, S.; Czajkowski, N. Resilience trajectories to full recovery in first-episode schizophrenia. *Eur. Psychiatry* **2018**, *52*, 54–60. [CrossRef] [PubMed]
129. Hovland, J.F.; Skogvang, B.O.; Ness, O.; Langeland, E. Development of salutogenic coping skills: Experiences with daily challenges among young adults suffering from serious mental illness. *Int. J. Qual. Stud. Health Well-Being* **2021**, *16*, 1879369. [CrossRef] [PubMed]
130. Pelikan, J.M. The Application of Salutogenesis in Healthcare Settings. In *The Handbook of Salutogenesis*; Mittelmark, M.B., Sagy, S., Eriksson, M., Bauer, G.F., Pelikan, J.M., Lindström, B., Espnes, G.A., Eds.; Springer: Berlin/Heidelberg, Germany, 2017; Chapter 25.
131. Price, O.; Baker, J.; Bee, P.; Lovell, K. The support-control continuum: An investigation of staff perspectives on factors influencing the success or failure of de-escalation techniques for the management of violence and aggression in mental health settings. *Int. J. Nurs. Stud.* **2018**, *77*, 197–206. [CrossRef]
132. Bhat, S.; Rentala, S.; Nanjegowda, R.B.; Chellappan, X.B. Effectiveness of Milieu Therapy in reducing conflicts and containment rates among schizophrenia patients. *Invest. Educ. Enferm.* **2020**, *38*, e06. [CrossRef]
133. Hasson-Ohayon, I. Integrating cognitive behavioral-based therapy with an intersubjective approach: Addressing metacognitive deficits among people with schizophrenia. *J. Psychother. Integr.* **2012**, *22*, 356–374. [CrossRef]
134. Bell, M.D.; Zito, W.Q.; Greig, T.; Wexler, B.E. Neurocognitive enhancement therapy with vocational services: Work outcomes at two-year follow-up. *Schizophr. Res.* **2008**, *105*, 18–29. [CrossRef]
135. Ahmed, A.O.; Hunter, K.M.; van Houten, E.G.; Monroe, J.M.; Bhat, I.A. Cognition and Other Targets for the Treatment of Aggression in People with Schizophrenia. *Ann. Psychiatry Ment. Health* **2014**, *2*, 1004.
136. Pinna, F.; Manchia, M.; Paribello, P.; Carpiniello, B. The Impact of Alexithymia on Treatment Response in Psychiatric Disorders: A Systematic Review. *Front. Psychiatry* **2020**, *11*, 311. [CrossRef]
137. Kennedy, M.; Franklin, J. Skills-based Treatment for Alexithymia: An Exploratory Case Series. *Behav. Chang.* **2002**, *19*, 158–171. [CrossRef]
138. Rathod, S.; Phiri, P.; Kingdon, D. Cognitive behavioral therapy for schizophrenia. *Psychiatr. Clin. North Am.* **2010**, *33*, 527–536. [CrossRef] [PubMed]
139. Dickerson, F.B.; Lehman, A.F. Evidence-based psychotherapy for schizophrenia. *J. Nerv. Ment. Dis.* **2006**, *194*, 3–9. [CrossRef] [PubMed]
140. Darmedru, C.; Demily, C.; Franck, N. Cognitive remediation and social cognitive training for violence in schizophrenia: A systematic review. *Psychiatry Res.* **2017**, *251*, 266–274. [CrossRef] [PubMed]
141. Quinn, J.; Kolla, N.J. From Clozapine to Cognitive Remediation. *Can. J. Psychiatry* **2017**, *62*, 94–101. [CrossRef] [PubMed]

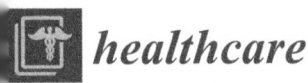 healthcare

Article

Mental Health Nurses' Tacit Knowledge of Strategies for Improving Medication Adherence for Schizophrenia: A Qualitative Study

Yao-Yu Lin [1], Wen-Jiuan Yen [2], Wen-Li Hou [3,4], Wei-Chou Liao [5] and Mei-Ling Lin [6,*]

1. Department of Nursing, Tsaotun Psychiatric Center, Ministry of Health and Welfare, Nantou 542, Taiwan; yylin@ttpc.mohw.gov.tw
2. College of Nursing, Chung Shan Medical University Hospital, Taichung 402, Taiwan; wyen@csmu.edu.tw
3. College of Nursing, Kaohsiung Medical University, Kaohsiung 807, Taiwan; wlhou422@gmail.com
4. Department of Medical Research, Kaohsiung Medical University Hospital, Kaohsiung 807, Taiwan
5. Internship Counselling Office, Taichung School for the Visually Impaired, Taichung 421, Taiwan; jou@cmsb.tc.edu.tw
6. Department of Nursing, HungKuang University, Taichung 433, Taiwan
* Correspondence: linml@sunrise.hk.edu.tw

Abstract: Non-adherence to medication among patients with schizophrenia is an important clinical issue with very complex reasons. Since medication administration is an essential nursing responsibility, improving strategies for patient medication compliance must be fully understood. This study aimed to explore the strategies mental health nurses (MHNs) implement in clinically improving patients with schizophrenia and to describe the nurses' tacit knowledge of application strategies. A qualitative study with purposeful sampling was used. Twenty-five experienced MHNs in a psychiatric hospital in central Taiwan were given an in-depth interview. The texts were content-analyzed using NVivo 12 Pro software. MHNs promote medication adherence among patients with schizophrenia using the following strategies: establishing a conversational relationship, overall assessment of non-adherence to medication, understanding the disease and adjusting the concept of medication, incorporating interpersonal connection feedback, and building supportive resources. This study explored the strategies of MHNs that incorporated knowledge in managing treatment adherence in patients with schizophrenia. The findings add knowledge to clinical nursing practice about medication adherence among patients with schizophrenia.

Keywords: medication adherence; mental health nurses; tacit knowledge; schizophrenia

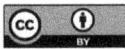

1. Introduction

Adherence to medication is essential but challenging in the psychiatric profession [1,2]. A meta-analysis including 35 studies that reported a pooled estimate of medication non-adherence found that the non-adherence rate in schizophrenia, major depression, and bipolar disorder was 56%, 50%, and 44%, respectively [3]. Antipsychotic medications are effective in successfully preventing relapses if taken regularly [4,5]. Schizophrenia is a lifelong disease with the lowest adherence to medication.

Non-adherence to medication in schizophrenia is a multifaceted issue. Previous studies have found that this non-adherence is associated with first onset, young age, lack of insight, negative attitude to medication, side effects of the medication, social support, medication alliance, alcohol, and substance abuse, among others [6,7]. In addition, a poorly planned discharge, post-discharge environment, and poor therapeutic alliances, among others, can also contribute to non-adherence [8–10].

Antipsychotic adverse effects may also occur more in compliant patients because patients with poor adherence are not regularly taking their medications and do not, therefore, experience side effects [5,11]. A study interviewed pharmacists, psychiatrists, and nurses to explore how they help patients manage their medication and found that the topmost concerns were understanding patients' beliefs about medication and systematically monitoring side effects [12]. The findings indicate the need for a regular follow-up evaluation to simplify medication treatment and reduce the problem of patients taking complex medications to increase adherence [13].

Building a good relationship with the patient is very important in improving medication adherence. A good therapeutic alliance or therapeutic interpersonal relationship between mental health professionals and patients is positively related to improved adherence [5,14,15]. The connotation of a therapeutic alliance includes cooperation, an emotional connection between the therapist and the patient, and common goal setting [16]. Building a trusting relationship with the patient is also the most commonly used strategy used by nurses, which involves listening to and interpreting their needs and concerns [17]. However, many patients with schizophrenia are not hospitalized voluntarily, and their relationship with medical professionals is not spontaneously established, which makes implementing measures to enhance adherence with medications difficult for nurses. Furthermore, no relevant studies have been conducted.

In order to improve medication adherence among patients with schizophrenia, MHNs (mental health nurses) provide psychological education to increase patients' understanding of the characteristics of the disease and recognition of medications [18], cognitive behavior therapy [19], and adopted motivation interviewing to increase motivation to take medications [20] in the clinical setting. Otherwise, long-acting antipsychotic injections can be administered to assist oral medication to decrease relapse [21]. Healthcare professionals encourage patient involvement in shared decision making with their physician to express their preference and opinion in treatment selection to increase their adherence to medication [22]. Inviting family caregivers involved in the treatment of patients with schizophrenia is one strategy to increase adherence to medication [9]. Some studies suggest that social support is also related to medication adherence [5,9,11], but some studies report that it is unrelated [14]. Nurses have frequently conducted psychoeducation for families in practice [23], which means that social networks can support patients and encourage them to adhere to their treatment. Involving family for social support may vary with culture. Therefore, the patient's condition or preference during the intervention should be considered before involving the family.

Nurses have a positive influence and can help patients change their attitudes toward disease and enhance their insights to increase medication adherence [24]. Previous studies aimed to clarify the factors that influence medication adherence in psychiatric patients. However, there are two problematic aspects in clinical practice. First, the quantitative study separates the variables into a part of medication adherence that cannot be understood in the whole view context of increasing medication adherence. Second, previous studies rarely demonstrated the "how" aspect; specifically, how the influences on medication adherence embody nurses' experiences. The 3D creativity management theory considers the within-discipline expertise, out-of-discipline knowledge, and a disciplined creative process to explain how creativity and innovation are manifested throughout information processes [25,26]. Nurses have the longest and most frequent contact with patients. Moreover, patients' adherence to medicine must consider the overall context in clinical practice. The experiences of MHNs may embody the tacit knowledge gained in actual practice; however, these experiences have not been highlighted and consolidated in previous studies.

Aim

This study has two goals. First, it sought to explore the strategies employed by MHNs to improve medication adherence in clinical practice. Second, it aimed to describe MHNs' knowledge of facilitation strategies in medication.

2. Methods

This study was based on qualitative exploratory methodology and used in-depth interviews to collect information on nursing experiences and strategies for medication adherence in mental illness. Ethical approval was obtained from the research ethics committee (TTPC 108026) and the administrative committee of a psychiatric hospital in Taiwan. All participants provided signed informed consent on their understanding of the study and to the audio recording of their interviews.

2.1. Sample

All participants were selected from a psychiatric hospital in central Taiwan. The corresponding author conducted all interviews. The participants were accompanied by MHNs who were over the age of 20 years and had at least 1 year of nursing experience. One-on-one interviews were conducted for data collection. The interview began with questions on the participant's recognition and experience of non-adherence, followed by questions that elucidated how they dealt with those situations.

2.2. Data Collection

Purposeful sampling was conducted on 25 MHNs in this study. The researcher kept the interview questions in mind and used them flexibly to avoid interfering with the interview process. The interviews were conducted from February to July 2020. An in-depth interview included questions focusing on the strategies employed by MHNs to improve medication adherence and describe the knowledge of facilitation strategies in medication. These interviews used an interview guide with questions that were developed a priori by the authors based on their review of the literature and clinical experience: "Could you describe care experience about non-adherence medication of schizophrenia?", "Based on your clinical experience, could you describe the reasons for the non-adherence medication for schizophrenia?", and "Could you give me some examples of how to increase non-adherence medication for schizophrenia?". Additionally, the following questions were asked about the context, in order to elicit tacit knowledge of medication adherence in nurses' experiences: "How does this happen?" or "What causes this to happen?".

Each participant was interviewed one to two times. The interviews lasted for 45–65 min. All interviews were audio-recorded and transcribed verbatim. Possible identifying information was deleted from the data, and codes were used to replace the names of participants. Data were kept anonymous, and coding numbers were used during analysis to ensure they could not be linked to any personal information.

2.3. Data Analysis

A 7-step inductive qualitative content analysis was performed [27]. Data analysis began after the first interview and simultaneously continued with subsequent interviews until data saturation was reached for the purpose of this research and no new relevant information could be obtained [28,29]. The data were saved in Word files before being uploaded to NVivo 12 Pro software (QSR International, Melbourne Australia) for analysis.

Each unit of analysis was given meaning units from the text. Descriptions of participants who used strategies to increase medication adherence for mental illness were as detailed as possible. Preliminary labels were given to the meaning units and were grouped based on similarities and differences. The codes from the data were divided into subthemes, and these themes were labeled according to the content. The subthemes were further compared and grouped based on similarities and differences. The themes were named based on content characteristics. The researchers continued to analyze the data until data saturation had been reached.

2.4. Rigor and Credibility

To ensure rigor [30], purposive sampling was conducted, and the participants enrolled all had experience of promoting medication adherence in psychiatric mental illness. The researcher (M.L.L.) had a background in phenomenology and experience in qualitative research in the field of mental health nursing. The researcher established a relationship of respect and trust with each participant and maintained intersubjectivity. All participants provided rich, diverse perspectives of the phenomena in this study. To enhance transferability, interview questions were used to assist the researcher to encourage the participants to recall their caring experience of medication non-adherence with detailed descriptions to obtain extensive data. Regular research meetings among researchers were held to examine the verbatim transcriptions to ensure the quality of the interviews. The text was preliminarily coded and categorized independently and manually (MLL). The codes, subthemes, and themes were checked and discussed (WCL). If the subthemes or themes varied, the authors modified the list and read the transcripts to confirm the participants' views until an agreement of categorization among researchers was achieved. The participants provided their comments after reviewing the summary of the theme, sub-theme, and summary of the final results. Regular meetings with the authors were held. To ensure confirmability, peer debriefings among researchers were adopted to discuss the findings, emerging themes, and interpretations of data. Reflective diaries were kept to assist the researcher to maintain neutrality during the data analysis process.

3. Results

The demographic characteristics of the 25 MHNs are presented in Table 1. The following were identified as the strategies MHNs used to promote medication among patients with schizophrenia: establishing a conversational relationship, overall assessment of non-adherence to medication, understanding the disease and adjusting the concept of medication, incorporating interpersonal connection feedback, and building supportive resources (Table 2).

3.1. Establishing a Conversational Relationship

Establishing a conversational relationship means that nurses create a feeling of safety and trust for patients and establish a basis for dialog with patients about taking medication. Subthemes of this topic include concerning daily life, expressing care nonverbally, lenience and being-with, and handling patients' characters.

Table 1. Sociodemographic characteristics of the participants.

Demographics			$n = 25$
Sex		Female (%)	23 (92%)
		Male (%)	2 (8%)
	Age (years)	Mean (SD)	39.6 years old (SD 6.1)
	Education	College/university	11 (44%)
		postgraduate	14 (56%)
	Marital status	Married	19 (76%)
		Single	5 (20%)
		Divorced	1 (4%)
Psychiatric work experience		Mean (SD)	13.4 years (SD 5.9)
Current psychiatric work department		Acute ward	15 (60%)
		Chronic ward	5 (20%)
		Community	5 (20%)

Table 2. Summary strategies of MHNs to promote medication adherence in schizophrenia.

Themes	Subthemes
1. Establishing a conversational relationship	1.1. Concerning daily life 1.2. Express care nonverbally 1.3. Lenience and being-with 1.4. Handling patients' characters
2. Overall assessment of non-adherence to medication	2.1. Evaluating beliefs about taking medication from the context 2.2. Tactfully confirm side effects 2.3. Assessing ability to support medication from family
3. Understanding the disease and adjusting the concept of medication	3.1. Analogy to an acceptable disease 3.2. The pros and cons of taking medication 3.3. Identifying and managing medications 3.4. Reducing influence from side effects
4. Incorporate interpersonal connection feedback	4.1. Positive affirmations for taking medication 4.2. Describing illness anecdotes from peers 4.3. Consideration of the burden on their loved ones
5. Building supportive resources	5.1. Encourage shared decision making 5.2. Using long-acting antipsychotics 5.3. Inviting family to monitor symptoms and promote medication adherence 5.4. Referral to related resources

3.1.1. Concerning Daily Life

Nurses interact with patients in their daily lives to reduce the sensitivity of patients and to create a starting point for interactions. Only by gaining trust can MHNs further discuss the core problems of the disease. Participant 17 thinks that providing care in daily life is not intrusive and avoids the patient's symptoms. She said:

> "If his (patient) symptoms are really bad, or he has delusions, don't be too deliberate. Continue providing routine care every day. You can ask: How are you (patient) sleeping lately or how are you eating? He may feel that this is just a common concern. The patient may be willing to talk about why he doesn't (want to) take his medication further."

MHNs start with normal contact, and only after establishing trust can they talk to the patient about problems with their disease and medication status.

3.1.2. Express Care Nonverbally

Non-verbal communication of care acknowledges that patients are more sensitive to non-verbal expressions of care. MHNs can convey their concern for patients through non-verbal communication, which helps to build relationships. Participant 9 discusses this as follows:

> "Actually, language is a secondary form of communication. What's more important is the nurse's attitude, expression in the nurse's eyes, tone of voice, and spending time with them. That can help the patient feel safe to talk about their illness."

Given the importance of non-verbal communication in relationship building, MHNs thus try to communicate nonverbally.

3.1.3. Lenience and Being-With

Containment and being-with mean that nurses respond to the patient's negative emotions through listening and empathy to convey understanding and acceptance to the patient. Participant 9 recalled facing psychiatric patients complaining about medication problems:

"When he (patient) may have some complaints, I just comfort him. He was complaining about the discomfort of taking medicine. First, I listened to his complaints. After he complained, he talked about taking medicine slowly."

Participant 10 thought that, given enough time, the patient will gradually vent out their emotions, which will help to establish the relationship. He said:

"You should give the patient plenty of time to talk nonsense or complain and vent the accumulated emotions and pressure. He (the patient), in this way, will more likely develop trust in you."

Nurses can show empathy, listen, and accept behaviors to deal with patient's negative emotions and earn the patient's trust in order to talk about medications.

3.1.4. Handling Patients' Characters

Handling patients' characters means nurses should appropriately adjust the interaction according to the different personalities and situations with the patients to maintain a friendly interaction. At the beginning of the interaction between Participant 11 and a patient, an adjustment of the interaction according to the patient's characteristics facilitated the patient's cooperation in therapeutic activities after the relationship was established. She said:

"There are some patients who are more perceptive. It is better to give him a little flexibility rather than confront him. Then, he will be more willing to accept and cooperate in the follow-up. We learn how to use the patient's traits to take care of him."

Nurses should have sensitivity during the interaction. Participant 17 thought that they should not talk about medication too directly. She said:

"At the beginning, you can't directly talk about medicine. No! Otherwise, you will not be received well. The patient may instead say that they don't use it anymore. Patients will disagree with you. You will be rejected."

The nurse is unable to carry out the follow-up treatment plan if it triggers negative emotions in this case.

3.2. Overall Assessment of Non-Adherence to Medication

Non-adherence to medication involves various factors, and the nurse should assess the medication status and difficulties. The subthemes of this include evaluating beliefs about taking medication from the context, tactfully confirming side effects, and assessing the ability of the family to support medication.

3.2.1. Evaluating Beliefs about Taking Medication from the Context

Evaluating the beliefs about taking medication from the context means that the nurses evaluate the reasons why the patient is disinclined to take medication to use as a reference for intervention. Participant 21 described a clear reason:

"The patient's lack of desire to take medicine must be based on reasons. If the patient can specify his reasons, we can assist him in eliminating them to improve his motivation to take medicines."

The nurse should also confirm the medication status from the patient's relatives and friends. In this regard, Participant 12 said:

"I listened to the patients and the family members to see if there are any points of fit because they actually live together."

In addition to assessing medication, the nurse should also confirm from their relatives observervations whether patients take medication. The assessment status is used as the basis for interventional medication by understanding the context.

3.2.2. Tactfully Confirm Side Effects

Nurses know that side effects are one of the reasons for non-adherence to medication. They take indirect or tactful methods to clarify the side effects experienced by patients. Participant 6 described an example using postural hypotension:

> "If the patient is taking medicine that causes postural hypotension, we will ask: 'Do you usually have it?' or 'In addition to the uncomfortable things you said, do you still feel dizzy?' We will not directly say that this is a side effect of the medicine."

Participant 19 also mentioned:

> "We will avoid saying we notice the patient's worry, such as tremor of hands. I will not ask him directly, 'Do your hands tremor?' Instead, I will ask, 'Do you feel uncomfortable after taking the medicine?'"

MHNs use euphemistic methods to clarify and evaluate to prevent patients from hesitating or ceasing to take medicine due to side effects.

3.2.3. Assessing Ability to Support Medication from Family

To determine the knowledge of family members in supporting medication adherence, the family's ability and individual problems of the family members as medication supervisors are assessed to confirm the patient's medication problems. Participant 16 described the assessment of the family members' ability and concern about medication adherence:

> "Sometimes family members have to work and can only prepare medicines for him to take. Sometimes family members are afraid of the patient's anger, fearing that the patient will be upset by being urged to take the medicine. Nurses need to evaluate the abilities and attitudes of family in supervising the patient in adhering to medication."

The family members are the main caregivers of patients with mental illness, and nurses need to evaluate the ability of a family as a resource in medication adherence.

3.3. Understanding Disease and Adjusting the Concept of Medication

Nurses use different viewpoints to help patients understand disease, explain the pros and cons of medication, and improve patients' willingness to take medication. Subthemes include an analogy to an acceptable disease, the pros and cons of taking medication, identifying and managing medications, and reducing influence from side effects.

3.3.1. Analogy to an Acceptable Disease

Creating an analogy to an acceptable disease means that the nurse compares the treatment of psychiatric medication to a generalized disease that can be accepted to increase the patient's willingness to take medicines. Participant 3 explained that taking psychiatric drugs is similar to taking medication for a general physical illness to increase motivation in taking medication:

> "Some patients have no insight. I use analogy to physical diseases. I will tell patients: 'Taking this medicine (antipsychotic) is just like taking medications if you have high blood pressure or heart disease.' I also tell the patient, 'Even us nurses have to take medicines when we are sick.'"

Participant 12 used acceptable generalized symptoms as a starting point for the explanation:

> "I think that discussing symptoms of the disease that are acceptable to the patient, such as insomnia, and asking them to confirm with continued treatment whether the symptoms improve can persuade him to take the medicine."

MHNs can help improve the patient's acceptance of symptoms and medications by comparing the treatment process to those of general illnesses.

3.3.2. The Pros and Cons of Taking Medication

The nurse discusses the pros and cons of taking medication to emphasize that failure to do so will cause the return of symptoms and relapse. The nurse reminds the client of the consequences and losses of not taking medication. Participant 9 positively reminded a patient of the changes after the medication:

> "Let the patient compare the results of adherence and non-adherence, and ask them to think about what is good for them."

To encourage continuous medication treatment, Participants 21 said:

> "Let the patient know that with treatment, their situation would be more stable. Without treatment, they may be sick or hospitalized all the time, unable to work, unable to maintain their marriage, and the family will eventually be affected."

The nurse can enumerate the benefits of taking the medicine to avoid losing one's well-being due to the influence of symptoms.

3.3.3. Identifying and Managing Medications

Identifying and managing medications refers to improving motivation to take medications by understanding the benefits of drugs for disease control. The improvement in symptoms after patients administer the medicine is used as the premise to increase their awareness regarding medications. Participant 20 stated:

> "I will inform patients about the effects and side effects of medications. The main purpose is to let the patients know how medicine can help stabilize the disease."

MHNs can also assist in the administration of medicines so that patients can take medicines conveniently. Participant 12 said:

> "There are some patients who will still be unable to identify their medicines clearly. I can help them concentrate the medicine and tell them: 'this package is your after-breakfast medication."

MHNs can assist patients in organizing medications to improve medication adherence behaviors and convenience.

3.3.4. Reducing Influence from Side Effects

Side effects are one of the reasons that cause patients to stop adhering. One of the strategies used by nurses to improve patients' medication adherence is to help reduce the side effects via providing information or assisting the physicians to adjust the medications that affect patients' confidence in taking the medication. Participant 5 provided suggestions to alleviate side effects after speaking with the patient:

> "I will provide nursing knowledge and inform patients that if side effects are present, the medication can be adjusted to relieve discomfort."

MHNs can act as agents for the patient. Nurses can communicate with the physician the need to adjust medication and reduce the impact of side effects. Participant 2 said:

> "Some patients need to work, and the drugs make them groggy and sleepy. I can ask the doctor to make some adjustments in the medication regimen."

MHNs can provide information on reducing side effects and also serve as a communication bridge between patients and physicians to increase patient willingness to take medication while helping decrease the influence of side effects.

3.4. Incorporate Interpersonal Connection Feedback

Incorporating interpersonal connection feedback means helping patients perceive the benefits and responsibilities of taking medications through feedback of the wellness associated with taking medications as prescribed. Subthemes include positive affirmations for taking medication, describing illness anecdotes from peers, and consideration of the burden on their loved ones.

3.4.1. Positive Affirmations for Taking Medication

Positive affirmations for taking medication means providing encouragement to the patient to boost the patient's willingness to continue taking medication. Participant 4 provided patients with feedback on taking medication through affirmation cards:

> "The patient likes the star. I made cards and wrote blessings on the back of the cards. After the patient takes the medicine, I give them the card as positive affirmation for adhering to medication."

Positive feedback improves the motivation of patients to adhere to medication, thereby enhancing medication compliance.

3.4.2. Describing Illness Anecdotes from Peers

The nurse invites the patient's peers to describe their experiences of the benefits of taking the medicine to enhance the patient's motivation to do the same. Participant 12 described her experience:

> "I invited patients with the same disease to talk about their experiences of taking the medicine. The invitees told the hesitant patient, 'You must take it! I can sleep better and I don't have a bee in my bonnet.' Hearing anecdotes from peers has a significant effect on persuading patients to do the same."

Hearing the experiences of peers with the same can increase motivation for adherence to medication.

3.4.3. Consideration of the Burden on Their Loved Ones

Consideration of the burden of the disease on their loved ones entails the nurse reminding the patient to pay attention to the effort of their caregivers in helping them manage their illness. Participant 7 recalled:

> "Tell the patient that if they take their medicine, they will be less likely to be hospitalized and that they can also make their mother feel more at ease."

Participant 16 further reminded patients to value the hard work of their family members in helping them manage their illnesses. Only stabilizing their symptoms can reduce the burden on their family. She said:

> "I tell the patient: 'Your mother is worried about your health, but she is also getting older. If you are willing to take the medicine and to manage your symptoms, then you will be also helping unburden you mother."

MHNs can remind patients that their illness not only affects themselves, but also increases the burden on their family. Taking medications as directed helps to stabilize symptoms and reduce caregiver burden.

3.5. Building Supportive Resources

The nurse evaluates how to help the patient comply with the medication regimen by changing the patient's participation in medical care and/or oral medication status or using family and community resources. The subthemes of this intervention include encouraging shared decision making, using long-acting antipsychotics, inviting family to monitor symptoms and promote medication adherence, and referral to related resources.

3.5.1. Encourage Shared Decision-Making

MHNs encourage patients to communicate with their physicians in order to talk about medicine and fight for their best interests. Participant 19 said:

"You can adjust the medication during the hospitalization, and you can talk to the attending doctor. You can also communicate with your doctor and make adjustments during outpatient visits."

Nurses can encourage patients to express their thoughts on the medications prescribed to them and to get involved in consultation with doctors to find the most suitable medical treatments for themselves.

3.5.2. Using Long-Acting Antipsychotics

The use of long-acting antipsychotic injections can help stabilize the illness and its symptoms for a longer duration. Participant 1 mentioned that changing the drug dosage form is one of the strategies to improve medication:

"I will tell the patient during the hospitalization: 'Long-acting antipsychotics can be injected once a month. If you forget to take the oral medicine, you will not relapse too quickly which can cause you to be hospitalized.' Oral medications are more prone to non-adherence. Long-acting injections help remedy this and/or increase compliance."

3.5.3. Inviting Family to Monitor Symptoms and Promote Medication Adherence

Families can help to monitor the patient's symptoms and medication adherence at home. Therefore, improving family members' knowledge of symptoms and drugs is helpful. The nurse can remind and assist family members in this. Participant 16 let the family members know about the symptoms and medication status:

"I will tell the family to pay attention to the signs of the patient's illness, for example, to see if the patient is starting to suffer from insomnia or emotional instability, and to pay attention to his medication status."

Family members confirm that medication and illness status contribute to adjuvant treatment. Participant 22 said:

"I will mention to the family that you have to observe the patient's medication status and confirm the remaining amount of medication to prevent any disruptions."

Family members have an important supporting role in enhancing medication compliance. Nurses can teach family members to identify the signs of onset and confirm medication.

3.5.4. Referral to Related Resources

A pre-hospital search for related resources can help stabilize the patient's condition and improve compliance with medications. Participant 2 mentioned that when assessing patients for poor drug compliance, follow-up resources should be considered to continue care. She said:

"If the patient does not cooperate with the medication, he may prepare for referral to a home care, daycare, or another sheltered environment and find a place that can help them supervise medication adherence before leaving the hospital."

From the perspective of resource linking, patients can continue to take medication after discharge from the hospital.

4. Discussion

This study explored the strategies of MHNs that incorporated tacit knowledge in managing treatment adherence in patients with schizophrenia in clinical work. MHNs choose medication adherence strategies based on a judgement that considers patient attitude, side effects, and related resources. The first conditions need to be fulfilled in building a trusting relationship between nurses and patients. There is a complex process based on the patient's response in the next step. Nurses consider "act" to be a viable and preferable option in terms of the patient's response that is similar to 3D creativity management theory to explain how creativity and innovations from nurses are involved in promoting adherence to medication in patients with schizophrenia [25]. Nurses nonverbally express sincerity and safety, provide psychoeducation, and go on to build a trustworthy relationship with patients. The core tenet of medication adherence strategies is to avoid ruining relationships with patients. The results indicate that nurses will often select strategies from patients' feedback, which is a dynamic process, and consider the best benefits for patients. Nurses euphemistically and thoughtfully adjust their behavior to the attitude of the patient, make sure the information is available, evaluate information, and provide related resources to increase medication adherence.

4.1. Trust Building

A high level of trust helps facilitate information reception and acceptance. A previous study promoted medication adherence and acknowledged that patients' beliefs about medications play an important role [12]. The authors agree with this opinion. MHNs, as the first-line psychiatric professionals in the management of mental illness, are well aware that the relationship with the patient can constitute the basis of drug beliefs. It is critical for psychiatric patients to take medications as prescribed. Research has shown that establishing therapeutic alliances with patients can increase the benefit of medications [16]. However, in the early stages of the treatment relationship, few patients are voluntarily hospitalized, and the positions of nurses and patients tend to differ. The key to the role of nurses in enhancing compliance with medications depends on whether the patient can trust the nurse as a starting point for cooperation that maintains dialog and interaction with patients.

MHNs' "tacit knowledge" is different from "explicit knowledge" of improving mediation adherence in patients with schizophrenia. Explicit knowledge can be easily expressed, written, and transferred from one person to another. In this study, nurses accumulate tacit knowledge that is obtained from the experience and intuition gained during interpersonal interaction based on hands-on experience and in-depth practice analysis, observation, etc. The term "tacit knowledge" was coined by Michael Polanyi [31] to refer to the knowledge that cannot be transferred through formalization (writing or verbalization). Similar to previous research, MHNs also think that good interpersonal relationships between mental health professionals and patients can improve adherence [5,14,15]. Moreover, MHNs strive for cooperation and alliance with patients and avoid triggering negative emotions in the patient that may cause the patient to distance themselves from or reject the nurse in clinical practice. It could be based on the concept of the disease, and the cognition of medications is different between the patient and the nurse at the beginning of the contact. In this regard, the MHNs used a careful probing attitude to confirm the problem of the patient's adherence to the prescribed medication. Establishing an interpersonal strategy for maintaining conversational relationships to improve compliance with medications cannot be applied as a whole. Given the wide variety of patient personalities, nurses need to flexibly use their experience to slowly grasp the essentials in an interaction.

4.2. Information Availability

Nurses help patients identify what information is needed and to deal with side effects to increase medication adherence. MHNs know that patients encounter side effects and this may cause them to stop taking the medication [5,11]. The nurses use tactful methods to assess the patient's feelings about the side effects in the identification process. They express a caring attitude to ask generalizing questions for the assessment of side effects and symptoms, but they avoid directly mentioning the side effect to the patients. Nurses are concerned about highlighting the side effects that may cause patients to stop taking the medication. Nurses try to lead patients to receive medication and improve medication compliance, but nurses using their knowledge as power should maintain a high degree of self-awareness and caution while using this "invisible" power in professional roles [32]. The MHNs assess side effects in indirect ways to avoid worsening the patient's apprehension and reluctance to take medication. However, MHNs may neglect to inform patients about side effects.

4.3. Information Evaluation

Nurses understand that the patients' perceptions of medication depend on what subjective values they attach to that concept. Generalization of the disease and making analogies can help the patient to understand the purpose of adhering to medication and help soften or change the patient's perceptions of antipsychotic medications due to the social stigma of mental illness [33,34]. MHNs can provide positive affirmations and invite family members to support medication adherence, as also suggested in previous studies [5,11]. The authors found that nurses can enlist the help of peers with similar illnesses and more insight to share positive experiences of medication adherence and provide anecdotes that are relevant to the patient. Research plans previously proposed to improve medication adherence are similar [35,36]. However, nurses who have accumulated experience and information through interpersonal exchange can persuade patients to willingly take medication as prescribed by doctors.

The nurse reminds the patient that disease stability can reduce the burden on their loved ones to motivate them to take their medication. This has not been mentioned in previous studies. Even good support from relatives and professionals also motivates patients to continue taking medication [37]. It may be because Confucianism is deeply rooted in Taiwanese society and has expectations of the relationships between people in society [38]. Although this approach may increase the patient's awareness of taking medicine for others, how long can the effect last? What is the benefit to the patient? Further research is still needed to explore these questions.

4.4. Resource Management

A patient's willingness to adhere to medication is based on a complex system of interlocking. The patient can best understand his body and the improvement of symptoms after taking the medicine, as well as his preferences. The nurse encourages the patient to discuss their treatment with the doctor for shared decision making [39]. The patient advocates for their needs, which can positively affect compliance with medication. Medication management can facilitate patient recovery. Nurses will consider relevant resources for promoting patient adherence to medication. There are several resources available to support patients' adherence to medication, including inviting family members to monitor symptoms and promote medication adherence, discussing with the physician the provision of long-acting antipsychotics as an injection, and the referral to related community systems. MHNs' cognition of adherence to medication is not the patient's business, but needs a system for support.

This study expects to gather information relevant to an increase in medication adherence strategies from MHNs, which can serve as a reference for new colleagues and psychiatric nurses to continue education. Additionally, considering the positive impacts of medical research on not only the patients but also the whole society, MHNs' strategies for medication adherence need to further comprehensively consider the role of the institution in assisting patients to adhere to medication. The value of this study as a scientific enterprise brings integrity and self-correction in social evolution [40]. Furthermore, it is necessary to provide nurses with sufficient education, training, and counseling. It should be ensured that nurses can receive adequate support. The related systems should also be sufficient for supporting patient adherence medication tracking after discharge, thereby preventing patients from constantly swinging through the revolving door of hospitalization.

The advantage of this study is that way in which samples were selected was a fair and adequate reflection of the study purpose, which maximizes the potential transferability of the study. More qualitative research needs to be undertaken in various contexts and among patients with similar economic statuses to widen the current understanding of the factors that influence medication adherence. While the analysis attempted to remain as close to the interview data as possible, the selection of extracts and analyses inevitably involved subjective interpretation; thus, other interpretations may also exist concurrently.

5. Conclusions

This study has responded to how nurses increase medication adherence in patients with schizophrenia from the internalized experiences and practice of nurses through practical exercises. Because there are diverse reasons for nonadherence in patients with schizophrenia, nurses cannot use the same methods in the increased medication adherence process, and need to consider patients' situations in order to adopt fitting strategies. The establishment of a conversational relationship is the starting point in the overall assessment of the causes of non-compliance with medications, the adjustment of attitudes toward disease and medication, and the promotion of participation with medication. This method of connecting with patients with schizophrenia allows them to better understand their symptoms and achieve medication compliance, which in turn will help stabilize their symptoms and reduce the burden on loved ones. Side effects are an important factor affecting patients' willingness to take medications. MHNs can actively intervene in reducing side effects and thus reduce non-compliance with medications.

6. Relevance for Clinical Practice

This study discusses the strategies used by experienced nurses to improve medication compliance in patients with schizophrenia. The use of seminars and problem-based learning contributed to the rich experience of nurses in medication adherence. To enable nurses to exchange experience, they should be encouraged to continue learning and use their accumulated knowledge when interacting with patients to complement the static clinical guidelines.

Author Contributions: Y.-Y.L., M.-L.L. and W.-L.H. contributed to the design and implementation of the research. W.-J.Y., W.-C.L. and M.-L.L. contributed to the analysis of the results and to the writing of the manuscript. All authors have read and agreed to the published version of the manuscript.

Funding: This work was supported by the Ministry of Health and Welfare of Taiwan funding for independent analysis of the data (grant number 10956).

Institutional Review Board Statement: The study was conducted in accordance with the guidelines of the Declaration of Helsinki and was approved by the Institutional Review Board of Tsaotun Psychiatric Center (protocol code 108026).

Informed Consent Statement: Written informed consent was obtained from all subjects involved in the study.

Data Availability Statement: All data were generated at the Tsao Psychiatric Center, Taiwan. The derived data supporting the findings of this study are available from the corresponding author Lin, M.-L. on request.

Acknowledgments: The authors thank all participants for their contributions to these data.

Conflicts of Interest: The authors declare that they received no financial or relationship support that could pose a conflict of interest with this manuscript.

References

1. Gray, R.; White, J.; Schulz, M.; Abderhalden, C. Enhancing medication adherence in people with schizophrenia: An international programme of research. *Int. J. Ment. Health Nurs.* **2010**, *19*, 36–44. [CrossRef]
2. Lauriello, J.; Perkins, D.O. Enhancing the treatment of patients with schizophrenia through continuous care. *J. Clin. Psychiatry* **2019**, *80*, al18010ah2c. [CrossRef] [PubMed]
3. Semahegn, A.; Torpey, K.; Manu, A.; Assefa, N.; Tesfaye, G.; Ankomah, A. Psychotropic medication non-adherence and its associated factors among patients with major psychiatric disorders: A systematic review and meta-analysis. *Syst. Rev.* **2020**, *9*, 17. [CrossRef] [PubMed]
4. Kane, J.M.; Correll, C.U. Optimizing treatment choices to improve adherence and outcomes in schizophrenia. *J. Clin. Psychiatry* **2019**, *80*, 13505. [CrossRef]

5. Tham, X.C.; Xie, H.; Chng, C.M.L.; Seah, X.Y.; Lopez, V.; Klainin-Yobas, P. Exploring predictors of medication adherence among inpatients with schizophrenia in Singapore's mental health settings: A non-experimental study. *Arch. Psychiatr. Nurs.* **2018**, *32*, 536–548. [CrossRef]
6. Bright, C.E. Measuring medication adherence in patients with schizophrenia: An integrative review. *Arch. Psychiatr. Nurs.* **2017**, *31*, 99–110. [CrossRef]
7. Ngui, A.N.; Vasiliadis, H.-M.; Tempier, R. Factors associated with adherence over time to antipsychotic drug treatment. *Clin. Epidemiol. Glob. Health* **2015**, *3*, 3–9. [CrossRef]
8. Lacro, J.P.; Dunn, L.B.; Dolder, C.R.; Leckband, S.G.; Jeste, D.V. Prevalence of and risk factors for medication nonadherence in patients with schizophrenia: A comprehensive review of recent literature. *J. Clin. Psychiatry* **2002**, *63*, 892–909. [CrossRef]
9. Tham, X.C.; Xie, H.; Chng, C.M.; Seah, X.Y.; Lopez, V.; Klainin-Yobas, P. Factors affecting medication adherence among adults with schizophrenia: A literature review. *Arch. Psychiatr. Nurs.* **2016**, *30*, 797–809. [CrossRef]
10. Velligan, D.I.; Sajatovic, M.; Hatch, A.; Kramata, P.; Docherty, J.P. Why do psychiatric patients stop antipsychotic medication? A systematic review of reasons for nonadherence to medication in patients with serious mental illness. *Patient Prefer. Adherence* **2017**, *11*, 449–468. [CrossRef]
11. Sendt, K.V.; Tracy, D.K.; Bhattacharyya, S. A systematic review of factors influencing adherence to antipsychotic medication in schizophrenia-spectrum disorders. *Psychiatry Res.* **2015**, *225*, 14–30. [CrossRef] [PubMed]
12. Brown, E.; Gray, R. Tackling medication non-adherence in severe mental illness: Where are we going wrong? *J. Psychiatr. Ment. Health Nurs.* **2015**, *22*, 192–198. [CrossRef] [PubMed]
13. Pfeiffer, P.N.; Ganoczy, D.; Valenstein, M. Dosing frequency and adherence to antipsychotic medications. *Psychiatr. Serv.* **2008**, *59*, 1207–1210. [CrossRef] [PubMed]
14. Rungruangsiripan, M.; Sitthimongkol, Y.; Maneesriwongul, W.; Talley, S.; Vorapongsathorn, T. Mediating role of illness representation among social support, therapeutic alliance, experience of medication side effects, and medication adherence in persons with schizophrenia. *Arch. Psychiatr. Nurs.* **2011**, *25*, 269–283. [CrossRef]
15. Tessier, A.; Boyer, L.; Husky, M.; Baylé, F.; Llorca, P.M.; Misdrahi, D. Medication adherence in schizophrenia: The role of insight, therapeutic alliance and perceived trauma associated with psychiatric care. *Psychiatry Res.* **2017**, *257*, 315–321. [CrossRef]
16. Martin, D.J.; Garske, J.P.; Davis, M.K. Relation of the therapeutic alliance with outcome and other variables: A meta-analytic review. *J. Consult. Clin. Psychol.* **2000**, *68*, 438–450. [CrossRef]
17. Emsley, R.; Alptekin, K.; Azorin, J.M.; Cañas, F.; Dubois, V.; Gorwood, P.; Haddad, P.M.; Naber, D.; Olivares, J.M.; Papageorgiou, G.; et al. EMEA ADHES group Nurses' perceptions of medication adherence in schizophrenia: Results of the ADHES cross-sectional questionnaire survey. *Ther. Adv. Psychopharmacol.* **2015**, *5*, 339–350. [CrossRef]
18. Bauml, J.; Pitschel-Walz, G.; Volz, A.; Lüscher, S.; Rentrop, M.; Kissling, W.; Jahn, T. Psychoeducation improves compliance and outcome in schizophrenia without an increase of adverse side effects: A 7-year follow-up of the Munich PIP-study. *Schizophr. Bull.* **2016**, *42* (Suppl. 1), S62–S70. [CrossRef]
19. Siddle, R.; Kingdon, D. The management of schizophrenia: Cognitive behavioural therapy. *Br. J. Community Nurs.* **2000**, *5*, 20–25. [CrossRef]
20. Fiszdon, J.M.; Kurtz, M.M.; Choi, J.; Bell, M.D.; Martino, S. Motivational interviewing to increase cognitive rehabilitation adherence in schizophrenia. *Schizophr. Bull.* **2016**, *42*, 327–334. [CrossRef]
21. Verdoux, H.; Pambrun, E.; Tournier, M.; Bezin, J.; Pariente, A. Risk of discontinuation of antipsychotic long-acting injections vs. oral antipsychotics in real-life prescribing practice: A community-based study. *Acta Psychiatr. Scand.* **2017**, *135*, 429–438. [CrossRef] [PubMed]
22. Hamann, J.; Parchmann, A.; Sassenberg, N.; Bronner, K.; Albus, M.; Richter, A.; Hoppstock, S.; Kissling, W. Training patients with schizophrenia to share decisions with their psychiatrists: A randomized-controlled trial. *Soc. Psychiatry Psychiatr. Epidemiol.* **2017**, *52*, 175–182. [CrossRef] [PubMed]
23. Kauppi, K.; Hätönen, H.; Adams, C.E.; Välimäki, M. Perceptions of treatment adherence among people with mental health problems and health care professionals. *J. Adv. Nurs.* **2015**, *71*, 777–788. [CrossRef] [PubMed]
24. Clifford, L.; Crabb, S.; Turnbull, D.; Hahn, L.; Galletly, C. A qualitative study of medication adherence amongst people with schizophrenia. *Arch. Psychiatr. Nurs.* **2020**, *34*, 194–199. [CrossRef]
25. Vuong, Q.H.; Le, T.T.; La, V.P.; Nguyen, H.T.T.; Ho, M.T.; Khuc, Q.V.; Nguyen, M.H. COVID-19 vaccines production and societal immunization under the serendipity-mindsponge-3D knowledge management theory and conceptual framework. *Humanit. Soc. Sci. Commun.* **2022**, *9*, 22. [CrossRef]
26. Vuong, Q.H.; Napier, N.K. Anatomy of the 3D innovation production with the Cobb-Douglas specification. *Sociol. Study* **2013**, *3*, 69–78.
27. Graneheim, U.H.; Lundman, B. Qualitative content analysis in nursing research: Concepts, procedures and measures to achieve trustworthiness. *Nurse Educ. Today* **2004**, *24*, 105–112. [CrossRef]
28. Burns, N.; Grove, S. *The Practice of Nursing Research: Appraisal, Synthesis and Generation of Evidence*; Elsevier: Amsterdam, The Netherlands, 2009.
29. Saunders, B.; Sim, J.; Kingstone, T.; Baker, S.; Waterfield, J.; Bartlam, B.; Burroughs, H.; Jinks, C. Saturation in qualitative research: Exploring its conceptualization and operationalization. *Qual. Quant.* **2018**, *52*, 1893–1907. [CrossRef]
30. Lincoln, Y.S.; Guba, E.G. *Naturalistic Inquiry*; SAGE: Thousand Oaks, CA, USA, 1985.

31. Polanyi, M. *Personal Knowledge: Towards a Post-Critical Philosophy*; University of Chicago Press: Chicago, IL, USA, 1958.
32. Cutcliffe, J.; Happell, B. Psychiatry, mental health nurses, and invisible power: Exploring a perturbed relationship within contemporary mental health care. *Int. J. Ment. Health Nurs.* **2009**, *18*, 116–125. [CrossRef]
33. Fadipe, B.; Olagunju, A.T.; Ogunwale, A.; Fadipe, Y.O.; Adebowale, T.O. Self-stigma and decision about medication use among a sample of Nigerian outpatients with schizophrenia. *Psychiatr. Rehabil. J.* **2020**, *43*, 214–224. [CrossRef]
34. Yilmaz, E.; Okanli, A. The effect of internalized stigma on the adherence to treatment in patients with schizophrenia. *Arch. Psychiatr. Nurs.* **2015**, *29*, 297–301. [CrossRef] [PubMed]
35. Boardman, G.; McCann, T.; Kerr, D. A peer support programme for enhancing adherence to oral antipsychotic medication in consumers with schizophrenia. *J. Adv. Nurs.* **2014**, *70*, 2293–2302. [CrossRef] [PubMed]
36. Jones, N.; Corrigan, P.W.; James, D.; Parker, J.; Larson, N. Peer support, self-determination, and treatment engagement: A qualitative investigation. *Psychiatr. Rehabil. J.* **2013**, *36*, 209–214. [CrossRef] [PubMed]
37. Salzmann-Erikson, M.; Sjödin, M. A narrative meta-synthesis of how people with schizophrenia experience facilitators and barriers in using antipsychotic medication: Implications for healthcare professionals. *Int. J. Nurs. Stud.* **2018**, *85*, 7–18. [CrossRef] [PubMed]
38. Tsai, D.F. Reflecting on the nature of Confucian ethics. *Am. J. Bioeth.* **2010**, *10*, 84–86. [CrossRef] [PubMed]
39. Mahone, I.H.; Maphis, C.F.; Snow, D.E. Effective strategies for nurses empowering clients with schizophrenia: Medication use as a tool in recovery. *Issues Ment. Health Nurs.* **2016**, *37*, 372–379. [CrossRef] [PubMed]
40. Vuong, Q.H. The (ir)rational consideration of the cost of science in transition economies. *Nat. Hum. Behav.* **2018**, *2*, 5. [CrossRef]

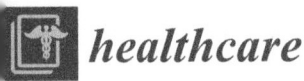 healthcare

Article

Impact of Multiple Sclerosis and Its Association with Depression: An Analytical Case-Control Investigation

Francisco Javier Ruiz-Sánchez [1], Maria do Rosário Martins [2], Salete Soares [2], Carlos Romero-Morales [3], Daniel López-López [1,*], Juan Gómez-Salgado [4,5] and Ana María Jiménez-Cebrián [6]

1. Research, Health and Podiatry Group, Department of Health Sciences, Faculty of Nursing and Podiatry, Industrial Campus of Ferrol, Universidade da Coruña, 15403 Ferrol, Spain
2. UICISA:E, Escola Superior de Saúde, Instituto Politécnico de Viana do Castelo, Rua D. Moisés Alves Pinho 190, 4900-314 Viana do Castelo, Portugal
3. Faculty of Sport Sciences, Universidad Europea de Madrid, Villaviciosa de Odón, 28670 Madrid, Spain
4. Department of Sociology, Social Work and Public Health, Faculty of Labor Sciences, University of Huelva, 21007 Huelva, Spain
5. Safety and Health Postgraduate Program, Universidad Espíritu Santo, Guayaquil 092301, Ecuador
6. Nursing and Podiatry Department, Faculty of Health Sciences, Instituto de Investigación Biomédica de Málaga (IBIMA), University of Malaga, 29071 Malaga, Spain
* Correspondence: daniellopez@udc.gal

Abstract: Multiple sclerosis (MS) is a neurological, chronic, inflammatory, and progressive disease with musculoskeletal problems and neurodegenerative disorders that causes worsening of the health status of patients. The aim of this study was to determine the level of depression in MS patients compared to a population of healthy subjects. The established sample size was 116 subjects matched with the same age, sex, and body mass index. The subjects were recruited from different multiple sclerosis associations and neurology clinics in different public health areas (case group $n = 58$) and healthy subjects from the same locality (control group $n = 58$). The scores and categories of the Beck Depression Inventory (BDI) in its Spanish version were collected. There was a clear statistically significant difference ($p < 0.05$) in the BDI scores between both groups. As a result, we found that the subjects with MS presented worse results with BDI = 9.52 ± 7.70 points compared to the healthy subjects with a BDI score = 5.03 ± 5.14. Within the BDI categories, there were statistically significant differences ($p < 0.001$), which were greater for the MS group. Depression is a dangerous factor for MS patients, being a trigger for a poorer quality of life.

Keywords: multiple sclerosis; depression; Beck depression inventory

1. Introduction

Multiple sclerosis (MS) is a chronic inflammatory neurodegenerative disease of the central nervous system. MS presents sexual dimorphism showing importance in the incidence and severity of the disease. The female sex shows a higher incidence of the disease and the male sex shows faster clinical progression [1,2]. Numerous epidemiological studies in the Spanish population indicate that it is a region of medium-high prevalence of the disease throughout the whole country. The cases have been increasing progressively and have reached 80–180 cases per 100,000 inhabitants with the frequency being higher in women [3].

This pathology is characterized by the spread of spatio-temporal lesions, with frequent exacerbations and remissions [4]. In addition to psychomotor signs and symptoms, demyelination has psychological and psychiatric consequences, presenting depressive symptoms in 50% of people with MS [5–7].

The discovery of biomarkers in the blood is a fundamental tool for predicting, diagnosing, and monitoring the efficacy of depression treatment [8]. Biomarkers are present in depressive patients with autoimmune diseases, in whom, in turn, there is a development of the proinflammatory state of cytokines IL-1β, IL-6, and TNF-α [9]. Recent studies have identified that the inflammatory process is closely related to the neurodegenerative pathways associated with depression, with proinflammatory cytokines being important in its pathophysiology [10]. In autonomic diseases such as MS, proinflammatory cytokine production triggers episodes of depression [11]. Another way to measure depression-related biomarkers is through saliva where the anti-inflammatory cytokine IL-10 is significantly associated with depression severity in MS patients [12].

The diagnosis of depression in people with MS is complex as it can have a multifactorial etiology and can be associated with clinical manifestations including euphoria, anxiety, emotional lability, and psychosis [4]. A series of atypical symptoms also must be taken into account, such as peripheral facial paralysis, painless optic neuritis, and encephalopathy [13]. Histological inflammatory changes are also implicated in the etiology [14]. The state of depression represents one of the main determinants of quality of life in MS and can lead to suicidal intent [15,16] as it is related to the intake of interferon alpha and beta [17]. In addition, within the clinical picture, there are motor disorders (spasticity, ataxia, foot drop), sensory disorders (paresthesia, pain), cerebral disorders (dysarthria, gait ataxia, fear, lack of coordination of limbs), alterations of the cranial nerves (decreased visual acuity, facial muscle weakness), disorders of the autonomic nervous system (urinary and intestinal incontinence), and cognitive disorders (decreased attention) [18,19]. A study using magnetic resonance imaging (MRI) in 46 acute MS patients showed that there was a significant correlation between frontal periventricular or non-periventricular white matter lesions and psychopathological conditions such as depression [20].

Cases of depression in subjects with MS are higher in women, tending to decrease with increasing age, with 16.7% of women and 13.1% of men being affected [21]. Depression is significantly related to education, and 89.9% of MS subjects in a recent sample had mild to severe depressive symptoms [22]. There is a significant relationship between the type of MS and depression, where subjects with progressive relapsing MS have a higher risk (100%) of developing depression [23]. Likewise, there were higher depression scores in subjects with relapsing–remitting and secondary progressive MS [24].

However, there are few studies on the Spanish population that evaluate the significance of the resulting levels of depression in its three domains (affective, behavioral, and cognitive) and anxiety in patients with multiple sclerosis. Therefore, after reviewing the published literature, we found that levels of depression have not been described in previous studies comparing subjects with MS and healthy subjects. The objective of this study is to help to improve their well-being and quality of life.

Finally, the study tries to ascertain relative depression risk in people with multiple sclerosis and healthy subjects, thus making it a case-control study.

2. Materials and Methods
2.1. Design and Sample

To develop this study, a total sample of 116 subjects was recruited for an analytical, observational, and multicenter study of cases and controls carried out in different MS associations in the province of Malaga and Granada and in the neurology area of the "Hospital de Serrania de Ronda". This research was performed according to the criteria of the Strengthening the Reporting of Observational Studies in Epidemiology guidelines [25].

The subjects who participated were patients with MS (case group n = 58) and without MS (control group n = 58) with similar socio-economic status. The patients were recruited using a convenience sampling method. Multiple sclerosis patients were taken from reference associations and healthy subjects from the same locality as the cases.

The subjects with MS were chosen once their association and neurologist had informed them of the study on depression and quality of life and they had decided to participate voluntarily.

The inclusion criteria were as follows: Between 18 and 88 years, of both sexes, able to walk, and who authorized their participation in the signing of the consent form.

The exclusion criteria of the subjects were another neurodegenerative disease other than MS, cognitive impairment, and severe mental disorder (measured with the Expanded Disability Status Scale (EDSS)). Cases and controls were matched for age, gender, and BMI.

2.2. Sample Size Calculation

To calculate the sample size, we used Epidat 4.2 software (Epidemiology Service of the General Directorate of Public Health of the Consellería de Sanidade (Xunta de Galicia) with the support of the Pan American Health Organization (PAHO-WHO) and the University CES of Colombia, thus obtaining specific levels of trust, power, and groups of equal size. A sample of 102 participants (51 per group) was obtained with a confidence level of 70%, an odds ratio of 2.0, a power of 0.80, and an exposure value of 66.67% for the MS group and 50% in the control group. Finally, for operational and safety reasons, a total of 58 patients (in each group) were used in this study.

2.3. Procedure

Data collection included general health questions associated with demographic variables (age, weight, height, sex, and BMI) and comorbid characteristics such as diabetes, arterial hypertension/hypotension, and ischemic heart disease. In addition, health questions related to the disease were recorded, such as the type of MS, degree of spasticity, years diagnosed, and medication administered.

Next, the participants were given the Spanish version of the Beck Depression Inventory (BDI) questionnaire [26–28]. This questionnaire was validated and translated into Spanish and is one of the instruments used to establish depression levels [29,30]. This version of the instrument consists of a total of 21 items with four alternatives each, which are classified from 0 to 3 points, giving a possible total of 63 points. The results obtained are measured in four ranges: The first category goes from 0 to 13 points (no signs of depression), the second from 14 to 19 points (mild depression), the third from 20 to 28 points (moderate depression), and the fourth from 29 to 63 points (severe depression). This instrument is one of the fastest and most efficient for the correct assessment of signs of depression with a Cronbach's alpha coefficient of 0.889 [31].

2.4. Ethics Procedure

A favorable assessment was obtained from the Ethics Committee of the University of Malaga (CEUMA) with registration number 32-2021-H and the Ethics Committee of the Provincial Research of Malaga with code 5002V01. Likewise, the participants in this study completed and signed an informed consent form detailing the entire procedure and the protection of their data. This study respected all the ethical principles for experimentation and clinical research in humans of the Declaration of Helsinki (World Medical Association) and other organizations [32].

2.5. Statistics

SPSS 25.0v software (IBM Corp., Armonk, NY, USA) was used to perform the statistical analysis, reporting an alpha error of 0.05 for a confidence interval (CI) of 95%.

The normality of the quantitative data was demonstrated using the Kolmogorov–Smirnov test showing a p-value of less than 0.05 and was described as mean ± standard deviation (SD) and range (minimum–maximum). The contrasts were compared with Student's t-test or the Mann–Whitney U test for independent samples. The differences between both groups were contrasted with the Chi square test (BDI category).

3. Results

The data obtained showed a normal distribution ($p > 0.05$) except in the ranges of depression. The investigation was completed with a sample of 102 subjects divided into

$n = 51$ for the case group and $n = 51$ for the control group, being divided and matched according to age, sex, and BMI. As can be seen in Table 1, there were no statistically significant differences ($p > 0.05$) between both groups for the descriptive data.

Table 1. Descriptive and socio-demographic data of the sample.

Demographic and Descriptive Data		Total Group $n=116$ Mean ± SD (IC95%)	MS $n = 58$ Mean ± SD (IC95%)	Healthy $n= 58$ Mean ± SD (IC95%)	p Value *
Age (Years)		47.38 ± 10.62 (24–66)	47.38 ± 10.68 (24–66)	47.38 ± 10.65 (24–66)	1.000 †
Weight (kg)		71.36 ± 12.75 (46–105)	70.19 ± 13.31 (46–105)	72.53 ± 12.16 (47–100)	0.324 †
Height (cm)		167.68 ± 8.43 (150–188)	167.24 ± 8.49 (150–183)	168.12 ± 8.43 (154–188)	0.577 †
BMI (Kg/m^2)		25.32 ± 4.14 (18.0–37.5)	24.98 ± 3.94 (18.0–37.5)	25.65 ± 4.34 (18.4–37.2)	0.391 †
Time since MS diagnosis (years)		N/A	12.55 ± 8.53 (1–33)	N/A	<0.001 †
Sex (%)	Male	34 (29.3 %)	17 (29.3 %)	17 (29.3 %)	1.000 ‡
	Female	82 (70.7 %)	41 (70.7 %)	41 (70.7 %)	

Comparison of the demographic characteristics of the total sample, MS with foot pain and healthy matched MS with normalized reference values BMI: Body mass index; * Mean ± standard deviation, range (min–max), and Student's t test were applied for independent samples. In all analyses, $p < 0.05$ (with a 95% confidence interval) was considered statistically significant and † Student' t-test was applied for independent samples. ‡ The Chi-square test was used.

All the participants ($n = 116$) presented the characteristics described in Table 1. It can be seen that the years of evolution of MS were high according to the mean (12.55 ± 8.53), and the type of MS that was most present in the study was remittent–recurring (93.1%).

Table 2 shows a statistically significant difference ($p < 0.05$) in the BDI scores between both groups. The highest scores correspond to subjects with MS (BDI = 9.52 ± 7.70 points) and the lowest scores for the control group (BDI = 5.03 ± 5.14). Statistically significant differences ($p < 0.001$) were found for the BDI categories in the MS group compared to the non-MS group (Table 2).

Table 2. Relationship of scores and categories of the BDI between patients with MS and healthy controls.

Outcome Measurements		Total Group Mean ± SD ($n = 116$)	Cases Mean ± SD ($n = 58$)	Controls Mean ± SD ($n = 58$)	p-Value (Cases vs. Controls)
BDI Category *	No	82 (70.7%)	34 (58.6%)	48 (82.8%)	0.022 *
	Mild	18 (15.5%)	11 (19%)	7 (12.1%)	
	Moderate	12 (10.3%)	10 (17.2%)	2 (3.4%)	
	Severe	4 (3.4%)	3 (5.2%)	1 (1.7%)	
BDI scores		7.28 ± 6.90 (0–28)	9.52 ± 7.70 (0–28)	5.03 ± 5.14 (0–24)	0.001 †

* BDI, Beck depression inventory. Frequency, percentage (%), and Chi-square test (x^2) were utilized. BDI domains were divided as follows: (1) 0 to 9 points: Without depression, (2) 10 to 15 points: Mild depression, (3) 16 to 23 points: Moderate depression, and (4) 24 to 57 points: Severe depression. † BDI scores, Median ± interquartile range, range (min–max), and Mann–Whitney U test were used. In all the analyses, $p < 0.05$ (with a 95% confidence interval) was considered statistically significant (bold).

4. Discussion

This research studied depression in 58 patients with MS compared to 58 healthy subjects, the first case-control study of this type carried out on the Spanish population. The results obtained showed that many of the people with MS (41.4%) are at risk of suffering from depression in at least some range of the BDI.

According to a recent study, treating depression in MS patients significantly improves fatigue [33]. Therefore, it is important for these patients to be evaluated by a multidisciplinary team in order to improve their quality of life.

Depression tends to be related to other symptoms such as pain and fatigue exacerbated by the psychomotor degeneration of these patients [34]. The prevalence of depression in patients with MS is remarkably high, although it is still not properly diagnosed, leading to cognitive impairment causing the risk of suicide [35]. In the review by Claudio Solaro et al., it is stated that for the correct management of depression in subjects with MS, it is necessary to understand the damage in the central nervous system using MRI and relate fatigue and pain with depression [16].

In agreement with our study, patients with MS (51%) present clinically significant depressive symptoms [36]. Thus, we compared the control group with the case group, taking all the patients without considering depression as an inclusion criterion, and when reviewing the data obtained, we found that many people with MS (19%) present a mild level of depression.

For our study, the range of depression was obtained with the Beck Depression Inventory (BDI) questionnaire. This document was validated by other authors as having optimal characteristics to establish depression in subjects with MS [27], and furthermore, this questionnaire correlates with other types of questionnaires used to study depression, fatigue, and affect (Hamilton Rating Scale, Yale Single Questionnaire and PDQ) in patients with MS [37–39]. For this reason, studies conducted on depression in MS tend to have different results due to the use of other types of questionnaires and different types of samples.

Other studies carried out on depression in chronic pathologies also recommend the BDI as a good self-assessment tool for screening and evaluation in clinical practice of depression, its intensity, and its evolution in patients with chronic kidney disease [40]. As depression not only affects patients with MS or other chronic diseases but also their family environment, the BDI proved to be a valid and reliable instrument to measure depression in the family caregivers of children with chronic diseases [41]. Shelby et al., in their study on Parkinson's disease, showed that the BDI in clinical practice is suitable for additional psychiatric evaluation and for adopting different therapeutic interventions [42]. This agrees with the study by Ana María Jiménez-Cebrián et al. where, for the first time, it was shown in a sample of subjects with Parkinson's compared to healthy subjects that depression represents a significant potential risk for the increase in symptoms and has a negative impact on these patients compared to healthy subjects [43]. We can, thus, based on previous studies and our results, consider that depression and chronic pathologies have an unwanted effect on the quality of life of people with MS, especially in somatic-vegetative aspects such as fewer hours of sleep, loss of energy, greater tiredness, and loss of appetite [6,24,44].

Taking into account our findings and the bibliographic review, it is necessary for patients with MS to be aware of the importance of depression on their quality of life and to offer them a multidisciplinary team to establish good management of this pathology. In addition, biomarkers have been studied in some research with MS subjects, but all of them refer to the need for a larger sample for better consistency to thus complete the aspects of depressive studies and their possible causes in MS [11,40].

To correctly manage MS and depression, it would be important to use other biomarkers tools (blood or salivary) together with the BDI to provide more consistency and more treatment possibilities for this group of patients, determine the triggers involved, and improve their quality of life.

5. Conclusions

The results obtained show us that people with MS have higher scores on all levels of depression compared to healthy subjects, with greater differences at the mild and moderate levels.

Author Contributions: Conceptualization, F.J.R.-S., M.d.R.M., S.S., C.R.-M., D.L.-L., J.G.-S. and A.M.J.-C.; Data Curation, F.J.R.-S., M.d.R.M., S.S, methodology, F.J.R.-S., M.d.R.M., S.S., C.R.-M., D.L.-L., J.G.-S. and A.M.J.-C.; formal analysis, F.J.R.-S., M.d.R.M., S.S., C.R.-M., D.L.-L., J.G.-S. and A.M.J.-C.; investigation, F.J.R.-S., M.d.R.M., S.S., C.R.-M., D.L.-L., J.G.-S. and A.M.J.-C.; writing—original draft preparation, F.J.R.-S., M.d.R.M., S.S., C.R.-M., D.L.-L., J.G.-S. and A.M.J.-C.; writing—review and editing, F.J.R.-S., M.d.R.M., S.S., C.R.-M., D.L.-L., J.G.-S. and A.M.J.-C. All authors have read and agreed to the published version of the manuscript.

Funding: This research received no external funding.

Institutional Review Board Statement: The study was conducted according to the guidelines of the Declaration of Helsinki and approved by the Ethics Committee of the University of Malaga (CEUMA) with registration number 32-2021-H and the Ethics Committee of the Provincial Research of Malaga with code 5002V01.

Informed Consent Statement: Written informed consent was obtained from all subjects involved in the study.

Data Availability Statement: The dataset supporting the conclusions of this article is available upon request to f.ruiz@udc.es in the Research, Health and Podiatry Group, Department of Health Sciences, Faculty of Nursing and Podiatry. Industrial Campus of Ferrol, Universidade da Coruña, 15403 Ferrol, Spain.

Acknowledgments: We would like to thank the people who participated in this research.

Conflicts of Interest: The authors declare no conflict of interest.

References

1. Baranzini, S.E.; Oksenberg, J.R. The Genetics of Multiple Sclerosis: From 0 to 200 in 50 Years. *Trends Genet.* **2017**, *33*, 960–970. [CrossRef] [PubMed]
2. Mallucci, G.; Peruzzotti-Jametti, L.; Bernstock, J.D.; Pluchino, S. The role of immune cells, glia and neurons in white and gray matter pathology in multiple sclerosis. *Prog. Neurobiol.* **2015**, *127–128*, 1–22. [CrossRef] [PubMed]
3. De Sá, J. Epidemiology of multiple sclerosis in Portugal and Spain. *Rev. Neurol.* **2010**, *51*, 387–392. [CrossRef] [PubMed]
4. Soares, M. *de la Qualidade de vida e Esclerose Múltipla*; Universidade do Porto: Porto, Portugal, 2002.
5. Feinstein, A. Multiple sclerosis and depression. *Mult. Scler. J.* **2011**, *17*, 1276–1281. [CrossRef] [PubMed]
6. Solaro, C.; Trabucco, E.; Signori, A.; Martinelli, V.; Radaelli, M.; Centonze, D.; Rossi, S.; Grasso, M.G.; Clemenzi, A.; Bonavita, S.; et al. Depressive symptoms correlate with disability and disease course in multiple sclerosis patients: An Italian multi-center study using the Beck Depression Inventory. *PLoS ONE* **2016**, *11*, e0160261. [CrossRef] [PubMed]
7. Amtmann, D.; Kim, J.; Chung, H.; Bamer, A.M.; Askew, R.L.; Wu, S.; Cook, K.F.; Johnson, K.L. Comparing CESD-10, PHQ-9, and PROMIS depression instruments in individuals with multiple sclerosis. *Rehabil. Psychol.* **2014**, *59*, 220–229. [CrossRef] [PubMed]
8. Aspesi, D.; Pinna, G. Could a blood test for PTSD and depression be on the horizon? *Expert Rev. Proteom.* **2018**, *15*, 983–1006. [CrossRef] [PubMed]
9. Grygiel-Górniak, B.; Limphaibool, N.; Puszczewicz, M. Cytokine secretion and the risk of depression development in patients with connective tissue diseases. *Psychiatry Clin. Neurosci.* **2019**, *73*, 302–316. [CrossRef] [PubMed]
10. Chen, W.W.; Zhang, X.; Huang, W.J. Role of neuroinflammation in neurodegenerative diseases (Review). *Mol. Med. Rep.* **2016**, *13*, 3391–3396. [CrossRef] [PubMed]
11. Tauil, C.B.; da Rocha Lima, A.D.; Ferrari, B.B.; da Silva, V.A.G.; Moraes, A.S.; da Silva, F.M.; Melo-Silva, C.A.; Farias, A.S.; Brandão, C.O.; dos Santos Leonilda, M.B.; et al. Depression and anxiety in patients with multiple sclerosis treated with interferon-beta or fingolimod: Role of indoleamine 2,3-dioxygenase and pro-inflammatory cytokines. *Brain Behav. Immun. Health* **2020**, *9*, 100162. [CrossRef] [PubMed]
12. Newland, P.; Basan, Y.; Chen, L.; Wu, G. Depression and Inflammatory Markers in Veterans With Multiple Sclerosis. *Biol. Res. Nurs.* **2022**, *24*, 123–127. [CrossRef] [PubMed]
13. Pita, M.C.; Alonso, R.N.; Cohen, L.; Garcea, O.; Silva, B.A. Atypical clinical manifestations as a form of presentation in multiple sclerosis. *Medicina* **2021**, *81*, 972–977.
14. Miller, A.H.; Raison, C.L. The role of inflammation in depression: From evolutionary imperative to modern treatment target. *Nat. Rev. Immunol.* **2016**, *16*, 22–34. [CrossRef] [PubMed]
15. Göksel Karatepe, A.; Kaya, T.; Günaydn, R.; Demirhan, A.; Çe, P.; Gedizlioğlu, M. Quality of life in patients with multiple sclerosis: The impact of depression, fatigue, and disability. *Int. J. Rehabil. Res.* **2011**, *34*, 290–298. [CrossRef] [PubMed]
16. Solaro, C.; Gamberini, G.; Masuccio, F.G. Depression in Multiple Sclerosis: Epidemiology, Aetiology, Diagnosis and Treatment. *CNS Drugs* **2018**, *32*, 117–133. [CrossRef]
17. Patten, S.B.; Francis, G.; Metz, L.M.; Lopez-Bresnahan, M.; Chang, P.; Curtin, F. The relationship between depression and interferon beta-1a therapy in patients with multiple sclerosis. *Mult. Scler.* **2005**, *11*, 175–181. [CrossRef] [PubMed]
18. Frankel, D. Esclerose Múltipla. In *Reabilitação Neurológica*; Umpred, D., Ed.; Manole: São Paulo, 2004; pp. 529–546.

19. Peyser, J.N.; Poser, M.C. Neuropsychological Correlates of Multiple Sclerosis. *Hndb. Clin. Neuropsychol.* **1986**, *2*, 364–396.
20. Allen, D.N.; Goreczny, A.J. Assessment and Treatment of Multiples Sclerosis. In *Handbook of Health and Rehabilitation Psychology*; Plenum Press: New York, NY, USA, 1995; pp. 389–429.
21. Patten, S.B.; Beck, C.A.; Williams, J.V.A.; Barbui, C.; Metz, L.M. Major depression in multiple sclerosis: A population-based perspective. *Neurology* **2003**, *61*, 1524–1527. [CrossRef] [PubMed]
22. Alhussain, H.; Aldayel, A.A.; Alenazi, A.; Alowain, F. Multiple Sclerosis Patients in Saudi Arabia: Prevalence of Depression and its Extent of Severity. *Cureus* **2020**, *12*, e7005. [CrossRef] [PubMed]
23. Aljishi, R.H.; Almatrafi, R.J.; Alzayer, Z.A.; Alkhamis, B.A.; Yaseen, E.E.; Alkhotani, A.M. Prevalence of Anxiety and Depression in Patients With Multiple Sclerosis in Saudi Arabia: A Cross-Sectional Study. *Cureus* **2021**, *13*, e20792. [CrossRef] [PubMed]
24. Patten, S.B.; Marrie, R.A.; Carta, M.G. Depression in multiple sclerosis. *Int. Rev. Psychiatry* **2017**, *29*, 463–472. [CrossRef] [PubMed]
25. Vandenbroucke, J.P.; von Elm, E.; Altman, D.G.; Gøtzsche, P.C.; Mulrow, C.D.; Pocock, S.J.; Poole, C.; Schlesselman, J.J.; Egger, M. STROBE Initiative Strengthening the Reporting of Observational Studies in Epidemiology (STROBE): Explanation and elaboration. *Int. J. Surg.* **2014**, *12*, W163–W194. [CrossRef] [PubMed]
26. Richter, W.; Joachim, A.H.; Alfred, K.; Heinrich, S. On the Validity of the Beck Depression. *Psychopathology* **1998**, *31*, 160–168. [CrossRef] [PubMed]
27. Fishman, I.; Mcclellan, M.M.; Bakshi, R. Multiple Sclerosis Validity o f the Beck Depressio n Invento ry-Fast Screen in multiple. *Int. Sch. Res. Not.* **2003**, *9*, 393–396.
28. Beck, A.T.; Ward, C.H.; Mendelson, M.; Mock, J.; Erbaugh, J. An Inventory for Measuring Depression The difficulties inherent in obtaining. *Arch. Gen. Psychiatry* **1960**, *4*, 561–571. [CrossRef]
29. Vazquez, C.; Sanz, J. Fiabilidad y valores normativos de la versión española del inventario para la depresión de Beck de 1978. *Clínica y Salud* **1997**, *8*, 403–422.
30. Sanz, J.; Vázquez, C. Fiabilidad, validez y datos normativosdel inventario para la depresiónde beck. *Psicothema* **1998**, *10*, 303–318.
31. Vega-Dienstmaier, J.; Coronado-Molina, Ó.; Mazzotti, G. Validez de una versión en español del Inventario de Depresión de Beck en pacientes hospitalizados de medicina general. *Rev. Neuropsiquiatr.* **2014**, *77*, 95. [CrossRef]
32. Holt, G.R. Declaration of Helsinki-the world's document of conscience and responsibility. *South. Med. J.* **2014**, *107*, 407. [CrossRef]
33. Solaro, C.; Bergamaschi, R.; Rezzani, C.; Mueller, M.; Trabucco, E.; Bargiggia, V.; Dematteis, F.; Mattioda, A.; Cimino, V.; Restivo, D.; et al. Duloxetine is effective in treating depression in multiple sclerosis patients: An open-label multicenter study. *Clin. Neuropharmacol.* **2013**, *36*, 114–116. [CrossRef]
34. Alschuler, K.N.; Ehde, D.M.; Jensen, M.P. The co-occurrence of pain and depression in adults with multiple sclerosis. *Rehabil. Psychol.* **2013**, *58*, 217–221. [CrossRef] [PubMed]
35. Skokou, M.; Soubasi, E.; Gourzis, P. Depression in Multiple Sclerosis: A Review of Assessment and Treatment Approaches in Adult and Pediatric Populations. *ISRN Neurol.* **2012**, *2012*, 427102. [CrossRef] [PubMed]
36. Cetin, K.; Johnson, K.L.; Ehde, D.M.; Kuehn, C.M.; Amtmann, D.; Kraft, G.H. Antidepressant use in multiple sclerosis: Epidemiologic study of a large community sample. *Mult. Scler.* **2007**, *13*, 1046–1053. [CrossRef]
37. Moran, P.J.; Mohr, D.C. The validity of Beck Depression Inventory and Hamilton Rating Scale for Depression items in the assessment of depression among patients with multiple sclerosis. *J. Behav. Med.* **2005**, *28*, 35–41. [CrossRef] [PubMed]
38. Avasarala, J.R.; Cross, A.H.; Trinkaus, K. Comparative assessment of Yale Single Question and Beck Depression Inventory Scale in screening for depression in multiple sclerosis. *Mult. Scler.* **2003**, *9*, 307–310. [CrossRef]
39. Lovera, J.; Bagert, B.; Smoot, K.H.; Wild, K.; Frank, R.; Bogardus, K.; Oken, B.S.; Whitham, R.H.; Bourdette, D.N. Correlations of Perceived Deficits Questionnaire of multiple sclerosis quality of life inventory with Beck Depression Inventory and neuropsychological tests. *J. Rehabil. Res. Dev.* **2006**, *43*, 73–82. [CrossRef] [PubMed]
40. Alsaleh, M.; Videloup, L.; Lobbedez, T.; Lebreuilly, J.; Morello, R.; Thuillier Lecouf, A. Improved Detection and Evaluation of Depression in Patients with Chronic Kidney Disease: Validity and Reliability of Screening (PHQ-2) and Diagnostic (BDI-FS-Fr) Tests of Depression in Chronic Kidney Disease. *Kidney Dis.* **2019**, *5*, 228–238. [CrossRef]
41. Contreras-valdez, J.A.; Toledano-Toledano, F. Validity and reliability of the Beck Depression Inventory II (BDI-II) in family caregivers of children with chronic diseases. *PLoS ONE* **2018**, *13*, e0206917.
42. Stohlman, S.L.; Barrett, M.J.; Sperling, S.A.; Stohlman, S.L.; Barrett, M.J.; Sperling, S.A. Neuropsychology Factor Structure of the BDI-II in Parkinson's Disease. *Neuropsychology* **2021**, *35*, 540–546. [CrossRef]
43. Jiménez-Cebrián, A.M.; Becerro-De-bengoa-vallejo, R.; Losa-Iglesias, M.E.; López-López, D.; Calvo-Lobo, C.; Palomo-López, P.; Romero-Morales, C.; Navarro-Flores, E. The impact of depression symptoms in patients with parkinson's disease: A novel case-control investigation. *Int. J. Environ. Res. Public Health* **2021**, *18*, 2369. [CrossRef]
44. Julian, L.J.; Mohr, D.C. Cognitive predictors of response to treatment for depression in multiple sclerosis. *J. Neuropsychiatry Clin. Neurosci.* **2006**, *18*, 356–363. [CrossRef] [PubMed]

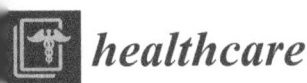

Article

Association of Depression, Anxiety, Stress and Stress-Coping Strategies with Somatization and Number of Diseases According to Sex in the Mexican General Population

Aniel Jessica Leticia Brambila-Tapia [1,*], Fabiola Macías-Espinoza [2,*], Yesica Arlae Reyes-Domínguez [3], María Luisa Ramírez-García [3], Aris Judit Miranda-Lavastida [4], Blanca Estela Ríos-González [5], Ana Miriam Saldaña-Cruz [6], Yussef Esparza-Guerrero [7], Francisco Fabián Mora-Moreno [4] and Ingrid Patricia Dávalos-Rodríguez [8]

1. Departamento de Psicología Básica, Centro Universitario de Ciencias de la Salud (CUCS), Universidad de Guadalajara, Guadalajara 44340, Mexico
2. Departamento de Psicología Aplicada, Centro Universitario de Ciencias de la Salud (CUCS), Universidad de Guadalajara, Guadalajara 44340, Mexico
3. Maestría en Psicología de la Salud, Centro Universitario de Ciencias de la Salud (CUCS), Universidad de Guadalajara, Guadalajara 44340, Mexico; yesica.reyes2393@alumnos.udg.mx (Y.A.R.-D.); maria.ramirez4357@alumnos.udg.mx (M.L.R.-G.)
4. Centro de Estudios sobre el Aprendizaje y Desarrollo (CEAD), Departamento de Psicología Básica, Centro Universitario de Ciencias de la Salud (CUCS), Universidad de Guadalajara, Guadalajara 44340, Mexico; aris.miranda@academicos.udg.mx (A.J.M.-L.); fabian.mora@academicos.udg.mx (F.F.M.-M.)
5. Unidad Médico Familiar #92, Instituto Mexicano del Seguro Social (IMSS), Guadalajara 44340, Mexico; blanca2282@hotmail.com
6. Departamento de Fisiología, Centro Universitario de Ciencias de la Salud (CUCS), Universidad de Guadalajara, Guadalajara 44340, Mexico; ana.saldanac@academicos.udg.mx
7. Doctorado en Farmacología, Centro Universitario de Ciencias de la Salud (CUCS), Universidad de Guadalajara, Guadalajara 44340, Mexico; yuss.tkd16@gmail.com
8. Centro de Investigación Biomédica de Occidente (CIBO), Instituto Mexicano del Seguro Social (IMSS), Guadalajara 44340, Mexico; ingriddavalos@hotmail.com
* Correspondence: aniel.brambila@academicos.udg.mx (A.J.L.B.-T.); fabiola.macias@academicos.udg.mx (F.M.-E.)

Abstract: Somatization and number of diseases are interrelated variables, whose association with stress-coping strategies, according to sex, has not been investigated. Therefore, the aim of this study was to investigate such association in a sample of the Mexican general population. The general population was invited to answer an electronic questionnaire via the social networks—e-mail, WhatsApp and Facebook—by the research team. A sample of 1008 adults was obtained, of which 62.2% were women, in whom we detected higher levels of negative psychological variables, somatization and number of diseases and lower levels of sleep quality. Positive moderate correlations were found between depression, anxiety and stress with somatization, on one hand, and with the number of diseases, on the other, and negative moderate correlations were found between sleep quality and the two dependent variables. As for the coping strategies, self-blame, behavioral disengagement, denial, self-distraction and substance use were positively correlated with somatization. Of these, self-blame, substance use, and self-distraction also showed a positive correlation with number of diseases in both sexes. Negative correlations were detected for active coping and the two dependent variables in men and for religion and planning with somatization in women. In conclusion, the coping strategies showed significant correlations with somatization and number of diseases in both sexes.

Keywords: somatization; number of diseases; coping strategies; sex

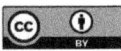

1. Introduction

Somatization, described as the "tendency to experience and communicate somatic stress and to seek medical help for it" [1], has been associated with a variety of positive and negative psychological factors, with different tendencies in women compared to men [2] and with more of these psychological and sociodemographic factors associated in women, in whom somatization is also present at higher levels in comparison with men [2–4]. In addition, we found that the number of diseases has been significantly associated with somatization in previous reports in both genders [2,5].

The number of diseases is also increased in women when compared with men [2,6], which suggests that the increased number of negative psychological factors in women [7,8] could be related to the higher frequencies of somatization and number of diseases in this sex [2]. However, among the factors studied in association with somatization and number of diseases, no reports were found in relation to stress-coping strategies, which are defined as an individual's attempts to use cognitive and behavioral strategies to manage and regulate pressures, demands and emotions in response to stress [9].

In a previous report, we showed that anxiety, depression and sleep quality were factors related to somatization in both sexes. Therefore, the aim of this study was to determine the association between coping strategies and both somatization and number of diseases, considering the previously associated variables of anxiety, depression and sleep quality. The study was performed in order to detect the coping strategies that are positively or negatively correlated with these two factors in each sex, which would permit the design of future preventing programs.

2. Subjects and Methods

An electronic questionnaire with sociodemographic and psychological instruments was sent via social networks, including WhatsApp, Facebook and e-mail, to the general population by the research team; this population included university students, relatives, friends, colleagues and acquaintances, many of whom re-sent the questionnaire.

The study was approved by the ethics and research committee of the Health Sciences University Center of the University of Guadalajara, and the participants gave their consent to participate in the questionnaire.

The socio-demographic data included sex, age, whether the participants had a romantic partner, schooling, whether they had children, whether they had a job, socioeconomic level (which represents the social and income level), monthly extra money (excluding necessary expenses), daily free hours and weekly physical activity hours, the presence of 21 different diseases (diabetes, hypertension, overweight, cancer, respiratory infections, gastrointestinal infections, allergies/asthma, gastritis/gastric ulcer, colitis/irritable colon, rheumatic diseases (rheumatoid arthritis, systemic lupus erythematosus, etc.), thyroid diseases, migraine, skin diseases (acne/neurodermatitis, etc.), sinusitis, kidney/bladder problems, anorexia/bulimia, hearth attack/angina pectoris, cerebral stroke, high cholesterol levels, anxiety and depression problems that require medication) and any additional disease in the last 6 months.

Sleep quality was measured with item 2 (which consists of 5 items) of the OVIEDO sleep questionnaire; these 5 questions were related to sleep problems and had 5 frequency options, from never to 6–7 days in a week [10]. Finally, smoking frequency and alcohol consumption frequency were measured with 6 options, i.e., from never to many times in a week.

The psychological measures included were: somatization, measured with the Patient Health Questionnaire 15 (PHQ-15), which evaluates 15 somatic symptoms with 3 frequency options for each symptom, i.e., not at all, bothered a little, bothered a lot [11]; stress, measured with the Cohen perceived stress scale (CPSS), which evaluates 14 phrases related to stress with 5 frequency options, i.e., from never to very frequent [12,13]; depression, measured with the CES-D scale, which consists of 10 questions related to depressive symptoms with 4 frequency options, i.e., from 0 days to 5–7 days in a week [14,15]; anxiety, measured with the GAD-7 scale, which consists of 7 phrases related to anxious symptoms with 4 frequency options, i.e., from never to almost all days [16,17]; and coping strategies, measured with the brief-COPE scale, which consists of 28 questions that evaluate 14 subscales (different coping strategies), each question having 4 frequency options, i.e., from "I never do it" to "I always do it" [18,19].

Statistical Analysis

To describe the qualitative variables, we used frequencies and percentages, and for the quantitative ones, we used means and standard deviation. In order to compare the number of diseases and somatization between sexes, the Man–Whitney U test was used, considering the non-parametric distribution of the variables. Alpha Cronbach test was used to determine the reliability of each scale and sub-scale utilized. To perform comparisons between the psychological variables and sleep quality with the two dependent variables, we used the Spearman correlation test, considering the non-parametric distribution of the variables. In order to detect the distribution of the data, the Kolmogorov–Smirnov test was used. Finally, a multiple regression analysis, with the stepwise method, for both dependent variables by each sex was performed, in order to determine the variables most associated with somatization and number of diseases in men and women. All analyses were carried out with the software SPSS v. 25, and a *p* value < 0.05 was considered significant.

3. Results

We estimate that the questionnaire was sent to about 5000 persons through the different social networks, achieving a response rate of 20%. After excluding the questionnaires submitted by underage persons (24 persons), a total of 1008 participants were included, of which 62.2% were women. The socio-demographic data of the participants are reported in Table 1. Both sexes were comparable in age, schooling, whether they had children and socioeconomic level. Nevertheless, men showed significantly higher levels of daily free hours, weekly physical activity hours, smoking frequency and alcohol consumption frequency than women ($p < 0.05$).

Table 1. Sociodemographic variables in the studied population.

Variable	Women, n = 627	Men, n = 381
Age, mean ± SD	29.89 ± 11.08	30.13 ± 11.36
With romantic partner, n (%)	382 (60.90)	205 (53.80)
With children, n (%)	192 (30.60)	102 (26.80)
With job, n (%)	376 (60.00)	259 (68.00)
Educational level		
- Elementary school	2 (0.30)	0 (0.0)
- High school	10 (1.60)	7 (1.84)
- Preparatory	136 (21.70)	92 (24.14)
- Bachelor's degree	352 (56.10)	205 (53.81)
- Technical career	30 (4.80)	21 (5.51)
- Master's degree	74 (11.80)	36 (9.45)
- Ph.D. degree	23 (3.70)	20 (5.25)
Socioeconomic level		
- Very low	0 (0.00)	4 (1.10)
- Low	106 (16.90)	61 (16.00)
- Medium	501 (79.90)	308 (80.80)
- High	20 (3.20)	8 (2.10)

Table 1. Cont.

Variable	Women, $n = 627$	Men, $n = 381$
Daily free hours, mean ± SD	4.08 ± 2.68	4.53 ± 2.80
Weekly physical activity hours, median (range)	2 (0–20)	3 (0–35)
Smoking frequency, mean ± SD	1.63 ± 1.42	1.97 ± 1.74
Alcohol consumption, mean ± SD	2.70 ± 1.40	3.07 ± 1.55

SD: Standard deviation. Smoking and alcohol consumption were measured from 1, never, to 6, many times, in a week.

The most frequent reported diseases in both sexes were anxiety, depression, skin problems, overweight, migraine and colitis/irritable colon, while the least frequent were cancer, cerebral stroke and heart attack (Table 2).

Table 2. Frequency of the self-reported diseases in each sex.

Disease, n (%)	Women, $n = 627$	Men, $n = 381$
Anxiety problems	364 (58.05)	144 (37.80)
Depression problems	204 (32.54)	98 (25.72)
Skin diseases	213 (33.97)	60 (15.75)
Overweight	176 (28.07)	93 (24.41)
Migraine	190 (30.30)	59 (15.49)
Colitis/Irritable colon	192 (30.62)	48 (12.60)
Gastritis/gastric ulcer	145 (23.13)	51 (13.39)
Allergies/asthma	99 (15.79)	36 (9.45)
Gastrointestinal infections	75 (11.96)	45 (11.81)
Respiratory infections	65 (10.37)	28 (7.35)
Sinusitis	34 (5.42)	13 (3.41)
Thyroid problems	30 (4.78)	5 (1.31)
Hypertension	19 (3.03)	27 (7.09)
Anorexia/bulimia	27 (4.30)	2 (0.52)
High cholesterol	21 (3.35)	15 (3.94)
kidney/bladder problems	17 (2.71)	8 (2.10)
Diabetes	16 (2.56)	8 (2.10)
Rheumatic diseases	15 (2.39)	6 (1.57)
hearth attack/angina pectoris	1 (0.16)	2 (0.52)
Cerebral stroke	0 (0.00)	0 (0.00)
Cancer	0 (0.00)	0 (0.00)

3.1. Bivariate Correlations between Psychological Variables and Both Somatization and Number of Diseases

The Cronbach alpha test for all the instruments used was above 0.7. In the case of the sub-scales of the brief COPE, most of them had scores above 0.6, with the exception of self-distraction, behavioral disengagement, denial and acceptance, which had scores above 0.5. In the case of the sub-scale venting, the Cronbach alpha was low, i.e., 0.35; therefore, we did not use this sub-scale in order to perform correlations and comparisons.

When we compared the somatization and number of diseases between sexes, women reported significantly higher somatization, number of diseases, stress, depression and anxiety than men; likewise, women reported lower sleep quality than men (Table 3).

Table 3. Comparison of psychological variables and number of diseases between sexes.

Variable	Men (n = 381) Mean ± SD	Women (n = 627) Mean ± SD	p Value
Somatization	1.47 ± 0.30	1.75 ± 0.36	<0.001
Number of diseases	2.02 ± 1.80	3.11 ± 2.18	<0.001
Sleep quality	3.75 ± 0.89	3.55 ± 0.93	0.001
Stress	2.71 ± 0.68	3.03 ± 0.65	<0.001
Depression	1.01 ± 0.61	1.27 ± 0.64	<0.001
Anxiety	0.99 ± 0.76	1.35 ± 0.81	<0.001

SD: Standard deviation, somatization scale (PHQ-15), range: 1–3, Number of diseases, range: 0–22, sleep quality (OVIEDO scale) range: 1–5, stress scale (CPSS) range of 1–5; depression scale (CES-D) range: 0–3 and anxiety scale (GAD-7) range: 0–3.

3.1.1. Correlations with Stress, Depression, Anxiety and Sleep Quality

In the bivariate correlations, both sexes showed significant positive moderate correlations between stress, anxiety and depression with somatization, on one hand, and with the number of diseases, on the other, with higher correlations for depression in women and for anxiety in men. In addition, sleep quality showed significant negative moderate correlations with both dependent variables (Table 4).

Table 4. Bivariate correlations between psychological variables and coping strategies and somatization and number of diseases in each sex.

	Men, n = 381		Women, n = 627	
Variable	Somatization	Number of Diseases	Somatization	Number of Diseases
Depression	0.566 **	0.423 **	0.631 **	0.449 **
Anxiety	0.604 **	0.462 **	0.622 **	0.444 **
Stress	0.496 **	0.383 **	0.525 **	0.365 **
Sleep quality	−0.571 **	−0.348 **	−0.589 **	−0.430 **
Coping strategies				
Religion	−0.090	−0.035	−0.101 *	−0.044
Substance use	0.108 *	0.122 *	0.212 **	0.188 **
Self-blame	0.353 **	0.204 **	0.340 **	0.278 **
Behavioral disengagement	0.193 **	0.098	0.216 **	0.106 **
Emotional support	0.019	−0.038	0.018	0.055
Instrumental support	0.045	−0.070	0.057	0.079
Active coping	−0.112 *	−0.114 *	−0.075	0.007
Planning	−0.036	0.073	−0.106 **	−0.010
Self-distraction	0.167 **	0.105 *	0.197 **	0.098 *
Denial	0.168 **	0.019	0.267 **	0.146 **
Positive reframing	−0.042	−0.089	−0.045	−0.002
Acceptance	−0.061	−0.087	−0.062	−0.003
Humor	0.047	−0.115 *	0.156 **	0.092 *

* $p < 0.05$, ** $p < 0.01$. p value obtained with Spearman correlation test.

When anxiety and depression problems were not included in the number of diseases, the correlations between the three psychological variables diminished, but were still significant for both sexes. The correlation of number of diseases with anxiety was as follow: for men, r = 0.380, p <0.01; for women, r = 0.313, p < 0.01. The same correlation with depression was, for men, r = 0.311, p < 0.01; for women, r = 0.306, p < 0.01. The correlation with stress was, for men, r = 0.290, p < 0.01; for women, r = 0.237, p < 0.01. The correlation with sleep quality was, for men, r = −0.262, p < 0.01; for women, r = −0.328, p < 0.01. When overweight was also excluded from the number of diseases, the correlations remained similar as those found when excluding anxiety and depression problems. Somatization and number of diseases showed significant positive moderate correlations between them in both sexes: men: r = 0.545, p < 0.001, and women: r = 0.547, p < 0.001.

3.1.2. Correlations with Coping Strategies

In relation to coping strategies, women showed significant low positive correlations between somatization and self-blame, denial, behavioral disengagement, substance use, self-distraction and humor, and significant low negative correlations between somatization and planning and religion. For the number of diseases, women showed significant low positive correlations with self-blame, substance use, denial, behavioral disengagement, self-distraction, humor and instrumental support.

Men showed significant low positive correlations between somatization and self-blame, behavioral disengagement, denial, self-distraction and substance use. For the number of diseases, men showed significant low positive correlations with self-blame, substance use and self-distraction, and significant low negative correlations with humor and active coping.

3.1.3. Bivariate Correlations between Socio-Demographic Variables and Somatization and Number of Diseases

Correlations with Somatization

Sociodemographic variables also showed low but significant negative correlations with somatization and number of diseases. In women, we found negative correlations between somatization and age (r = −0.256, p < 0.01), weekly physical activity hours (r = −0.214, p < 0.01), monthly extra money (r = −0.182, p < 0.01), whether they had children (r = −0.158, p < 0.01), schooling (r = −0.134, p < 0.01), socioeconomic level (r = −0.129, p < 0.01), daily free hours (r = −0.085, p < 0.05) and whether they worked (r = −0.080, p < 0.05), and a low positive correlation with smoking frequency (r = 0.093, p < 0.05).

In men, we found negative correlations between somatization and monthly extra money (r = −0.164, p < 0.01), weekly physical activity hours (r = −0.149, p < 0.01) and whether they had children (r = −0.115, p < 0.01).

Correlations with Number of Diseases

For the number of diseases, in women, we found low but significant negative correlations with whether they had children (r = −0.143, p < 0.01), socioeconomic level (r = −0.112, p < 0.01) and weekly physical activity hours (r = −0.101, p < 0.01), and a low positive correlation with smoking frequency (r =0.110 p < 0.05). In men, we found low but significant negative correlations between the number of diseases and weekly physical activity hours (r = −0.132, p < 0.05), and a low positive correlation with age (r = 0.105, p < 0.05) and smoking frequency (r = 0.105, p < 0.05).

3.2. Multiple Regression Analysis for Somatization and Number of Diseases

In the multiple regression analysis for somatization in men and women, adjusting for the sociodemographic variables, the most associated variable was depression followed by number of diseases, sleep quality (negatively associated) and anxiety. In contrast, for number of diseases, the most associated variables were sleep quality (negatively associated), anxiety and schooling (Tables 5 and 6).

Table 5. Multivariate regression analysis for somatization.

Variable	Not Standardized Coefficient B	Coefficient B CI 95% (Lower and Upper Limits)		Standardized Beta Coefficient	p Value	Change in R^2
Men						
Constant	1.372	1.214	1.528	-	0.000	-
Depression	0.064	0.002	0.126	0.126	0.043	0.349
Number of diseases	0.059	0.045	0.073	0.348	0.000	0.115
Sleep quality	−0.066	−0.097	−0.036	−0.195	0.000	0.039
Anxiety	0.091	0.045	0.138	0.225	0.000	0.016
Denial	0.052	0.016	0.089	0.106	0.005	0.009
Humor	0.032	0.009	0.056	0.100	0.007	0.005
Women						
Constant	1.826	1.675	1.977	-	0.000	-
Depression	0.109	0.058	0.159	0.195	0.000	0.395
Number of diseases	0.038	0.028	0.048	0.232	0.000	0.079
Sleep quality	−0.091	−0.118	−0.065	−0.238	0.000	0.043
Anxiety	0.091	0.053	0.129	0.208	0.000	0.022
Monthly extra money	−0.020	−0.038	0.002	−0.063	0.029	0.006
Age	−0.002	−0.004	−0.0003	−0.070	0.019	0.004
Weekly physical activity hours	−0.007	−0.014	−0.001	−0.065	0.022	0.004

The unstandardized coefficient B represents the direct contribution of each variable to the dependent variable, while the standardized beta coefficient is obtained by converting the direct contributions to typical contributions (standard deviations of the dependent variable), which permits to determine the relative value of each variable in relation to the dependent variable. R of the model for men: 0.729, R^2 = 0.532. R of the model for women: 0.743, R^2 = 0.553.

Table 6. Multivariate regression analysis for number of diseases.

Variable	Not Standardized Coefficient B	Coefficient B CI 95% (Lower and Upper Limits)		Standardized Beta Coefficient	p Value	Change in R^2
Men						
Constant	1.674	0.468	2.880	-	0.007	-
Sleep quality	−0.389	−0.596	−0.182	−0.194	0.000	0.192
Anxiety	0.861	0.612	1.110	0.360	0.000	0.029
Schooling	0.253	0.103	0.403	0.151	0.001	0.022
Instrumental support	−0.274	−0.497	−0.050	−0.111	0.017	0.012
Women						
Constant	2.815	1.552	4.077	-	0.000	-
Sleep quality	−0.621	−0.821	−0.421	−0.264	0.000	0.196
Anxiety	0.477	0.188	0.767	0.178	0.001	0.054
Schooling	0.225	0.082	0.369	0.110	0.002	0.010
Depression	0.490	0.098	0.881	0.143	0.014	0.009
Substance use	0.261	0.025	0.498	0.079	0.030	0.006

The unstandardized coefficient B represents the direct contribution of each variable to the dependent variable, while the standardized beta coefficient is obtained when the direct contributions are converted to typical contributions (standard deviations of the dependent variable), which permits to determine the relative value of each variable in relation to the dependent variable. R of the model for men: 0.505, R^2 = 0.255. R of the model for women: 0.524, R^2 = 0.275. * Somatization was not included in these analyses, considering that this variable, rather than a cause, is a consequence of the number of diseases.

4. Discussion

We found that somatization and number of diseases were associated and that they were also associated with the main negative psychological variables, i.e., anxiety, depression and stress. Likewise, they were negatively correlated with sleep quality, in both sexes. We also showed that typical maladaptive coping patterns were positively correlated with somatization and number of diseases (mainly self-blame) in both sexes and that active coping correlated negatively with somatization and number of diseases only in men.

As previously shown, negative psychological variables, somatization and number of diseases reached higher levels in women than in men [2–5]. We also detected that sleep quality was lower in women than in men, which can be related to the increased frequency of the negative psychological variables in this sex, considering that sleep quality is negatively correlated with anxiety, stress and depression [2,7]. Interestingly, the most frequent diseases in both sexes were anxiety and depression problems that required medication (58% and 33% in women, and 38% and 26% in men), which were more frequent in women than in men. This is an unexpected finding, together with the relatively low frequency of diabetes and hypertension, which were reported as the most frequent diseases in Mexico (~10% for diabetes, and 30% for hypertension) [20].

These differences can be explained by considering that the population studied was mainly young and could present more psychological problems and less metabolic ones.

With respect to the correlation analysis, we found that the variables most associated with somatization in both sexes were anxiety, depression and stress, with moderate positive correlations, as well as sleep quality, with moderate negative correlations.

The coping strategies showed lower correlations with somatization in both sexes. It is of interest that self-blame showed the highest correlations in both sexes, followed by behavioral disengagement, denial, self-distraction and substance use; these correlations indicate a possible indirect correlation between these coping strategies and somatization, considering that these strategies were positively correlated with the negative psychological variables in both sexes (data not shown) and are typically considered as maladaptive coping strategies [21,22]. Additionally, women showed a low positive correlation between the coping strategy humor and both somatization and number of diseases, which suggests that this coping strategy may be maladaptive only in women. This is supported by the fact that humor also showed very low positive correlations with stress, depression and anxiety in women (data not shown).

The coping strategies negatively correlated with somatization were active coping in men, and religion and planning in women, which coincides with the fact that these strategies have been classified as adaptive [21,22]. However, the positive correlations were stronger than the negative correlations, which suggests that maladaptive coping strategies may contribute to somatization more than adaptive ones.

As previously shown, a positive moderate correlation was found between somatization and number of diseases in both sexes [2]. This suggests that somatization is also a consequence of disease presence. For the number of diseases, the three negative psychological variables showed moderate positive correlations, and sleep quality showed moderate negative correlations with this variable in both sexes. These results coincide with our previous report showing a significant positive correlation between anxiety and depression with number of diseases in women, and a negative correlation between sleep quality and number of diseases also in women [2]. However, in the case of men, we now detected a positive correlation between anxiety and depression and number of diseases, and a negative correlation between sleep quality and number of diseases that had not been previously identified, which can be explained by the increased sample size and the higher number of diseases considered in this study, which permitted us to better evaluate these associations. These correlations are in concordance with psychoneuroendocrinology findings, which correlate negative psychological variables with inflammation and oxidative stress that contribute to disease development [23,24]. In addition, the importance of sleep quality in order to maintain a good health condition, with no or less diseases, has been highlighted; however, bilateral relationships are also possible, and only longitudinal designs can clarify this. In this sense, a recent report showed that sleep promotes the activity of DNA damage response proteins in zebrafish [25], relating sleep with DNA repair, which could be a protective factor for disease development.

In addition, self-blame and substance use were the only coping strategies positively associated (low correlation) with number of diseases in both sexes; women also showed low positive correlations with behavioral disengagement, denial and humor, while men showed low negative correlations with humor and active coping. These results confirm the correlations found for somatization, although for this variable, a decreased number of associated coping strategies and a diminishment in the strength of the associations were observed. These changes were expected, considering that disease presence is a variable related to more causes than somatization, which, in turn, is more associated with psychological variables.

The multivariate analysis confirmed the results of the bivariate analysis, indicating that depression, number of diseases, sleep quality and anxiety were the variables that most explained the variability of somatization. Likewise, sleep quality and anxiety were the variables that most explained the number of diseases. These findings coincide with our previous report [2] where sleep quality was included in the multivariate analysis for the number of diseases in both sexes. However, differently from this previous report, we suggest that the negative psychological variables studied, i.e., anxiety, depression and stress, together with sleep quality, equally contribute to disease development in both sexes.

This study has the following limitations: the sample was predominantly young and was not randomly selected, which could decrease the representativeness of the Mexican population, restricting it to young and educated people, from a medium socioeconomic level, who have access to the internet and social networks, and not representing older people and those from lower socioeconomic levels. In addition, the cross-sectional design of the study did not permit us to demonstrate causality between the studied variables, being bilateral relationships plausible, mainly between sleep quality and somatization and number of diseases. Finally, the estimated response rate of the questionnaire was low (20%), which can represent a bias by considering that it could be answered by people who had more interest in the theme and/or who presented more emotional problems/concerns.

In conclusion, somatization and number of diseases showed a higher frequency in women than in men. These variables were mainly related (positively) with the negative psychological variables of depression, anxiety and stress, as well as with sleep quality (negatively) in both sexes. Likewise, these variables showed lower but significant positive correlations with some maladaptive strategies, mainly, self-blame, in both sexes. Additionally, some of these strategies, considered as adaptive, showed negative correlations with somatization and number of diseases, being more constant in the case of men, where active coping was negatively correlated with these two variables. Humor showed different correlations in men and women, suggesting that this strategy is adaptive in men but maladaptive in women. Further studies with larger sample sizes, longitudinal designs and performed in different populations should be performed to confirm these results.

Author Contributions: Conceptualization, A.J.L.B.-T., F.M.-E., Y.A.R.-D. and M.L.R.-G.; investigation, A.J.L.B.-T., F.M.-E., Y.A.R.-D., M.L.R.-G., A.J.M.-L., B.E.R.-G., A.M.S.-C., Y.E.-G., F.F.M.-M. and I.P.D.-R.; writing—original draft preparation, A.J.L.B.-T.; project administration, A.J.L.B.-T. and F.M.-E. All authors have read and agreed to the published version of the manuscript.

Funding: This research received no external funding.

Institutional Review Board Statement: The study was approved by the ethics and research committee of the Health Sciences University Center of the University of Guadalajara, with the number CI-06821.

Informed Consent Statement: Informed consent was obtained from all subjects involved in the study.

Data Availability Statement: Data that support the findings of the study are available upon reasonable request.

Conflicts of Interest: The authors declare no conflict of interest.

References

1. Lipowski, Z.J. Somatization: The concept and its clinical application. *Am. J. Psychiatry* **1988**, *145*, 1358–1368. [PubMed]
2. Brambila-Tapia, A.J.L.; Saldaña-Cruz, A.M.; Meléndez-Monreal, K.C.; Esparza-Guerrero, Y.; Martínez-Hernández, A.; Rosales-Torres, B.G.; Ríos-González, B.E. Association of personal, behavioral and positive psychological variables with somatization and number of diseases in Mexican general population: The influence of gender. *Psychol. Health Med.* **2021**, 1–9. [CrossRef] [PubMed]
3. Ladwig, K.H.; Marten-Mittag, B.; Erazo, N.; Gündel, H. Identifying Somatization Disorder in a Population-Based Health Examination Survey: Psychosocial Burden and Gender Differences. *Psychosomatics* **2001**, *42*, 511–518. [CrossRef] [PubMed]
4. Vargas-Prada, S.; Coggon, D.; Ntani, G.; Walker-Bone, K.; Palmer, K.T.; Felli, V.E.; Harari, R.; Barrero, L.H.; Felknor, S.A.; Gimeno, D.; et al. Descriptive Epidemiology of Somatising Tendency: Findings from the CUPID Study. *PLoS ONE* **2016**, *11*, e0153748. [CrossRef]
5. Brambila-Tapia, A.J.L.; Meda-Lara, R.M.; Palomera-Chávez, A.; de-Santos-Ávila, F.; Hernández-Rivas, M.I.; Bórquez-Hernández, P.; Juárez-Rodríguez, P. Association between personal, medical and positive psychological variables with somatization in university health sciences students. *Psychol. Health Mes.* **2019**, *25*, 879–886. [CrossRef]
6. Case, A.; Paxson, C. Sex differences in morbidity and mortality. *Demography* **2005**, *42*, 189–214. [CrossRef]
7. Schlarb, A.A.; Claßen, M.; Hellmann, S.M.; Vögele, C.; Gulewitsch, M.D. Sleep and somatic complaints in university students. *J. Pain Res.* **2017**, *18*, 1189–1199. [CrossRef]
8. Garaigordobil, M.; Perez, J.I.; Mozaz, M. Self concept, self-esteem and psychopathological symptoms. *Psicothema* **2008**, *20*, 114–123.
9. Lazarus, R. Coping Strategies. In *Illness Behavior: A Multidisciplinary Model*; McHugh, S., Vallis, T.M., Eds.; Plenum Press: New York, NY, USA, 1986; pp. 303–308.
10. Bobes-García, J.; González, G.; Portilla, P.; Sáiz-Martínez, D.A.; Bascarán-Fdez, M.; Iglesias-Álvarez, G.; Fdez-Dominguez, J.M. Propiedades psicométricas del cuestionario de Oviedo de sueño. *Psicothema* **2000**, *12*, 107–112.
11. Ros-Montalbán, S.; Comas Vives, A.; Garcia-Garcia, M. Validation of the Spanish version of the PHQ-15 questionnaire for the evaluation of physical symptoms in patients with depression and/or anxiety disorders: DEPRE-SOMA study. *Actas Esp. Psyquiatr.* **2010**, *38*, 345–357.
12. Cohen, S.; Kamarck, T.; Mermelstein, R. A global measure of perceived stress. *J. Health Soc. Behav.* **1983**, *24*, 385–396. [CrossRef] [PubMed]
13. Remor, E. Psychometric properties of a European Spanish version of the perceived Stress Scale (PSS). *Span. J. Psychol.* **2006**, *9*, 86–93. [CrossRef] [PubMed]
14. Radloff, L. The CES-D Scale: A self-report depression scale for research in the general population. *Appl. Psychol. Meas.* **1977**, *1*, 385–401. [CrossRef]
15. González-Forteza, C.; Jiménez-Tapia, J.A.; Ramos-Lira, L.; Wagner, F.A. Aplicación de la Escala de Depresión del Center of Epidemiological Studies en adolescentes de la Ciudad de México. *Salud Publica Mex.* **2008**, *50*, 292–299. [CrossRef] [PubMed]
16. Spitzer, R.L.; Kroenke, K.; Williams, J.B.W.; Löwe, B. A Brief Measure for Assessing Generalized Anxiety Disorder. *Arch. Intern. Med.* **2006**, *166*, 1092. [CrossRef] [PubMed]
17. Garcia-Campayo, J.; Zamorano, E.; Ruiz, M.A.; Pardo, A.; Perez-Paramo, M.; Lopez-Gomez, V.; Freire, O.; Rejas, J. Cultural adaptation into Spanish of the generalized anxiety disorder-7 (GAD-7) scale as a screening tool. *Health Qual. Life Outcomes* **2010**, *8*, 8. [CrossRef]
18. Carver, C.S. You want to measure coping but your protocol' too long: Consider the brief cope. *Int. J. Behav. Med.* **1997**, *4*, 92–100. [CrossRef]
19. Morán, C.; Landero, R.; González, M.T. COPE-28: Un análisis psicométrico de la versión en español del BriefCOPE. *Univ. Psychol.* **2010**, *9*, 543–552. [CrossRef]
20. Tapia-Conyer, R.; Gallardo-Rincón, H.; Saucedo-Martinez, R. CASALUD: An innovative health-care system to control and prevent non-communicable diseases in Mexico. *Perspect. Public Health* **2013**, *135*, 180–190. [CrossRef]
21. Cooper, C.; Katona, C.; Orrell, M.; Livingston, G. Coping strategies and anxiety in caregivers of people with Alzheimer's disease: The LASER-AD study. *J. Affect. Disord.* **2006**, *90*, 15–20. [CrossRef]
22. Meyer, B. Coping with severe mental illness: Relations of the brief COPE with symptoms, functioning, and well-being. *J. Psychopathol. Behav. Assess.* **2006**, *23*, 265–277. [CrossRef]
23. Furman, D.; Campisi, J.; Verdin, E.; Carrera-Bastos, P.; Targ, S.; Franceschi, C.; Ferrucci, L.; Gilroy, D.W.; Fasano, A.; Miller, G.W.; et al. Chronic inflammation in the etiology of disease across the life span. *Nat. Med.* **2019**, *25*, 1822–1832. [CrossRef] [PubMed]
24. Liguori, I.; Russo, G.; Curcio, F.; Bulli, G.; Aran, L.; Della-Morte, D.; Gargiulo, G.; Testa, G.; Cacciatore, F.; Bonaduce, D.; et al. Oxidative stress, aging, and diseases. *Clin. Interv. Aging* **2018**, *13*, 757–772. [CrossRef] [PubMed]
25. Zada, D.; Sela, Y.; Matosevich, N.; Monsonego, A.; Lerer-Goldshtein, T.; Nir, Y.; Appelbaum, L. Parp1 promotes sleep, which enhances DNA repair in neurons. *Mol. Cell* **2021**, *81*, 4979–4993.e7. [CrossRef]

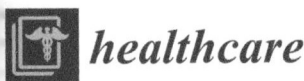

Article

Association between Alexithymia and Depression among King Khalid University Medical Students: An Analytical Cross-Sectional Study

Mohammed Ahmed Aleisa [1,*], Naif Saud Abdullah [2], Amar Abdullah A. Alqahtani [3], Jaber Ahmed J Aleisa [4], Mohammed R. Algethami [5] and Najim Z. Alshahrani [6,*]

1. Preventive Medicine Department, Armed Forces Hospitals Southern Region, Khamis Mushit 61961, Saudi Arabia
2. Consultant of Preventive Medicine and Public Health, Ministry of Health, Abha 62585, Saudi Arabia
3. College of Medicine, King Khalid University, Abha 61421, Saudi Arabia
4. Senior Specialist of Health Services Administration, Ministry of Health, Abha 62585, Saudi Arabia
5. Preventive Medicine and Public Health Resident, Ministry of Health, Jeddah 21577, Saudi Arabia
6. Department of Family and Community Medicine, Faculty of Medicine, University of Jeddah, Jeddah 21589, Saudi Arabia
* Correspondence: abuaadi077@gmail.com (M.A.A.); nalshahrani@uj.edu.sa (N.Z.A.); Tel.: +966-569-228-222 (M.A.A.); +966-544-404-833 (N.Z.A.)

Abstract: Alexithymia is a condition in which a person is unable to explain his/her emotions, bodily sensations, or discuss sentiments. This study aims to determine the prevalence of alexithymia and its relationships with socio-demographics and depression among medical students. A cross-sectional survey was conducted among medical students at King Khalid University (KKU), Saudi Arabia. A stratified random sampling technique was utilized for data collection using the Toronto Alexithymia Scale (TAS-20) and the Patient Health Questionnaire-9 (PHQ-9). A multiple logistic regression model was used to identify the factors associated with alexithymia. A total of 333 students participated in this study, almost two-thirds (64.6%) were from clinical years, and 51.4% were females. The prevalence of alexithymia and depression was 47.4% and 88.9%, respectively. Regression analysis showed females had a doubled risk (OR = 2.09), and students with high-income status showed less probability of having alexithymia (OR = 0.39), whereas people with chronic health problems showed a doubled risk for alexithymia (OR = 2.04). Moreover, depression was significantly associated with alexithymia (OR = 1.91). Our study revealed that the prevalence of alexithymia was high along with depression among studied samples. This raises attention towards finding measures to reduce it for the better performance of students and to avoid psychological problems in the future.

Keywords: alexithymia; depression; students; medical; psychological problem; undergraduate; Saudi Arabia

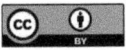

1. Introduction

Medical education is considered one of the most difficult professions of specialized training in terms of program duration, competition, and emotional demands [1]. Students transitioning from high school to medical college may suffer from a variety of challenges, including depression, alexithymia, burnout, and anxiety [2,3]. Alexithymia was identified to be one of the most common mental disorders among students [4]. The Greek term alexithymia means "lack of words for emotions" or "inability to discover words that identify and express feelings". It is described as a subclinical lack of emotional awareness, or more specifically, difficulties recognizing and defining feelings, as well as differentiating feelings from body sensations associated with emotional arousal [5,6]. As alexithymia is a symptom rather than a condition, it does not have any diagnostic criteria in the DSM-5 [7]. However, this symptom can worsen and lead to other mental illnesses such as depression, subjective distress, and burnout [7–9]. The prevalence of alexithymia varied between medical and non-medical students [10]. For example, a study carried out among Egyptian medical students showed the prevalence of alexithymia was 24.4% [11]. In addition, a study conducted by Velea et al. [12] showed the prevalence of alexithymia among Romanian medical students was 36.02%. In Arab countries, the prevalence of alexithymia was higher than in non-Arab countries, studies in Jordan and Saudi Arabia showed the prevalence among university students was 24.6% and 49%, respectively [4,13]. Medical students were found to be more prone to alexithymia due to their difficult curriculum and training [13]. According to studies, first- and fifth-year medical students had higher alexithymia scores than second-, third-, and fourth-year students [14,15]. In contrast, Morice-Ramat et al. [16] reported that there was no significant difference in alexithymia across medical students of different years of study. Nevertheless, students with alexithymia are more likely to participate in maladaptive behaviors such as suicide, substance misuse, poor academic performance, low self-efficacy, and poor self-care [7,17–19]. Although poor academic achievement, a lack of physical exercise, chronic illnesses, and cigarette smoking all seem to be related in some way to alexithymia, lack of family support among medical students is a crucial factor that needs to be investigated, especially its association with alexithymia [14,20]. In addition, several sociodemographic factors are associated with alexithymia among different sub-groups of the population (such as medical students, university students, or adults) including gender, advanced age, low educational level, marital status, and low socioeconomic status (see Figure 1) [4,14,21–23].

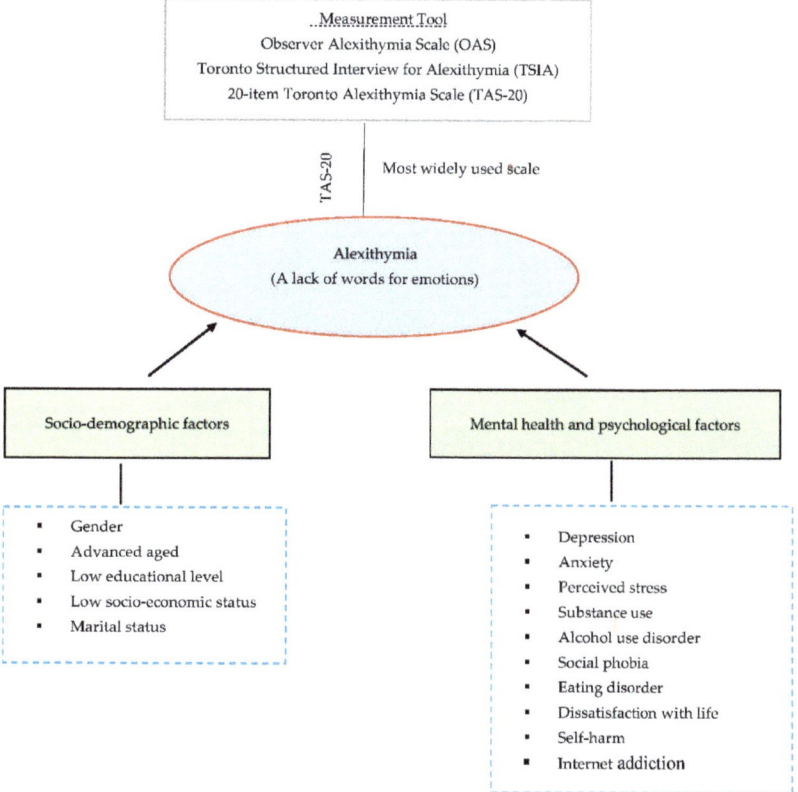

Figure 1. Framework indicating the social and other (such as psychological factors) determinants of alexithymia. (Note: The framework is prepared by the authors based on the literature.)

Additionally, medical students are susceptible to certain types of psychological distress, such as depression, anxiety, and stress, which can alter their emotional states and make it difficult or impossible for them to express and recognize their emotions [4,24,25]. According to a recent review study, depression is quite prevalent among Saudi Arabian medical students, showing the prevalence of depression varied from 30.9% to 77.6% with a mean prevalence of 51.5% [26]. Depression is a common form of mental suffering that can have a variety of clinical forms, is linked to numerous diseases, and can even lead to mortality [27]. Moreover, depression was found to be associated with alexithymia in several studies from non-Arabian countries [28,29]. Therefore, the relationship between alexithymia and depression among Saudi medical students needs to be investigated immediately because it has not been conducted yet given the extreme importance of these two issues. According to research evidence, Saudi people, similar to other Arab nations, have trouble identifying and explaining their emotions, particularly among men. Customs and cultural beliefs play a vital role in this fact, emotions are a private matter that should not be probed [13]. In Saudi Arabia, few studies have been conducted on alexithymia among medical students or university students, all of which evaluated the relationship with sociodemographic factors, students' academic factors, and internet addiction [13,20,30]. These studies acknowledged that depression was underreported in the studies and offered recommendations for further research. Moreover, since these studies were conducted at a single institution using data from various Saudi Arabian regions, their generalization to the entire country had limitations. The southern Saudi Arabian city of Abha has cultural and sociodemographic differences (such as capital city, tourist point, climatically vulnerable, and considerably high level of mental distress among different sub-groups [31,32]) than other Saudi Arabian cities (such as Jeddah), where studies on alexithymia have been undertaken. As a result, there may be variations in the prevalence and determinants of alexithymia among medical students from Abha. In order to fill the gap in the literature and consider the regional variability, the current study sought to determine the prevalence of alexithymia and its relationships with socio-demographics and depression among medical students at King Khalid University, Abha, Saudi Arabia. The outcomes of this study will be helpful to university authorities in proposing and establishing intervention programs to diagnose and treat alexithymia.

2. Materials and Methods

2.1. Study Design and Setting

An analytical cross-sectional study was carried out among undergraduate medical students at King Khalid University, Abha, Saudi Arabia, from 11 March to 11 June 2022. A structured, anonymous, and close-ended questionnaire was used in this study. Medical students from all levels "one to twelve" of King Khalid University were invited to take part in this study. Students from other colleges, rather than medical colleges, were barred from participating, as were medical students who refused to participate.

2.2. Sample Size

The sample size was calculated using the single proportion equation in the Raosoft software package (Raosoft Inc., Seattle, WA, USA) [31] with a margin of error of five percent at the 95% confidence range. Based on a study published in Saudi Arabia the estimated prevalence of alexithymia was 49% [13]. The required sample size was approximately 296 students. The sample size was expanded due to a predicted lower response to an online questionnaire.

2.3. Sampling Technique

A stratified sampling technique was used to choose the participants. We used Google Forms and Excel sheets for data collection and entry. In addition, we sent the questionnaire via students' university email to the participants. Prior to being asked to provide consent to participate, each participant was briefed on the study's goal and objectives. Participants were also given the assurance that their replies to the questionnaire would remain anonymous. The participants were also told that they could withdraw from the study at any time and that it was not a requirement for their course.

2.4. Survey

The questionnaire (see Supplementary Materials) consisted of three parts: the first one being the demographics section, where participants were asked to identify their age, gender, smoking status, BMI, academic phase, marital status, income, and type of housing. They were then asked if they have a chronic disease and how often they engage in physical activities. The variables included in the statistical analysis were determined through the literature, and their applicability to the Saudi Arabian setting was assessed. The second part consisted of the Toronto Alexithymia Scale (TAS-20), which is used to assess the prevalence of alexithymia [32]. The TAS-20 is a self-report scale comprising 20 items that are rated using a five-point Likert scale where 1 = strongly disagree and 5 = strongly agree. The cut-off scores on the TAS-20 are ≤ 51 for the low end (meaning no alexithymia) and ≥ 61 for the high end (alexithymia). Scores between 52 and 60 indicate possible alexithymia. There is no relevant validation and adaptation research of this scale for the population of Saudi Arabia based on statistics. However, this scale has been utilized in a number of studies in Saudi Arabia and has shown that they had an acceptable level of internal consistency for the Saudi population [13,20,30,33]. We also found an acceptable level of internal consistency in this part of the questionnaire (Cronbach's alpha: 0.77). The third part consisted of the Patient Health Questionnaire-9 (PHQ-9), which is a self-administered questionnaire used to screen for depression and assess its severity. The items were scored on a four-point scale rated from nil (not at all) to three (nearly every day) [34]. As for the PHQ-9, the overall score was obtained by totaling all discrete scores for the items that ranged from 0–27 points. The PHQ-9 scales indicated that those who had a score of 0–4 were considered normal, 5–9 was mild depression, 10–14 was moderate depression, 15–19 was moderately severe, and 20–27 was severe depression. This scale was adapted and validated in the Saudi population [35–38].

2.5. Ethical Consideration

All ethical considerations were assured before, during, and after conducting the study. Approval to conduct the study was obtained from the Institutional Review Board committee at the KKU (HAPO-06-B-001).

2.6. Statistical Analysis

The data were collected, reviewed, and then fed to the Statistical Package for Social Sciences version 21 (SPSS: An IBM Company). All statistical methods used were two-tailed with an alpha level of 0.05, considering significance if the p-value is less than or equal to 0.05. Descriptive analysis was conducted by prescribing frequency distribution and percentage for study variables including students' bio-demographic data, grade, Grade Point Average (GPA), medical data, TAS-20, and PHQ-9. Alexithymia and depression prevalence and severity were graphed. Crosstabulation for factors associated with alexithymia among medical students was determined with Pearson's chi-square test for significance and an exact probability test for small frequency distributions. A multiple logistic regression model was used to assess adjusted relationships with an odds ratio as effect size for relationships.

3. Results

3.1. Particpitants Demographic Chractristics

A total of 333 students were included. The students' ages ranged from 18 to 27 years with a mean age of 22.3 years old. A total of 215 (64.6%) students were in their clinical years, and 171 (51.4%) were females. A total of 290 (87.1%) were single. As for BMI, 80 (24%) complained of being overweight, 48 (14.4%) had class I obesity, 22 (6.6%) had class II obesity and 6 (1.8%) had class III obesity. A total of 94 (28.2%) students were smokers, and 108 (32.4%) exercised once weekly; however, 95 (28.5%) never exercised. A total of 67 (20.1%)

of students' parents were divorced. Ninety-one students (27.3%) had a monthly income of 10,000–15,000 Saudi Riyal (SAR), while 133 (39.9%) had a monthly income exceeding SAR 15,000. A total of 114 (34.2%) had chronic health problems (Table 1).

Table 1. Demographic data of medical students at King Khalid University, Saudi Arabia, 2022.

Demographic Data	N	%
Age in years		
18–20	53	15.9
21–23	202	60.7
24–27	78	23.4
Gender		
Male	162	48.6
Female	171	51.4
Academic phase		
Pre-clinical	118	35.4
Clinical	215	64.6
Marital status		
Single	290	87.1
Married	43	12.9
Body Mass Index (BMI)		
Underweight	32	9.6
Normal weight	145	43.5
Overweight	80	24
Obesity Class I	48	14.4
Obesity Class II	22	6.6
Obesity Class III	6	1.8
Smoking status		
Yes	94	28.2
No	239	71.8
How often do you take part in physical training per week?		
>3 times	47	14.1
3 times	83	24.9
1 time	108	32.4
Never	95	28.5
Parents' status		
Married	266	79.9
Divorced	67	20.1
Family monthly income		
SAR < 3000	20	6
SAR 3000–6000	41	12.3
SAR 6000–10,000	48	14.4
SAR 10,000–15,000	91	27.3
SAR>15,000	133	39.9
Housing		
Own house	235	70.6
Rented house	59	17.7
Students' dormitory	39	11.7
Do you have any chronic illnesses?		
Yes	114	34.2
No	219	65.8

SAR = Saudi Riyal (SAR 1 = USD 3.75).

3.2. Prevalence of Alexithymia and Depression

A total of 158 (47.4%) medical students had alexithymia, while 135 (40.5%) had possible alexithymia and only 40 (12%) had no alexithymia. A total of 88.9% of students had depression. The prevalence of mild, moderate, moderately severe, and severe depression was 15.3%, 41.7%, 26.4%, and 5.4%, respectively (Figure 2).

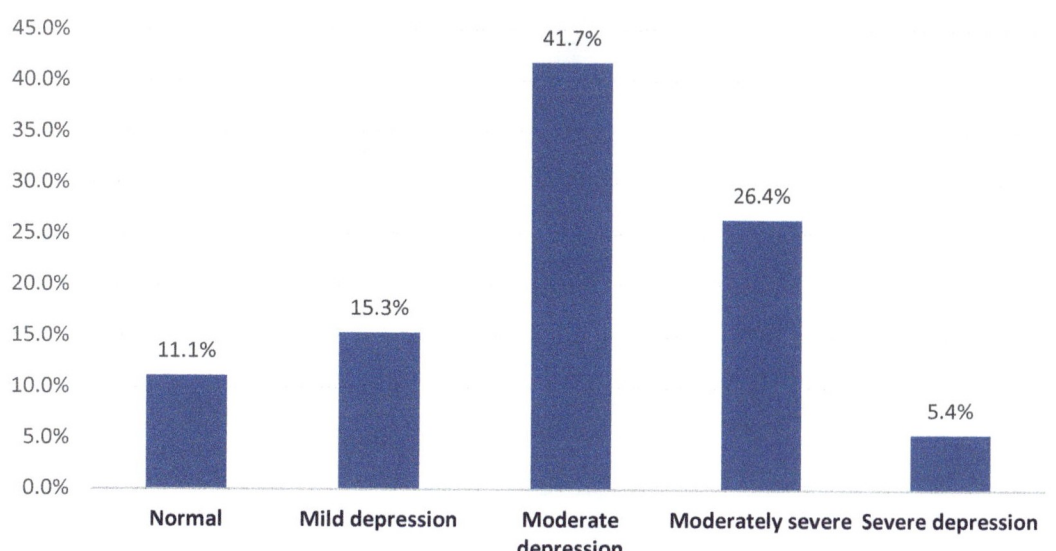

Figure 2. Depression severity among medical students at King Khalid University, Saudi Arabia.

3.3. Relationship between Alexithymia and Depression

A total of 94.3% of students with alexithymia showed depression symptoms compared to 86.7% of students with possible alexithymia and 75% of students with no alexithymia ($p = 0.001$) (Table 2).

Table 2. Relationship between alexithymia and depression among medical students at King Khalid University, Saudi Arabia, 2022.

TAS-20	Depression				p-Value
	Normal		Depression		
	N	%	N	%	
No alexithymia	10	25	30	75	
Possible alexithymia	18	13.3	117	86.7	0.001 *
Alexithymia	9	5.7	149	94.3	

p: Pearson X^2 test, * $p < 0.05$ (significant).

3.4. Factors Associated with Alexithymia

A total of 52.6% of female students had alexithymia compared to 42% of male students with a recorded statistical significance ($p = 0.048$). Additionally, 56.3% of students with a family monthly income of SAR 6000–10,000 had alexithymia versus 51.9% of students with an income of more than SAR 15,000, and 35% of those with a family income of less than SAR 3000 ($p = 0.011$). Other factors were insignificantly associated with students' alexithymia status (Table 3).

Table 3. Factors associated with Alexithymia among medical students at King Khalid University, Saudi Arabia, 2022.

Factors	Alexithymia						p-Value
	No Alexithymia		Possible Alexithymia		Alexithymia		
	N	%	N	%	N	%	
Academic phase							
Pre-clinical	11	9.3	52	44.1	55	46.6	0.430
Clinical	29	13.5	83	38.6	103	47.9	
Age in years							
18–20	6	11.3	19	35.8	28	52.8	0.216
21–23	30	14.9	81	40.1	91	45.0	
24–27	4	5.1	35	44.9	39	50	
Gender							
Male	20	12.3	74	45.7	68	42	0.048 *
Female	20	11.7	61	35.7	90	52.6	
Body mass index (BMI)							
Underweight	4	12.5	15	46.9	13	40.6	0.908 $
Normal weight	17	11.7	54	37.2	74	51	
Overweight	11	13.8	34	42.5	35	43.8	
Obese	8	10.5	32	42.1	36	47.4	
Smoking status							
Yes	14	14.9	41	43.6	39	41.5	0.334
No	26	10.9	94	39.3	119	49.8	
How often do you take part in physical training per week?							
>3 times	3	6.4	22	46.8	22	46.8	0.907 $
3 times	11	13.3	34	41	38	45.8	
1 time	14	13.0	42	38.9	52	48.1	
Never	12	12.6	37	38.9	46	48.4	
Parents' status							
Married	30	11.3	110	41.4	126	47.4	0.667
Divorced	10	14.9	25	37.3	32	47.8	
Family monthly income							
SAR < 3000	7	35.0	6	30.0	7	35	0.011 *
SAR 3000–6000	6	14.6	23	56.1	12	29.3	
SAR 6000–10,000	5	10.4	16	33.3	27	56.3	
SAR 10,000–15,000	12	13.2	36	39.6	43	47.3	
SAR >15,000	10	7.5	54	40.6	69	51.9	
Housing							
Own house	29	12.3	90	38.3	116	49.4	0.494 $
Rented house	7	11.9	24	40.7	28	47.5	
Students' dormitory	4	10.3	21	53.8	14	35.9	
Do you have any chronic illnesses?							
Yes	16	14.0	52	45.6	46	40.4	0.171
No	24	11	83	37.9	112	51.1	

p: Pearson X^2 test, $: Exact probability test, * $p < 0.05$ (significant).

A binary multivariate logistic regression to examine the factors related to alexithymia is shown in Table 4. Among included factors, female students showed an almost doubled risk for alexithymia compared to males (OR = 2.09; 95% CI: 1.18–4.78), students of families with a high income showed less probability for alexithymia (OR = 0.39; 95% CI: 0.17–0.97), and students with chronic health problems showed doubled risk for alexithymia (OR = 2.04; 95% CI: 1.23–7.11). In addition, depression was found to be associated with alexithymia (OR = 1.91; 95% CI: 1.11–3.34).

Table 4. Binary multivariate logistic regression of factors associated with alexithymia among medical students at King Khalid University, Saudi Arabia, 2022.

Factors	p-Value	OR	95% CI	
			Lower	Upper
Female gender	0.023 *	2.09	1.18	4.78
High income (>10,000 SAR)	0.044 *	0.39	0.17	0.97
Have chronic disease	0.041 *	2.04	1.23	7.11
Depression	0.012 *	1.91	1.11	3.34

OR: Odds ratio, CI: Confidence interval, * $p < 0.05$ (significant).

4. Discussion

The current study assessed the prevalence of alexithymia among medical students in Saudi Arabia and evidenced that alexithymia was associated with sociodemographic factors (such as female, having a chronic disease, and income) and depression. As per the TAS-20 scale, the sample of this study showed a lower prevalence of alexithymia (47.3%) than other studies among medical students in other Saudi cities such as Jeddah (49%) [14], and Makkah (56.5%) [30]. However, we found a higher prevalence of alexithymia than a previous study conducted in the Kingdom of Saudi Arabia, which reported that 30.2% of university students had alexithymia and 33.8% had possible alexithymia [39]. Using the same scale, Al-Eithan et al. [35] showed that Saudi mothers of disabled children had a significantly higher degree of alexithymia. Moreover, the prevalence of alexithymia differs from Arab regions to other countries [13]. In Chinese medical students, the prevalence was found to be 34% [14], and only 6.02% [12] among Romanian medical students. The high proportion of alexithymia among these participants, especially in Saudi Arabia, might be related to a number of variables that have been linked to an increased risk of mental problems in the literature [7]. These characteristics include beliefs and prior experiences with mental health concerns, a lack of information regarding official services, social stigma, uncertainties regarding the validity of mental diseases, and the utilization of indigenous informal resources [13,40]. However, the prevalence among non-medical students such as nursing students [41], university students [4], and high school students [29] was less when we compared it with medical students. Due to the higher proportions, medical students should be aware of alexithymia's prevalence and its consequences in their own lives as it might reflect on their performance which could influence their future as physicians [18].

Our study found significant gender differences in susceptibility to alexithymia. The current study reported female medical students had a higher risk of developing alexithymia compared to male students. This finding is consistent with the findings of several studies, including Hamaideh et al. [4] and Alharthi et al. [30], which state that females are more likely to develop emotional problems, which explains why they are more likely to develop alexithymia. In contrast, a study carried out by Zhu et al. [14] revealed that male medical students were at higher risk for alexithymia. Previous studies among young adults/general population reported that prevalence of alexithymia was higher in men than in women [21,22]. Our findings also demonstrated that students whose families have a high income were less likely to experience alexithymia. This finding is consistent with a study conducted among the Lebanese population by Obeid et al. [23], which showed that the prevalence of alexithymia decreased as income increased. Moreover, Kokkonean et al. found that alexithymia was associated with poor education and low-income status, and was common among unmarried people [21]. A previous study also found a strong association of alexithymia with increasing age among the general population [22]. However, in this study, we did not find any significant association between alexithymia and age.

In this study, we found medical students with chronic diseases were more likely to have alexithymia. Several studies revealed that chronic diseases have a high occurrence worldwide and psychological illnesses may impact patients' capacity to manage them, as a chronic disease is an age-related problem that will be with them to the end of their lives [42,43]. Generally, alexithymia is found to be associated with mortality and morbidity, for instance, a study reported the risk of cardiovascular disease death among middle-aged Finnish men was increased by 1.2% for each 1-point increase in TAS [44].

In our study, we found the prevalence of depression among medical students was 88.9%; nearly a third of them (31.8%) had moderate to severe depression, which is relatively high when compared to several studies carried out in Saudi Arabia [26,45]. A study conducted by Alamri et al. (2020) [46] reported that 28.9% of the general population in Saudi Arabia had depressive symptoms. As per a recent study, the rate of depression among the general population of the Jazan region in Saudi Arabia was nearly 26% during the COVID-19 pandemic [47]. However, Al Rashed and his colleagues [48] found a lower prevalence of depression (8.6%) among the general population in the Al-hasa region than in other parts of Saudi Arabia. Worldwide, mental health and psychological problems of university/medical students are recognized as serious public health issues [49,50]. Medical students are more likely to develop depressive symptoms since stress level is higher in medical students compared to the general population [3,51].

This study found a statistically significant difference among medical students with severe depression as they had the highest score of alexithymia in our sample. A meta-analysis of studies using both clinical and general population samples found that alexithymia scores were moderately correlated to scores for depression severity [51]. Our regression model showed that depression is a potential risk factor for alexithymia (OR = 1.91, 95% CI: 1.11–3.34). These findings were consistent with those of previous research that showed comparatively similar results [4,28,29]. A previous study undertaken among Jordanian university students reported that alexithymia was significantly correlated with depression, anxiety, and stress [4]. Another study conducted among Lebanese adolescents found higher levels of alexithymia were significantly associated with higher depression scores [52]. These results suggested that university officials would place the mental health and well-being of medical students at the top of their priority lists. Additionally, it is strongly recommended that future research examines the relationship between alexithymia and other psychological states such as stress, anxiety, and life satisfaction of medical students in Saudi Arabia.

Literature suggests that the higher the alexithymia scores, the higher the depression scores (i.e., positive association between the presentation of alexithymia and depression) [53]. A follow-up study also revealed that following the remission of depression, alexithymia persisted to some extent [54]. This implies that alexithymia has both state-dependent (e.g., mood but also general psychopathology) and trait-dependent characteristics [53]. If strong alexithymia hinders a consistent expression of emotional changes, for example, for patients who admit to a sad mood only erratically, a phenomenological form of depression may manifest without sadness [53,55].

Alexithymia and depression are often described as similar constructs; however, according to some researchers, the subscales of alexithymia only serve to measure the pre-defined concept of depression [56]. The evidence to date indicates that depression and alexithymia are distinct but closely linked entities [56–59]. One issue is still debatable whether alexithymia is a predisposing factor (vulnerability hypothesis) or the consequence of depression (reactivity hypothesis), or whether they coexist [56,58]. However, to date, most studies have provided support for the predisposition role of alexithymia (i.e., vulnerability hypothesis). For instance, Gilanifar and Delavar [59] found that women with alexithymia had a 2.6-fold higher risk of developing depressive symptoms.

Alexithymia is defined as a condition of poor emotional regulation that can lead to significant unpleasant feelings such as depression, anxiety, separation anxiety, and avoidance behaviors [11]. Medical students who scored highly for both alexithymia and depression in this study had more trouble with their experiences and feelings than those who did not. As a result, these students might practice harmful coping mechanisms such as smoking or risky actions such as suicidal behavior or social disengagement, leading a sedentary lifestyle, or even dropping out of college [60].

In this study, almost 40.5% of the participants had possible alexithymia, so it is necessary to keep reassessing these students to check if their scores are improving or declining over time, as some of them may be able to recover by using self-help coping methods such as spiritual coping mechanisms [13,61]. Further research should be conducted on the impact of customs and cultural beliefs on depressive symptoms and alexithymia among at-risk populations such as students, children, mothers, and the elderly.

Strength and Limitations of this Study

The present study has several drawbacks that should be acknowledged. First, the cross-sectional nature of this study does not allow to establish causal interferences, making it difficult to determine if alexithymia increases the incidence of depression among medical students or whether other risk factors are responsible. Secondly, the study participants (medical students) were recruited from a single medical institution; therefore, the findings cannot be generalized to the whole country. Thus, conducting a multi-centric study with an adequate sample size would enhance the generalizability of the results and could lead to significant improvements in other characteristics related to alexithymia. Finally, due to the self-report nature of the assessments utilized in this study, social desirability and reporting biases from the respondents may occur. Despite these, this study has a number of potential benefits. This was one of the first studies to assess the relationship between alexithymia and depression among medical students in Saudi Arabia. These results would add evidence to the existing body of literature, and serve as baseline data for policymakers, mental health professionals, and clinicians to assist with the development and implementation of evidence-based interventions and initiatives to improve alexithymia and mental health among medical students in Saudi Arabia. Moreover, methodological and analytical approaches represent another strength of this study.

5. Conclusions

This study reported nearly half of the participants (47.3%) had alexithymia, and several sociodemographic (such as being female, having chronic health problems, and income status) and psychological factors (depression) were found to be significantly associated with alexithymia. The findings imply the necessity for thorough screening for depression and alexithymia before the commencement of the first semester in order to prevent the usually harmful repercussions that come from it. Additionally, it is highly recommended to set up training, awareness programs, and psychological interventions for students who have alexithymia so that they can accurately identify and express their emotions and feelings. Since psychological factors such as depression are linked to alexithymia, students should be routinely monitored by mental health practitioners to prevent any psychological distress. Further longitudinal, follow-up, or interventional studies that may incorporate large and diverse samples are warranted to better understand the causal interactions between alexithymia and psychological distress such as stress, anxiety, and depression.

Supplementary Materials: The following supporting information can be downloaded at: https://www.mdpi.com/article/10.3390/healthcare10091703/s1, The study questionnaire.

Author Contributions: Conceptualization, M.A.A.; methodology, M.A.A., M.R.A. and N.Z.A.; software, M.A.A., A.A.A.A., J.A.J.A. and M.R.A.; validation, M.A.A., N.S.A. and N.Z.A.; formal analysis, M.A.A.; investigation, M.A.A., M.R.A. and N.Z.A.; resources, M.A.A., N.S.A., A.A.A.A., J.A.J.A. and M.R.A.; data curation, M.A.A.; writing—original draft preparation, M.A.A.; writing—review and editing, M.A.A., N.S.A., M.R.A. and N.Z.A.; visualization, N.Z.A.; supervision, N.S.A. and N.Z.A.;

project administration, M.A.A.; funding acquisition, M.A.A. All authors have read and agreed to the published version of the manuscript.

Funding: This research received no external funding.

Institutional Review Board Statement: This study was approved by the ethics and research committee at King Khalid University, with number (HAPO-06-B-001).

Informed Consent Statement: Informed consent was obtained from all subjects involved in the study.

Data Availability Statement: Not applicable.

Acknowledgments: The authors would like to thank Bharti Rishi and Fatima Riaz for their fruitful advice and their efforts in statistics consultation in preparing this manuscript.

Conflicts of Interest: The authors declare no conflict of interest.

References

1. Moffat, K.J.; McConnachie, A.; Ross, S.; Morrison, J.M. First year medical student stress and coping in a problem-based learning medical curriculum. *Med. Educ.* **2004**, *38*, 482–491. [CrossRef] [PubMed]
2. Messedi, N.; Feki, I.; Saguem, B.; Masmoudi, R.; Masmoudi, J. Alexithymia and coping strategies among medical students. *Eur. Psychiatry* **2017**, *41*, S695. [CrossRef]
3. Dyrbye, L.N.; West, C.P.; Satele, D.; Boone, S.; Tan, L.; Sloan, J.; Shanafelt, T.D. Burnout among US medical students, residents, and early career physicians relative to the general US population. *Acad. Med.* **2014**, *89*, 443–451. [CrossRef] [PubMed]
4. Hamaideh, S.H. Alexithymia among Jordanian university students: Its prevalence and correlates with depression, anxiety, stress, and demographics. *Perspect. Psychiatr. Care* **2017**, *54*, 274–280. [CrossRef]
5. Sifneos, P.E. The prevalence of 'alexithymic' characteristics in psychosomatic patients. *Psychother. Psychosom.* **1973**, *22*, 255–262. [CrossRef] [PubMed]
6. Nemiah, J.C. Alexithymia: A view of the psychosomatic process. *Mod. Trends Psychosom. Med.* **1976**, *3*, 430–439.
7. Dubey, A.; Pandey, R. Mental health problems in alexithymia: Role of positive and negative emotional experiences. *J. Proj. Psychol. Ment. Health* **2013**, *20*, 128–136.
8. Bratis, D.; Tselebis, A.; Sikaras, C.; Moulou, A.; Giotakis, K.; Zoumakis, E.; Ilias, I. Alexithymia and its association with burnout, depression and family support among Greek nursing staff. *Hum. Resour. Health* **2009**, *7*, 72. [CrossRef]
9. Reeves, R.R.; Johnson-Walker, D. Alexithymia: Should this personality disorder be considered during treatment of patients with mental illness? *J. Psychosoc. Nurs. Ment. Health Serv.* **2015**, *53*, 25–97. [CrossRef]
10. Gilbert, P.; McEwan, K.; Catarino, F.; Baião, R.; Palmeira, L. Fears of happiness and compassion in relationship with depression, alexithymia, and attachment security in a depressed sample. *Br. J. Clin. Psychol.* **2014**, *53*, 228–244. [CrossRef]
11. Essawy, H.I.; Hashem, N.Z.; El Hawary, Y.A.; Morsy, M.H.; El Awady, S.A. Prevalence of eating disorders and alexithymia among a sample of Egyptian medical students not attending psychiatric clinics. *QJM Int. J. Med.* **2021**, *114*, hcab102.024. [CrossRef]
12. Popa-Velea, O.; Diaconescu, L.; Mihăilescu, A.; Macarie, G.; Popescu, M.J. Burnout and its relationships with alexithymia, stress, and social support among Romanian medical students: A cross-sectional study. *Int. J. Environ. Res. Public Health* **2017**, *14*, 560. [CrossRef] [PubMed]
13. Alzahrani, S.H.; Coumaravelou, S.; Mahmoud, I.; Beshawri, J.; Algethami, M. Prevalence of alexithymia and associated factors among medical students at King Abdulaziz University: A cross-sectional study. *Ann. Saudi Med.* **2020**, *40*, 55–62. [CrossRef] [PubMed]
14. Zhu, Y.; Luo, T.; Liu, J.; Qu, B. Influencing factors of alexithymia in Chinese medical students: A cross-sectional study. *BMC Med. Educ.* **2017**, *17*, 66. [CrossRef]
15. Saravanan, C.; Wilks, R. Medical students' experience of and reaction to stress: The role of depression and anxiety. *Sci. World J.* **2014**, *2014*, 737382. [CrossRef]
16. Morice-Ramat, A.; Goronflot, L.; Guihard, G. Are alexithymia and empathy predicting factors of the resilience of medical residents in France? *Int. J. Med. Educ.* **2018**, *9*, 122. [CrossRef]
17. Abbasi, M.; Bagyan, M.J.; Dehghan, H. Cognitive failure and alexithymia and predicting high-risk behaviors of students with learning disabilities. *Int. J. High Risk Behav. Addict.* **2014**, *3*, e16948. [CrossRef]
18. Faramarzi, M.; Khafri, S. Role of alexithymia, anxiety, and depression in predicting self-efficacy in academic students. *Sci. World J.* **2017**, *2017*, 5798372. [CrossRef]
19. Schmitz, M.J. Alexithymia, Self-Care, and Satisfaction with Life in College Students. *Diss. Abstr. Int. Sect. B: Sci. Eng.* **2000**, *60*, 5790.
20. Soliman, M. Perception of stress and coping strategies by medical students at King Saud University, Riyadh, Saudi Arabia. *J. Taibah Univ. Med. Sci.* **2014**, *9*, 30–35. [CrossRef]
21. Kokkonen, P.; Karvonen, J.T.; Veijola, J.; Läksy, K.; Jokelainen, J.; Jarvelin, M.-R.; Joukamaa, M. Prevalence and sociodemographic correlates of alexithymia in a population sample of young adults. *Compr. Psychiatry* **2001**, *42*, 471–476. [CrossRef] [PubMed]

22. Mattila, A.K.; Salminen, J.K.; Nummi, T.; Joukamaa, M. Age is strongly associated with alexithymia in the general population. *J. Psychosom. Res.* **2006**, *61*, 629–635. [CrossRef] [PubMed]
23. Obeid, S.; Akel, M.; Haddad, C.; Fares, K.; Sacre, H.; Salameh, P.; Hallit, S. Factors associated with alexithymia among the Lebanese population: Results of a cross-sectional study. *BMC Psychol.* **2019**, *7*, 80. [CrossRef] [PubMed]
24. Alharbi, H.; Almalki, A.; Alabdan, F.; Haddad, B. Depression among medical students in Saudi medical colleges: A cross-sectional study. *Adv. Med. Educ. Pract.* **2018**, *9*, 887. [CrossRef]
25. Kulsoom, B.; Nasir, A.A. Stress, anxiety, and depression among medical students in a multiethnic setting. *Neuropsychiatr. Dis. Treat.* **2015**, *11*, 1713.
26. AlJaber, M.I. The prevalence and associated factors of depression among medical students of Saudi Arabia: A systematic review. *J. Fam. Med. Prim. Care* **2020**, *9*, 2608. [CrossRef]
27. Richards, D. Prevalence and clinical course of depression: A review. *Clin. Psychol. Rev.* **2011**, *31*, 1117–1125. [CrossRef]
28. Leweke, F.; Leichsenring, F.; Kruse, J.; Hermes, S. Is alexithymia associated with specific mental disorders. *Psychopathology* **2012**, *45*, 22–28. [CrossRef]
29. Scimeca, G.; Bruno, A.; Cava, L.; Pandolfo, G.; Muscatello, M.R.A.; Zoccali, R. The relationship between alexithymia, anxiety, depression, and internet addiction severity in a sample of Italian high school students. *Sci. World J.* **2014**, *2014*, 504376. [CrossRef]
30. Alharthi, A.M.; Almasoudi, M.A.; Alotaibi, M.B.; Jalaladdin, M.S.; Shatla, M.M. Prevalence of Alexithymia and the influencing factors among medical students at Umm Al-Qura University: A cross-sectional study. *Med. Sci.* **2022**, *26*, ms26e1947. [CrossRef]
31. Alenazi, S.F.; Hammad, S.M.; Mohamed, A.E. Prevalence of Depression, anxiety and stress among male secondary school students in Arar city, Saudi Arabia, during the school year 2018. *Electron. Physician* **2019**, *11*, 7522–7528. [CrossRef]
32. Alsaleem, M.A. Depression, Anxiety, Stress, and Obesity among Male Adolescents at Abha City, Southwestern Saudi Arabia. *J. Genet. Psychol.* **2021**, *182*, 488–494. [CrossRef] [PubMed]
33. Raosoft. Online Sample Size Calculator. Available online: https://www.raosoft.com/samplesize.html (accessed on 4 April 2017).
34. Bagby, R.M.; Parker, J.D.A.; Taylor, G.J. The twenty-item Toronto Alexithymia Scale—I. Item selection and cross-validation of the factor structure. *APA PsycTests* **1994**. [CrossRef]
35. Al-Eithan, M.H.; A Al Juban, H.; A Robert, A. Alexithymia among Arab mothers of disabled children and its correlation with mood disorders. *Saudi Med. J.* **2012**, *33*, 995–1000.
36. Alkhormi, A.H.; Mahfouz, M.S.; Alshahrani, N.Z.; Hummadi, A.; Hakami, W.A.; Alattas, D.H.; Alhafaf, H.Q.; Kardly, L.E.; Mashhoor, M.A. Psychological Health and Diabetes Self-Management among Patients with Type 2 Diabetes during COVID-19 in the Southwest of Saudi Arabia. *Medicina* **2022**, *58*, 675. [CrossRef]
37. Alzahrani, F.; Alshahrani, N.Z.; Abu Sabah, A.; Zarbah, A.; Abu Sabah, S.; Mamun, M.A. Prevalence and factors associated with mental health problems in Saudi general population during the coronavirus disease 2019 pandemic: A systematic review and meta-analysis. *PsyCh. J.* **2022**, *11*, 18–29. [CrossRef]
38. AlHadi, A.N.; AlAteeq, D.A.; Al-Sharif, E.; Bawazeer, H.M.; Alanazi, H.; AlShomrani, A.T.; Shuqdar, R.M.; AlOwaybil, R. An arabic translation, reliability, and validation of Patient Health Questionnaire in a Saudi sample. *Ann. Gen. Psychiatry* **2017**, *16*, 32. [CrossRef]
39. Soliman, E.S.; Allaboun, S.M.; Algenaimi, E.F.; Aldhuwayhi, R.H.; Almutairi, A.F.; Alwarthan, S.A. The relationship between alexithymia and internet addiction among university students in the Kingdom of Saudi Arabia. *Int. J. Med. Dev. Ctries.* **2021**, *5*, 433–438. [CrossRef]
40. Alamri, Y. Mental illness in Saudi Arabia: Stigma and acceptability. *Int. J. Soc. Psychiatry* **2016**, *62*, 306–307. [CrossRef]
41. Katsifaraki, M.; Tucker, P. Alexithymia and burnout in nursing students. *J. Nurs. Educ.* **2013**, *52*, 627–633. [CrossRef]
42. Van Houtum, L.; Rijken, M.; Groenewegen, P. Do everyday problems of people with chronic illness interfere with their disease management? *BMC Public Health* **2015**, *15*, 1000. [CrossRef] [PubMed]
43. Castelnuovo, G.; Pietrabissa, G.; Manzoni, G.M.; Corti, S.; Ceccarini, M.; Borrello, M.; Giusti, E.M.; Novelli, M.; Cattivelli, R.; Middleton, N.A.; et al. Chronic care management of globesity: Promoting healthier lifestyles in traditional and mHealth based settings. *Front. Psychol.* **2015**, *6*, 1557. [CrossRef] [PubMed]
44. Tolmunen, T.; Lehto, S.M.; Heliste, M.; Kurl, S.; Kauhanen, J. Alexithymia is associated with increased cardiovascular mortality in middle-aged Finnish men. *Psychosom. Med.* **2010**, *7*, 187–191. [CrossRef] [PubMed]
45. Al bajjar, M.A.; Bakarman, M.A. Prevalence and correlates of depression among male medical students and interns in Albaha University, Saudi Arabia. *J. Fam. Med. Prim. Care* **2019**, *8*, 1889.
46. Alamri, H.S.; Algarni, A.; Shehata, S.F.; Al Bshabshe, A.; Alshehri, N.N.; ALAsiri, A.M.; Hussain, A.H.; Alalmay, A.Y.; Alshehri, E.A.; Alqarni, Y.; et al. Prevalence of Depression, Anxiety, and Stress among the General Population in Saudi Arabia during COVID-19 Pandemic. *Int. J. Environ. Res. Public Health* **2020**, *17*, 9183. [CrossRef]
47. Alharbi, A. The Prevalence of Depression and Related Factors During the COVID-19 Pandemic Among the General Population of the Jazan Region of Saudi Arabia. *Cureus* **2022**, *2*, e21965. [CrossRef]
48. Al Rashed, A.S.; Al-Naim, A.F.; Almulhim, B.J.; Alhaddad, M.S.; Al-Thafar, A.I.; Alali, M.J.; Aleem, A.M.; Kashif, S.; Bougmiza, I. Prevalence and associated factors of depression among general population in Al-Ahsa, Kingdom of Saudi Arabia: A community-based survey. *Neurol. Psychiatry Brain Res.* **2019**, *31*, 32–36. [CrossRef]
49. Tian-Ci Quek, T.; Wai-San Tam, W.; Tran, B.X.; Zhang, M.; Zhang, Z.; Su-Hui Ho, C.; Chun-Man Ho, R. The Global Prevalence of Anxiety Among Medical Students: A Meta-Analysis. *Int. J. Environ. Res. Public Health* **2019**, *16*, 2735. [CrossRef]

50. Moir, F.; Yielder, J.; Sanson, J.; Chen, Y. Depression in medical students: Current insights. *Adv. Med. Educ. Pract.* **2018**, *9*, 323–333. [CrossRef]
51. Li, S.; Zhang, B.; Guo, Y.; Zhang, J. The association between alexithymia as assessed by the 20-item Toronto Alexithymia Scale and depression: A metaanalysis. *Psychiatry Res.* **2015**, *227*, 1–9. [CrossRef]
52. Sfeir, E.; Geara, C.; Hallit, S.; Obeid, S. Alexithymia, aggressive behavior and depression among Lebanese adolescents: A cross-sectional study. *Child Adolesc. Psychiatry Ment. Health* **2020**, *1*, 32. [CrossRef] [PubMed]
53. Messina, A.; Beadea, J.N.; Paradiso, S. Towards a classification of alexithymia: Primary, secondary and organic. *J. Psychopathol.* **2014**, *20*, 38–49.
54. Honkalampi, K.; Koivumaa-Honkanen, H.; Tanskanen, A.; Hintikka, J.; Lehtonen, J.; Viinamaki, H. Why do alexithymic features appear to be stable? A 12-month follow-up study of a general population. *Psychother. Psychosom.* **2001**, *5*, 247–253. [CrossRef] [PubMed]
55. Paradiso, S.; Caspers, K.; Tranel, D.; Coryell, W. Cognition and nondysphoric depression among adoptees at high risk for psychopathology. *Compr. Psychiatry* **2011**, *5*, 498–506. [CrossRef] [PubMed]
56. Hemming, L.; Haddock, G.; Shaw, J.; Pratt, D. Alexithymia and its associations with depression, suicidality, and aggression: An overview of the literature. *Front. Psychiatry* **2019**, *10*, 203. [CrossRef] [PubMed]
57. Hintikka, J.; Honkalampi, K.; Lehtonen, J.; Viinamäki, H. Are alexithymia and depression distinct or overlapping constructs?: A study in a general population. *Compr. Psychiatry* **2001**, *3*, 234–239. [CrossRef]
58. Honkalampi, K.; Hintikka, J.; Saarinen, P.; Lehtonen, J.; Viinamäki, H. Is alexithymia a permanent feature in depressed patients? Results from a 6-month follow-up study. *Psychother. Psychosom.* **2000**, *69*, 303–308. [CrossRef]
59. Gilanifar, M.; Delavar, M.A. Alexithymia in pregnant women: Its relationship with depression. *ASEAN J. Psychiatry* **2016**, *17*, 35–41.
60. De Berardis, D.; Fornaro, M.; Orsolini, L.; Valchera, A.; Carano, A.; Vellante, F.; Perna, G.; Serafini, G.; Gonda, X.; Pompili, M.; et al. Alexithymia and suicide risk in psychiatric disorders: A mini-review. *Front. Psychiatry* **2017**, *8*, 148. [CrossRef]
61. Zhang, H.; Fan, Q.; Sun, Y.; Qiu, J.; Song, L. A study of the characteristics of alexithymia and emotion regulation in patients with depression. *Shanghai Arch. Psychiatry* **2017**, *2*, 95. [CrossRef]

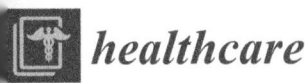

Article

Adaptation of the Highly Sensitive Person Scale (HSP) and Psychometric Properties of Reduced Versions of the Highly Sensitive Person Scale (R-HSP Scale) in Spanish Nursing Students

Alicia Ponce-Valencia [1], Diana Jiménez-Rodríguez [2,*], Agustín Javier Simonelli-Muñoz [2], Juana Inés Gallego-Gómez [1], Gracia Castro-Luna [2] and Paloma Echevarría Pérez [1]

[1] Faculty of Nursing, Campus de los Jerónimos s/n, Catholic University of Murcia, 30107 Murcia, Spain; aponce@ucam.edu (A.P.-V.); jigallego@ucam.edu (J.I.G.-G.); pechevarria@ucam.edu (P.E.P.)
[2] Department of Nursing, Physiotherapy and Medicine, University of Almeria, 04120 Almeria, Spain; sma147@ual.es (A.J.S.-M.); graciacl@ual.es (G.C.-L.)
* Correspondence: d.jimenez@ual.es

Citation: Ponce-Valencia, A.; Jiménez-Rodríguez, D.; Simonelli-Muñoz, A.J.; Gallego-Gómez, J.I.; Castro-Luna, G.; Echevarría Pérez, P. Adaptation of the Highly Sensitive Person Scale (HSP) and Psychometric Properties of Reduced Versions of the Highly Sensitive Person Scale (R-HSP Scale) in Spanish Nursing Students. *Healthcare* 2022, 10, 932. https://doi.org/10.3390/healthcare10050932

Academic Editors: Athanassios Tselebis and Argyro Pachi

Received: 8 April 2022
Accepted: 17 May 2022
Published: 18 May 2022

Publisher's Note: MDPI stays neutral with regard to jurisdictional claims in published maps and institutional affiliations.

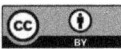

Copyright: © 2022 by the authors. Licensee MDPI, Basel, Switzerland. This article is an open access article distributed under the terms and conditions of the Creative Commons Attribution (CC BY) license (https://creativecommons.org/licenses/by/4.0/).

Abstract: Sensory processing sensitivity (SPS) can be defined as a personality characteristic that includes the individual characteristics of sensitivity towards endogenous and exogenous stimuli. The differences in environmental sensitivity can play a crucial role in the academic context of health professionals, thus defining it as an area of research that must be addressed. The reduced scale for highly sensitive people (HSP) is a short (16 items) and adapted version of the original scale for highly sensitive people (HSP). This study aims to analyze the psychometric properties of reduced versions of the Highly Sensitive Person Scale (r-HSP Scale) in Spanish nursing students. Once the questionnaire was translated, its psychometric characteristics were analyzed. The Spanish version of the r-HSP scale was administered to 284 university students enrolled in the Nursing Degree. The results from the factorial analysis confirmed the structure of sensitiveness of six factors in our sample. This structure included the following dimensions: (1) Instability, (2) Surroundings, (3) Interaction with others, (4) Sensoperception, (5) Sensitivity, and (6) Insecurity. Additionally, the Cronbach's α values indicated that the Spanish version of the r-HSP scale had an adequate reliability ($\alpha = 0.702$). The r-HSP scale is defined as a reliable, valid, and agile replica of the original structure of sensitivity in Spanish university students.

Keywords: sensory processing sensitivity; environmental sensitivity; university students; nursing; scale

1. Introduction

Sensory processing sensitivity (SPS) can be defined as a personality trait that includes the individual characteristics of sensitivity towards endogenous and exogenous stimuli [1]. It is colloquially called High Sensitivity, or Highly Sensitive Person (HSP), who are characterized by a high emotional and empathetic reactivity, and a greater depth in the processing of information [2], which makes them more vulnerable to external influences, more suggestible, and with a tendency towards sudden over-activation [3].

Sensory processing sensitivity is a non-pathological personality trait with a prevalence of 30% in the general population [4]. Initially, sensitivity was considered as a vulnerability [5]; however, recent studies have revealed adaptive traits of individuals with a high SPS, with more positive emotions in supporting environments [6,7]. In this sense, recent studies have proven that individuals with a high SPS have a greater ability to respond to positive and negative experiences [8,9]. This special sensitivity to the environment has implications on health, education, and work. Authors such as Costa-López et al. [10] and Aron et al. [3], believe that SPS is an important factor that has an influence not only on the well-being or quality of life, but also at the functional or physiological level.

It is well known that university students experience diverse stressful events [11]. Studies with samples of university students have systematically provided information on the positive correlation between SPS and symptoms of depression [12]. In the last few years, interest has also grown for studies on stress and the psychosocial factors associated with a position at work, given the repercussions they could have on the health of workers [13]. One of the groups of people that is more exposed to stress due to the characteristics of their day-to-day work is healthcare workers, with special emphasis on nursing personnel. Nevertheless, this physical and emotional overload begins previously at university, where future healthcare professionals are trained [14,15]. The sources of stress for health sciences students include balancing academic and clinical demands [16].

The 27-item Highly Sensitive Persons scale (HSP scale) was composed by Aron and Aron [1], and is the most utilized as an instrument for measuring the environmental sensitivity of students and adults. Based on this scale, others were developed for children (HSC scale) [4], as well as parents [17]. The HSP/HSC scales have been translated into various languages and their psychometric properties have been validated, although with respect to the factor structure, they revealed different solutions. Most of the results ranged from one to several structures. These authors suggested that they were closely related to neuroticism, a propensity to experience negative effects and positive openness to stimuli [18].

Sensory processing sensitivity (SPS) is a biologically based temperament trait associated with a greater awareness and ability to respond to environmental and social stimuli [19]. These individuals are characterized by being good observers and having a high creativity. However, they are introverted and can easily suffer from high levels of stress. The period at university is characterized by a greater vulnerability for a great range of mental health (MH) challenges [20], so the education context could have an important impact on the personal and professional development of students. During their university period, nursing students spend a large amount of their time in the classroom, clinical simulation rooms, and university hospitals, where they face different life experiences that can be emotionally challenging, and which can modulate their development and future well-being. In this sense, many studies consider that stress is generalized in every aspect of nursing university education [8,21,22], and that SPS increases the risk of problems related with stress as a response to negative environments [23], although it also provides a greater benefit from positive and supportive environments [24]. Therefore, the differences in environmental sensitivity play an important role in the education context, on which interventions could be made [25] to prevent the negative effects associated with SPS, and to promote its positive potential to improve the well-being and mental health of future nurses [2].

Considering the health training and education characteristics described, the differences in environmental sensitivity can play a crucial role in the academic context of health professionals, and is therefore defined as a field of research that must be addressed. For this, an abbreviated, reliable, and valid self-report is needed, that could be swiftly applied and which allows the identification of Highly Sensitive Persons among nursing students.

The general objective of the present article is to adapt the Highly Sensitive Person Scale (HSP) and to study the psychometric properties of a reduced version of the Highly Sensitive Person scale, which is widely used in Spain by the Association of Persons with High Sensitivity in Spain (Aspase), in sample of nursing students. As specific objectives, we set out to find out whether the reduced scale can be used to efficiently distinguish nursing students with HSP from those who are not, to study the prevalence, and to analyze the influence of socio-familial variables, gender and age.

2. Materials and Methods

2.1. Design

As this is an adaptation of a scale, a cross-sectional study was carried out including nursing students from the Catholic University of Murcia (UCAM, Murcia, Spain).

2.2. Participants

The study participants were enrolled in all four academic years in the Nursing Degree. The participants were informed about the characteristics of the study and aim of the data obtained from it. The participants provided their consent when completing the questionnaire. The final sample was composed of 284 students, enrolled in the 1st to 4th academic years within the Nursing Degree.

2.3. Data Collection

The study was conducted during the months of October and November, 2019. The data collection process took place during normal class hours, and the decision to participate was free and voluntary, without compensation, or disadvantages to the students who opted not to participate. Personal and academic variables were analyzed, such as gender, age, academic year, and previous healthcare education. The students were also asked whether their family, partner (if they had one at the time), and social relationships were satisfactory or unsatisfactory.

2.4. The Instruments for Data Colletion

Initially, the HSP scale developed by Aron and Aron (1997) was composed of 27 items. In Spain, the HSPS-S scale was validated in 2021 for an adult population, maintaining the 27 items from the original scale [26]. More recently, a reduced scale (HSC) was validated for an adolescent population [27]. Lastly, other authors at the international level also reduced the HSP scale for its use at the clinical level [28].

The values of the scale oscillate between 0 and 6 points. A higher score indicates a higher sensitivity. As a specific cut-off point does not exist for the questionnaire, the students who scored higher than the fourth quartile (4Q, ≥ 11 points) were defined as HSP.

2.5. Adaptation and Initial Validation of Instruments

For the process of translation and linguistic adaptation, the protocol suggested by Pluess [29] was followed. A committee of bilingual experts, who were educated in different disciplines, was convened. One was a physician, two were nurses, three were university professors, and two were clinical psychologists. A direct conceptual translation was made of the original in English to Spanish. Considering the cultural and university context, a provisional version was created of the reduced version of the highly sensitive person scale in Spanish, which was reviewed by a third expert. Of the 27 items from the original scale, 16 were kept in the r-HSP, as they had an item–total correlation coefficient > 0.30, considered useful for assessing the attribute under study, and a Cronbach's α value > 0.700. Items not fulfilling this condition were excluded. Lastly, cognitive interviews were given to 10 students. The interviewees did not have any difficulties with the answer alternatives, and their general assessment of the instrument was positive. None of the interviewees manifested having comprehension problems, or mentioned the need to include other elements. The transcultural adaptation of the original version of the HSP for a Spanish population (r-HSP) had a high degree of linguistic, cultural, and conceptual equivalence.

2.6. Statistical Analysis

The Kolmogorov–Smirnov test was utilized to confirm the normal distribution of the continuous data, with the result being <0.05, indicating that the data did not follow a normal distribution.

To analyze the reliability of the scale, a test–retest method was applied, with the calculation of the intraclass correlation coefficient (ICC) to evaluate the degree of consistency between the quantitative measurements obtained in the questionnaire. To examine the internal consistency, Cronbach's α was utilized, with a minimum value of 0.700 desired.

An exploratory factorial analysis (EFA) was performed. Before this, the Kaiser–Meyer–Olkin (KMO) and Bartlett's sphericity tests were performed to consider the adjustment of the values for the EFA. So that the factorial loads were consistent, the value had to be ≥ 0.40 for an item to be part of the factor selected [30].

Spearman's correlation coefficient, Welch's t-test and Welch's ANOVA were utilized. Values of $p < 0.05$ were considered significant. For the statistical analysis, the SPSS v21 software for Windows was utilized (SPSS, Inc., Chicago, IL, USA).

2.7. Ethical Considerations

Permission to use the English version of the 27-item standard research version was obtained via e-mail from Dr. Arthur Aron. The study was approved by the Ethics Board from the UCAM in June, 2019 (code CE 061902), considering the guidelines from the 1964 Declaration of Helsinki.

3. Results

Of the 284 students, 75% were women; 28.9% were enrolled in their first year, 25.4% in their second, 25% in their third, and lastly, 20.8% in their fourth year. The mean age was 21.6 ± 4.4 years. As for their training, 25.4% had some type of healthcare training. With respect to their family relationships, 8.8% described them as unsatisfactory. Additionally, 51.4% did not have a partner, and of those who did, 3.9% qualified their relationship as unsatisfactory. Lastly, 3.2% qualified their social relationships as very unsatisfactory.

Initial Validation of the Reduced Versions of the Highly Sensitive Person Scale (R-HSP Scale)

To verify the reliability of the scale, the consistency of the items was analyzed after repeating their measurement, through the application of the intraclass correlation coefficient. Table 1 shows the ICC value of all the items in the scale, with all of them being statistically significant, with a $p < 0.005$ value.

The reliability was also verified with the correlation analysis of the different measurements obtained after applying the scale multiple times, a procedure known as the split-halves method. Thus, in Table 1 we can verify a Spearman–Brown coefficient of $r = 0.886$, which indicates the high reliability of the questionnaire. Additionally, the Cronbach's α value was 0.705 on the initial test, and 0.760 on the retest, both of which were above 0.700, which verifies the reliability of the questionnaire (Table 1).

Table 2 shows the results from the correlation analysis of all the items on the questionnaire. Table 3 shows the results obtained in the homogeneity analysis of the items in the questionnaire. The Cronbach's α value obtained was 0.702. No items were eliminated, as the Cronbach's α value barely increased (Table 3).

As previously mentioned, the scale is composed of 16 items, with range in values between 0 and 16, with a higher score indicating a higher sensitivity. The mean was 9 ± 3.1 points, with 34.5% of the participants being HSP.

To analyze the validity of the construct, a factorial analysis was performed (Table 4). The Kaiser–Meyer–Olkin test provided a value of 0.729, with the Bartlett sphericity test being statistically significant, $p < 0.001$. The factorial analysis showed a structure composed of six factors, which as a set, explained up to 54.9% of the total variance of the results. Factor 1 with a value of 19.1%, factor 2 with 8.1%, factor 3 with 7.7%, factor 4 with 7%, factor 5 with 6.7%, and factor 6 with a value of 6.3%. Factor 1 included items 11, 12, 13, 14, and 16, which were considered related with "Instability". Factor 2 consisted of items 3, 9, 12, and 15, related with "Surroundings". Factor 3 was composed of items 1, 8, 10, and 13, "Interaction with others". Factor 4 was composed of items 5 and 6, "Sensoperception". Factor 5 included items 2 and 4, "Sensitivity". Lastly, factor 6 was composed of items 7 and 14, "Insecurity" (Table 4). Figure 1 provides a scree plot as a graphical representation of the extracted factors.

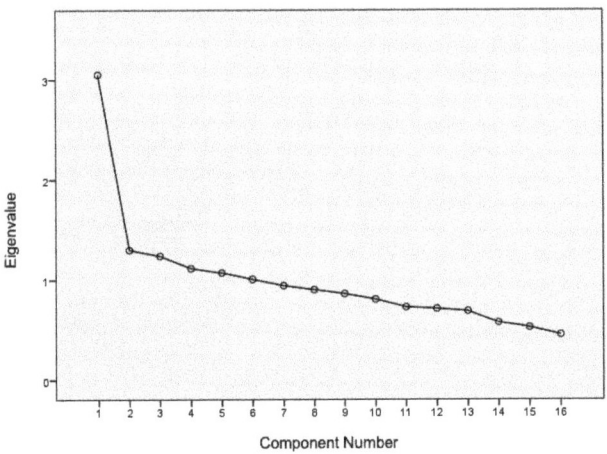

Figure 1. Scree Plot.

Table 1. Reliability test of the questionnaire in the pilot test study.

Questionnaire Items	ICC (CI 95%)	F (p)
Item 1 The behavior of others affects me.	0.735 (0.655–0.796)	3.767 (<0.001)
Item 2 I tend to be sensitive to pain.	0.719 (0.634–0.784)	3.554 (<0.001)
Item 3 On busy days, I tend to need to leave, to lay down in bed, and to look for a dark room or any other place where I can find peace and relief from stimulation.	0.569 (0.439–0.668)	2.318 (<0.001)
Item 4 I am particularly sensitive to the effects of caffeine.	0.811 (0.754–0.855)	5.290 (<0.001)
Item 5 I tend to be easily overwhelmed by things such as bright lights, strong odors, coarse fabrics, or police or ambulance sirens.	0.668 (0.568–0.745)	3.014 (<0.001)
Item 6 Loud noises make me feel uncomfortable.	0.720 (0.636–0.785)	3.569 (<0.001)
Item 7 I have a rich and complex inner life, I tend to overthink things.	0.527 (0.384–0.636)	2.113 (<0.001)
Item 8 I get scared easily.	0.813 (0.756–0.856)	5.339 (<0.001)
Item 9 I become overwhelmed when I have a lot of things to do and little time	0.723 (0.640–0.787)	3.610 (<0.001)
Item 10 I am bothered that the rest want me to do too many things at the same time.	0.564 (0.433–0.665)	2.296 (<0.001)
Item 11 I tend to avoid violent films and violent series on television.	0.788 (0.724–0.837)	4.714 (<0.001)
Item 12 The activation provoked by the hustle around me is unpleasant for me.	0.518 (0.373–0.629)	2.074 (<0.001)
Item 13 Life changes shock me (moving, work changes, separations, births, deaths . . .).	0.680 (0.584–0.754)	3.126 (<0.001)
Item 14 When I was a child, my parents or teachers tended to see me as a sensitive or shy person.	0.314 (0.107–0.472)	1.457 (=0.003)
Item 15 For me, it is important to have a life in which I can avoid perturbing or overwhelming situations.	0.357 (0.163–0.506)	1.555 (=0.001)
Item 16 When I have to compete or be observed as I perform a task, I become nervous and unsure, and I do it worse than what I could do.	0.531 (0.389–0.639)	2.131 (<0.001)
Split-halves analysis		
Cronbach's α		
Test	0.705	
Retest	0.760	
Correlation between parts	0.795	
Spearman's Brown coefficient	0.886	

F: Statistic's value. p: Significance level. ICC: Intraclass correlation coefficient. CI: Confidence interval.

With respect to the associations between the total HSP scale and the personal and academic factors of the university students, differences were only found in women (9.61 ± 2.99 vs. 7.1 ± 2.71; $p < 0.001$), and those who indicated having unsatisfactory family relations (10.16 ± 2.92 vs. 8.89 ± 3.10; $p = 0.049$) (Table 5).

Table 2. Correlation among the different questionnaire items.

ITEMS		Item 1	Item 2	Item 3	Item 4	Item 5	Item 6	Item 7	Item 8	Item 9	Item 10	Item 11	Item 12	Item 13	Item 14	Item 15	Item 16
Item 1 The behavior of others affects me.	rho	-															
	p																
Item 2 I tend to be sensitive to pain.	rho	0.162	-														
	p	0.015															
Item 3 On busy days, I tend to need to leave, to lay down in bed, and to look for a dark room or any other place where I can find peace and relief from stimulation.	rho	0.042	0.053	-													
	p	0.536	0.428														
Item 4 I am particularly sensitive to the effects of caffeine.	rho	0.062	0.165	0.027	-												
	p	0.360	0.013	0.684													
Item 5 I tend to be easily overwhelmed by things such as bright lights, strong odors, coarse fabrics, or police or ambulance sirens.	rho	0.183	0.053	0.034	0.191	-											
	p	0.006	0.430	0.616	0.004												
Item 6 Loud noises make me feel uncomfortable.	rho	0.129	0.210	0.156	0.147	0.456	-										
	p	0.053	0.002	0.019	0.028	<0.001											
Item 7 I have a rich and complex inner life, I tend to overthink things.	rho	0.165	−0.024	−0.019	0.095	0.131	0.068	-									
	p	0.013	0.724	0.780	0.156	0.051	0.311										
Item 8 I get scared easily.	rho	0.120	0.111	0.104	0.034	0.192	0.137	0.081	-								
	p	0.073	0.097	0.121	0.612	0.004	0.411	0.226									
Item 9 I become overwhelmed when I have a lot of things to do and little time	rho	0.103	0.074	0.191	−0.014	0.050	0.196	0.037	0.172	-							
	p	0.125	0.269	0.004	0.836	0.460	0.003	0.587	0.010								
Item 10 I am bothered that the rest want me to do too many things at the same time.	rho	0.158	0.007	0.023	0.007	0.110	0.133	0.073	0.077	0.087	-						
	p	0.018	0.912	0.737	0.991	0.100	0.047	0.279	0.250	0.193							
Item 11 I tend to avoid violent films and violent series on television.	rho	0.012	0.069	−0.005	−0.021	0.118	−0.033	−0.028	0.049	−0.068	0.114	-					
	p	0.855	0.306	0.935	0.754	0.079	0.623	0.674	0.469	0.310	0.088						
Item 12 The activation provoked by the hustle around me is unpleasant for me.	rho	0.008	0.185	0.070	0.103	0.261	0.127	0.068	0.173	0.132	0.101	0.126	-				
	p	0.990	0.005	0.298	0.124	<0.001	0.058	0.308	0.009	0.049	0.133	0.059					
Item 13 Life changes shock me (moving, work changes, separations, births, deaths...).	rho	0.034	0.087	0.218	−0.023	0.134	0.289	0.045	0.053	0.295	0.081	0.059	0.255	-			
	p	0.613	0.193	0.001	0.736	0.045	<0.001	0.506	0.433	<0.001	0.227	0.380	<0.001				
Item 14 When I was a child, my parents or teachers tended to see me as a sensitive or shy person.	rho	0.180	0.092	−0.025	0.056	0.137	0.156	0.030	0.249	0.171	0.214	0.125	0.218	0.138	-		
	p	0.007	0.168	0.709	0.403	0.041	0.019	0.651	<0.001	0.010	0.001	0.063	0.001	0.039			
Item 15 For me, it is important to have a life in which I can avoid perturbing or overwhelming situations.	rho	0.107	0.181	0.149	−0.007	0.124	0.205	0.194	0.166	0.210	0.196	0.127	0.146	0.271	0.192	-	
	p	0.110	0.007	0.026	0.913	0.065	0.002	0.004	0.013	0.002	0.003	0.058	0.029	<0.001	0.004		
Item 16 When I have to compete or be observed as I perform a task, I become nervous and unsure, and I do it worse than what I could do.	rho	0.059	0.173	0.140	0.161	0.153	0.242	0.171	0.096	0.243	0.149	0.006	0.241	0.172	0.214	0.196	-
	p	0.381	0.010	0.037	0.016	0.022	<0.001	0.011	0.154	<0.001	0.026	0.930	<0.001	0.010	0.001	0.003	

rho: Spearman's correlation coefficient. p: Significance level.

Table 3. Homogeneity analysis of the questionnaire.

Questionnaire Items	Mean ± Standard Deviation	Correlation of the Items with the Total Corrected Scale	Cronbach's α When an Item Is Eliminated
Item 1 The behavior of others affects me.	0.84 ± 0.36	0.285	0.690
Item 2 I tend to be sensitive to pain.	0.43 ± 0.49	0.276	0.691
Item 3 On busy days, I tend to need to leave, to lay down in bed, and to look for a dark room or any other place where I can find peace and relief from stimulation.	0.68 ± 0.46	0.178	0.702
Item 4 I am particularly sensitive to the effects of caffeine.	0.27 ± 0.44	0.157	0.703
Item 5 I tend to be easily overwhelmed by things such as bright lights, strong odors, coarse fabrics, or police or ambulance sirens.	0.23 ± 0.42	0.314	0.686
Item 6 Loud noises make me feel uncomfortable.	0.51 ± 0.50	0.437	0.670
Item 7 I have a rich and complex inner life, I tend to overthink things.	0.83 ± 0.37	0.185	0.699
Item 8 I get scared easily.	0.44 ± 0.49	0.275	0.691
Item 9 I become overwhelmed when I have a lot of things to do and little time	0.80 ± 0.40	0.380	0.680
Item 10 I am bothered that the rest want me to do too many things at the same time.	0.58 ± 0.49	0.229	0.696
Item 11 I tend to avoid violent films and violent series on television.	0.28 ± 0.45	0.296	0.688
Item 12 The activation provoked by the hustle around me is unpleasant for me.	0.47 ± 0.50	0.327	0.684
Item 13 Life changes shock me (moving, work changes, separations, births, deaths …).	0.75 ± 0.43	0.351	0.682
Item 14 When I was a child, my parents or teachers tended to see me as a sensitive or shy person.	0.50 ± 0.50	0.297	0.688
Item 15 For me, it is important to have a life in which I can avoid perturbing or overwhelming situations.	0.83 ± 0.37	0.377	0.681
Item 16 When I have to compete or be observed as I perform a task, I become nervous and unsure, and I do it worse than what I could do.	0.58 ± 0.49	0.421	0.672
Cronbach's α		0.702	

Table 4. Factor loading of the questionnaire items. Rotated components matrix.

Kaiser–Meyer–Olkin Test	0.729					
Bartlett Sphericity Test	<0.001					
ITEMS	Factor 1 Instability	Factor 2 Environment	Factor 3 Interaction with Others	Factor 4 Sensoperception	Factor 5 Sensitivity	Factor 6 Insecurity
Item 1 The behavior of others affects me.	−0.101	0.188	0.536	−0.040	0.228	0.361
Item 2 I tend to be sensitive to pain.	0.154	0.244	0.157	0.002	0.690	−0.108
Item 3 On busy days, I tend to need to leave, to lay down in bed, and to look for a dark room or any other place where I can find peace and relief from stimulation.	−0.120	0.738	0.006	0.010	0.110	−0.095
Item 4 I am particularly sensitive to the effects of caffeine.	−0.004	−0.136	−0.004	0.244	0.667	0.158
Item 5 I tend to be easily overwhelmed by things such as bright lights, strong odors, coarse fabrics, or police or ambulance sirens.	0.006	−0.050	0.170	0.835	0.094	0.053
Item 6 Loud noises make me feel uncomfortable.	0.260	0.221	0.031	0.672	0.118	0.101
Item 7 I have a rich and complex inner life, I tend to overthink things.	0.009	0.013	0.010	0.141	0.005	0.828
Item 8 I get scared easily.	0.052	0.054	0.607	0.136	0.103	−0.057
Item 9 I become overwhelmed when I have a lot of things to do and little time	0.345	0.501	0.279	−0.099	0.042	0.065

Table 4. Cont.

Kaiser–Meyer–Olkin Test	0.729					
Bartlett Sphericity Test	<0.001					
ITEMS	Factor 1 Instability	Factor 2 Environment	Factor 3 Interaction with Others	Factor 4 Sensoperception	Factor 5 Sensitivity	Factor 6 Insecurity
Item 10 I am bothered that the rest want me to do too many things at the same time.	0.008	0.155	0.538	0.214	−0.368	0.131
Item 11 I tend to avoid violent films and violent series on television.	0.610	−0.096	0.126	0.258	0.068	−0.204
Item 12 The activation provoked by the hustle around me is unpleasant for me.	0.564	0.444	−0.160	0.245	−0.145	−0.080
Item 13 Life changes shock me (moving, work changes, separations, births, deaths …).	0.465	−0.025	0.589	−0.034	0.045	−0.074
Item 14 When I was a child, my parents or teachers tended to see me as a sensitive or shy person.	0.598	−0.022	0.080	−0.107	0.055	0.428
Item 15 For me, it is important to have a life in which I can avoid perturbing or overwhelming situations.	0.119	0.527	0.205	0.199	−0.093	0.249
Item 16 When I have to compete or be observed as I perform a task, I become nervous and unsure, and I do it worse than what I could do.	0.454	0.265	0.056	0.138	0.273	0.194
Eigenvalue	3.051	1.300	1.241	1.118	1.073	1.006
Variance	19.1%	8.1%	7.7%	7%	6.7%	6.3%

Table 5. Association between each factor of the R-HSP scale and personal attribute of Spanish university students.

Variables Investigated	Factor 1	Factor 2	Factor 3	Factor 4	Factor 5	Factor 6	Total Scala HSP
Gender							
Female (n = 213)	2.79 ± 1.43	2.92 ± 1.03	2.82 ± 1.02	0.80 ± 0.79	0.72 ± 0.70	1.38 ± 0.65	9.61 ± 2.99
Male (n = 71)	1.94 ± 1.19	2.32 ± 1.22	1.94 ± 1.06	0.56 ± 0.69	0.62 ± 0.76	1.2 ± 0.68	7.1 ± 2.71
	$p < 0.001$	$p < 0.001$	$p < 0.001$	$p = 0.027$	$p = 0.298$	$p = 0.052$	$p < 0.001$
Academic year							
First (n = 82)	2.54 ± 1.44	2.80 ± 1.12	2.50 ± 1.25	0.65 ± 0.70	0.61 ± 0.68	1.30 ± 0.60	8.73 ± 3.19
Second (n = 72)	2.81 ± 1.49	2.81 ± 1.17	2.69 ± 1.03	0.78 ± 0.79	0.69 ± 0.70	1.40 ± 0.72	9.31 ± 3.42
Third (n = 71)	2.51 ± 1.29	2.72 ± 1.04	2.72 ± 0.97	0.75 ± 0.82	0.76 ± 0.74	1.38 ± 0.63	9.09 ± 2.59
Fourth (n = 59)	2.46 ± 1.47	2.76 ± 1.11	2.49 ± 1.10	0.81 ± 0.79	0.75 ± 0.77	1.22 ± 0.69	8.89 ± 3.18
	$p = 0.479$	$p = 0.959$	$p = 0.458$	$p = 0.596$	$p = 0.572$	$p = 0.401$	$p = 0.683$
Healthcare training							
No (n = 212)	2.58 ± 1.43	2.81 ± 1.11	2.67 ± 1.08	0.66 ± 0.74	0.68 ± 0.71	1.34 ± 0.65	9.01 ± 3.08
Yes (n = 72)	2.60 ± 1.42	2.67 ± 1.10	2.42 ± 1.13	0.99 ± 0.81	0.75 ± 0.74	1.31 ± 0.72	8.98 ± 3.19
	$p = 0.911$	$p = 0.339$	$p = 0.107$	$p = 0.003$	$p = 0.484$	$p = 0.724$	$p = 0.948$
Family relations							
Satisfactory (n = 259)	2.57 ± 1.42	2.75 ± 1.12	2.58 ± 1.09	0.71 ± 0.77	0.68 ± 0.71	1.33 ± 0.68	8.89 ± 3.10
Unsatisfactory (n = 25)	2.68 ± 1.52	3.08 ± 0.90	2.88 ± 1.09	1 ± 0.81	0.88 ± 0.78	1.32 ± 0.55	10.16 ± 2.92
	$p = 0.734$	$p = 0.151$	$p = 0.194$	$p = 0.104$	$p = 0.227$	$p = 0.920$	$p = 0.049$

Table 5. Cont.

Variables Investigated	Factor 1	Factor 2	Factor 3	Factor 4	Factor 5	Factor 6	Total Scala HSP
Relationship with partner							
No partner (n = 146)	2.58 ± 1.41	2.73 ± 1.09	2.57 ± 1.10	0.78 ± 0.77	0.71 ± 0.72	1.37 ± 0.65	9.03 ± 3.14
Satisfactory (n = 127)	2.64 ± 1.47	2.82 ± 1.14	2.61 ± 1.11	0.69 ± 0.77	0.68 ± 0.72	1.31 ± 0.68	8.97 ± 3.17
Unsatisfactory (n = 11)	2 ± 1	2.91 ± 1.04	2.91 ± 0.83	0.82 ± 0.87	0.73 ± 0.78	1.09 ± 0.70	9 ± 1.78
	p = 0.365	p = 0.727	p = 0.605	p = 0.564	p = 0.914	p = 0.357	p = 0.988
Social relations							
Satisfactory (n = 275)	2.59 ± 1.42	2.78 ± 1.10	2.59 ± 1.10	0.72 ± 0.76	0.69 ± 0.72	1.32 ± 0.67	8.97 ± 3.09
Unsatisfactory (n = 9)	2.33 ± 1.73	2.67 ± 1.50	3 ± 0.86	1.44 ± 0.88	0.78 ± 0.83	1.56 ± 0.52	10.11 ± 3.55
	p = 0.672	p = 0.830	p = 0.199	p = 0.005	p = 0.774	p = 0.231	p = 0.368
Age	rho = −0.055	rho = 0.062	rho = −0.129	rho = 0.172	rho = 0.159	rho = −0.026	rho = −0.008
	p = 0.352	p = 0.298	p = 0.030	p = 0.004	p = 0.007	p = 0.666	p = 0.899

rho: Spearman's correlation coefficient. p: statistical significance.

4. Discussion

To measure environmental sensitivity, the most utilized scale with university students or adults is the High Sensitivity Persons scale (HSP scale) developed by Aron and Aron [1]. However, for field studies in which time is highly prized, this original version of 27 items is inconvenient due to its length, and a need was detected to validate a Reduced High Sensitivity Persons scale (r-HSP) for nursing university students. This scale included the items that were habitually used in Spain by the Association of Persons with High Sensitivity (Aspase) for the diagnosis of Environmental Sensitivity, but it is necessary to show that the r-HSP is a simple tool that can be used to identify students who are highly sensitive.

The results showed that the tool had good psychometric characteristics. More specifically, the test and the retest showed a good reliability, with Cronbach's α values >0.700. Many studies related with the HSP scale showed one to three factors [1,28,31]. In the present study, six factors were identified. This structural model of the reduced HSP scale suggests that the general sensitivity score, as well as the scores of the six factors, are adequate for measuring the environmental sensitivity of Nursing students.

Aron and Aron [1] estimated that a high sensitivity was present in 20% of the general population. However, in the present study, 34.5% were identified, a value that is much higher than the one mentioned previously. In our study, we found significant differences, with women being much more sensitive than men. This finding is similar to the results from other authors. However, in these studies, the differences between gender groups were not statistically significant [4,32,33].

On the other hand, age was correlated with three of the six factors. The older the student, the fewer interactions with the rest, and more sensoperception and sensitivity. Costa-López et al. also found positive correlations between age and environmental sensitivity [27].

It has been described that individuals with a high level of environmental sensitivity can show over-stimulation, sensorial sensitivity, deep cognitive processing, and emotional reactivity [34]. In their social and personal relations, they are characterized as being empathetic and intuitive [3]. This means that these individuals relate better with others. These characteristics were not observed in our study, as a higher score in the scale was observed in those with unsatisfactory family relations.

Our study provides new evidence on the association between HSP and important aspects of the students, which could be considered as current life stressors, such as their relationships with their families and/or partner. The results show that those who had unsatisfactory family relations were HSP with higher scores on the scale. These results are similar to other studies, which verified that family problems of students increased their level of stress [21,22]. In other studies on HSP, research was not performed on current personal life aspects, and which directly influence their well-being. In general terms, the differential susceptibility of the adult subjects was not analyzed, including items in the questionnaires that were focused on the analysis of their childhood.

In summary, although the study used a small sample, the test–retest reliability showed ICC values (Table 1) ranging from poor (item 14, 15) to moderate and good. Furthermore, although the correlations between items were generally low, the reliability of the scale (Cronbach's alpha in Table 3) was acceptable.

Limitations

Just as the original scale, most of the items put emphasis on the negative traits ("I become overwhelmed when I have a lot of things to do and little time"). In future studies, it would be interesting to focus on the advantageous aspects of being an HSP, and to conduct a more in-depth analysis of other aspects such as processing ability, empathy, the emotional response ability, and the sensitivity to subtle aspects. Additionally, it would be positive to perform a multi-center study and broaden the sample to other university faculties. Due to the preliminary nature of this research, future studies are needed to confirm the results with a confirmatory factor analysis (CFA).

5. Conclusions

The adaptation of the reduced versions of the Highly Sensitive Person (r-HSP) scale is defined as a reliable, valid, and agile replica of the original structure of sensitivity in Spanish university students. The present initial validation of the reduced HSP scale is adequate for its application to university students, as it can distinguish between the HSP students and those who are not. The prevalence was found to be greater than the general population.

Author Contributions: Conceptualization, A.P.-V., D.J.-R. and P.E.P.; methodology, A.P.-V., D.J.-R. and P.E.P.; formal analysis, A.P.-V., A.J.S.-M. and G.C.-L.; investigation, A.P.-V., D.J.-R., P.E.P. and J.I.G.-G.; data curation, A.P.-V., A.J.S.-M. and G.C.-L.; writing—original draft preparation, A.P.-V., A.J.S.-M., J.I.G.-G., D.J.-R., P.E.P. and G.C.-L.; writing—review and editing, A.P.-V., J.I.G.-G., D.J.-R., A.J.S.-M. and P.E.P.; supervision, D.J.-R. All authors have read and agreed to the published version of the manuscript.

Funding: This research received no external funding.

Institutional Review Board Statement: The study was conducted according to the guidelines of the Declaration of Helsinki and approved by the Bioethics Committees of the Catholic University of Murcia (Approval no. CE 061902).

Informed Consent Statement: Informed consent was obtained from all participants involved in the study.

Data Availability Statement: The data presented in this study are available on request from the corresponding author.

Conflicts of Interest: The authors declare no conflict of interest.

References

1. Aron, E.N.; Aron, A. Sensory-processing sensitivity and its relation to introversion and emotionality. *J. Pers. Soc. Psychol.* **1997**, *73*, 345–368. [CrossRef] [PubMed]
2. Greven, C.U.; Lionetti, F.; Booth, C.; Aron, E.N.; Fox, E.; Schendan, H.E.; Pluess, M.; Bruining, H.; Acevedo, B.; Bijttebier, P.; et al. Sensory Processing Sensitivity in the context of Environmental Sensitivity: A critical review and development of research agenda. *Neurosci. Biobehav. Rev.* **2019**, *98*, 287–305. [CrossRef] [PubMed]
3. Aron, E.N.; Aron, A.; Jagiellowicz, J. Sensory Processing Sensitivity. *Pers. Soc. Psychol. Rev.* **2012**, *16*, 262–282. [CrossRef] [PubMed]
4. Pluess, M.; Assary, E.; Lionetti, F.; Lester, K.J.; Krapohl, E.; Aron, E.N.; Aron, A. Environmental sensitivity in children: Development of the Highly Sensitive Child Scale and identification of sensitivity groups. *Dev. Psychol.* **2018**, *54*, 51–70. [CrossRef]
5. Ellis, B.J.; Boyce, W.T.; Belsky, J.; Bakermans-Kranenburg, M.J.; van Ijzendoorn, M.H. Differential susceptibility to the environment: An evolutionary–neurodevelopmental theory. *Dev. Psychopathol.* **2011**, *23*, 7–28. [CrossRef]
6. Homberg, J.R.; Jagiellowicz, J. A neural model of vulnerability and resilience to stress-related disorders linked to differential susceptibility. *Mol. Psychiatry* **2021**, *27*, 514–524. [CrossRef]

7. Pluess, M. Vantage Sensitivity: Environmental Sensitivity to Positive Experiences as a Function of Genetic Differences. *J. Pers.* **2015**, *85*, 38–50. [CrossRef]
8. Lionetti, F.; Aron, A.; Aron, E.N.; Burns, G.L.; Jagiellowicz, J.; Pluess, M. Dandelions, tulips and orchids: Evidence for the existence of low-sensitive, medium-sensitive and high-sensitive individuals. *Transl. Psychiatry* **2018**, *8*, 24. [CrossRef]
9. Rubaltelli, E.; Scrimin, S.; Moscardino, U.; Priolo, G.; Buodo, G. Media exposure to terrorism and people's risk perception: The role of environmental sensitivity and psychophysiological response to stress. *Br. J. Psychol.* **2018**, *109*, 656–673. [CrossRef]
10. Costa-López, B.; Ferrer-Cascales, R.; Ruiz-Robledillo, N.; Albaladejo-Blázquez, N.; Baryła-Matejczuk, M. Relationship between Sensory Processing and Quality of Life: A Systematic Review. *J. Clin. Med.* **2021**, *10*, 3961. [CrossRef]
11. Ramón-Arbués, E.; Gea-Caballero, V.; Granada-López, J.M.; Juárez-Vela, R.; Pellicer-García, B.; Antón-Solanas, I. The Prevalence of Depression, Anxiety and Stress and Their Associated Factors in College Students. *Int. J. Environ. Res. Public Health* **2020**, *17*, 7001. [CrossRef] [PubMed]
12. Yano, K.; Kase, T.; Oishi, K. The effects of sensory-processing sensitivity and sense of coherence on depressive symptoms in university students. *Health Psychol. Open* **2019**, *6*, 1–5. [CrossRef] [PubMed]
13. Limone, P.; Zefferino, R.; Toto, G.A.; Tomei, G. Work Stress, Mental Health and Validation of Professional Stress Scale (PSS) in an Italian-Speaking Teachers Sample. *Healthcare* **2021**, *9*, 1434. [CrossRef]
14. Weed, P.L. *The Influence of Supervision on School Psychologists' Sense of Self-Efficacy*; Indiana University of Pennsylvania: Indiana, PA, USA, 2013.
15. Labrague, L.J.; McEnroe-Petitte, D.M.; Santos, J.A.D.L.; Edet, O. Examining stress perceptions and coping strategies among Saudi nursing students: A systematic review. *Nurse Educ. Today* **2018**, *65*, 192–200. [CrossRef] [PubMed]
16. Enns, A.; Eldridge, G.D.; Montgomery, C.; Gonzalez, V.M. Perceived stress, coping strategies, and emotional intelligence: A cross-sectional study of university students in helping disciplines. *Nurse Educ. Today* **2018**, *68*, 226–231. [CrossRef] [PubMed]
17. Boterberg, S.; Warreyn, P. Making sense of it all: The impact of sensory processing sensitivity on daily functioning of children. *Pers. Individ. Differ.* **2016**, *92*, 80–86. [CrossRef]
18. Tillmann, T.; Matany, E.K.; Duttweiler, H. Measuring Environmental Sensitivity in Educational Contexts: A Validation Study With German-Speaking Students. *J. Educ. Dev. Psychol.* **2018**, *8*, 17–28. [CrossRef]
19. Acevedo, B.P.; Santander, T.; Marhenke, R.; Aron, A.; Aron, E. Sensory Processing Sensitivity Predicts Individual Differences in Resting-State Functional Connectivity Associated with Depth of Processing. *Neuropsychobiology* **2021**, *80*, 185–200. [CrossRef]
20. Liu, C.H.; Stevens, C.; Wong, S.H.; Yasui, M.; Chen, J.A. The prevalence and predictors of mental health diagnoses and suicide among U.S. college students: Implications for addressing disparities in service use. *Depression Anxiety* **2018**, *36*, 8–17. [CrossRef]
21. Gallego-Gómez, J.I.; Campillo-Cano, M.; Carrión-Martínez, A.; Balanza, S.; Rodríguez-González-Moro, M.T.; Simonelli-Muñoz, A.J.; Rivera-Caravaca, J.M. The COVID-19 Pandemic and Its Impact on Homebound Nursing Students. *Int. J. Environ. Res. Public Health* **2020**, *17*, 7383. [CrossRef]
22. Simonelli-Muñoz, A.J.; Balanza, S.; Rivera-Caravaca, J.M.; Vera-Catalán, T.; Lorente, A.M.; Gallego-Gómez, J.I. Reliability and validity of the student stress inventory-stress manifestations questionnaire and its association with personal and academic factors in university students. *Nurse Educ. Today* **2018**, *64*, 156–160. [CrossRef]
23. McCarthy, B.; Trace, A.; O'Donovan, M.; Brady-Nevin, C.; Murphy, M.; O'Shea, M.; O'Regan, P. Nursing and midwifery students' stress and coping during their undergraduate education programmes: An integrative review. *Nurse Educ. Today* **2018**, *61*, 197–209. [CrossRef] [PubMed]
24. Slagt, M.; Dubas, J.S.; van Aken, M.A.G.; Ellis, B.J.; Deković, M. Sensory processing sensitivity as a marker of differential susceptibility to parenting. *Dev. Psychol.* **2018**, *54*, 543–558. [CrossRef] [PubMed]
25. Gallego-Gómez, J.I.; Balanza, S.; Leal-Llopis, J.; García-Méndez, J.A.; Oliva-Pérez, J.; Doménech-Tortosa, J.; Gómez-Gallego, M.; Simonelli-Muñoz, A.J.; Rivera-Caravaca, J. Effectiveness of music therapy and progressive muscle relaxation in reducing stress before exams and improving academic performance in Nursing students: A randomized trial. *Nurse Educ. Today* **2019**, *84*, 104217. [CrossRef] [PubMed]
26. Chacón, A.; Pérez-Chacón, M.; Borda-Mas, M.; Avargues-Navarro, M.L.; López-Jiménez, A.M. Cross-Cultural Adaptation and Validation of the Highly Sensitive Person Scale to the Adult Spanish Population (HSPS-S). *Psychol. Res. Behav. Manag.* **2021**, *14*, 1041–1052. [CrossRef]
27. Costa-López, B.; Ruiz-Robledillo, N.; Albaladejo-Blázquez, N.; Baryła-Matejczuk, M.; Ferrer-Cascales, R. Psychometric Properties of the Spanish Version of the Highly Sensitive Child Scale: The Parent Version. *Int. J. Environ. Res. Public Health* **2022**, *19*, 3101. [CrossRef]
28. Konrad, S.; Herzberg, P.Y. Psychometric Properties and Validation of a German High Sensitive Person Scale (HSPS-G). *Eur. J. Psychol. Assess.* **2019**, *35*, 364–378. [CrossRef]
29. Pluess, M. *Protocol for the Adaptation of Questionnaires*; Queen Mary University of London: London, UK, 2020.
30. de Winter, J.C.F.; Dodou, D.; Wieringa, P.A. Exploratory Factor Analysis with Small Sample Sizes. *Multivar. Behav. Res.* **2009**, *44*, 147–181. [CrossRef]
31. Evans, D.E.; Rothbart, M.K. Temperamental sensitivity: Two constructs or one? *Pers. Individ. Differ.* **2008**, *44*, 108–118. [CrossRef]
32. Weyn, S.; Van Leeuwen, K.; Pluess, M.; Lionetti, F.; Greven, C.U.; Goossens, L.; Colpin, H.; Van Den Noortgate, W.; Verschueren, K.; Bastin, M.; et al. Propiedades psicométricas de la escala de niños altamente sensibles a través de la etapa de desarrollo, el género y el país. *Actual Psicol.* **2021**, *40*, 3309–3325.

33. Assary, E.; Zavos, H.M.S.; Krapohl, E.; Keers, R.; Pluess, M. La arquitectura genética de la sensibilidad ambiental refleja múltiples componentes hereditarios: Un estudio de gemelos con adolescentes. *Mol. Psiquiatr.* **2020**, *26*, 4896–4904.
34. De la Serna, J.M.; Chacón, M.P.; Chacón, A. *Eres Altamente Sensible?* Descubre todas las claves: Litres, Spain, 2022.

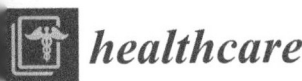

Article

Effectiveness of an Educational Filmmaking Project in Promoting the Psychological Well-Being of Adolescents with Emotive/Behavioural Problems

Antonella Gagliano [1], Carola Costanza [2], Marzia Bazzoni [3], Ludovica Falcioni [3], Micaela Rizzi [3], Costanza Scaffidi Abbate [4,*], Luigi Vetri [5], Michele Roccella [4], Massimo Guglielmi [1], Filippo Livio [6], Massimo Ingrassia [7] and Loredana Benedetto [7]

1. Department of Human and Pediatric Pathology "Gaetano Barresi", University of Messina, 98122 Messina, Italy; antonellagagliano.npi@gmail.com (A.G.)
2. Department of Sciences for Health Promotion and Mother and Child Care "G. D'Alessandro", University of Palermo, 90128 Palermo, Italy; carola.costanza@unipa.it
3. University of Cagliari & "A. Cao" Pediatric Hospital, Brotzu Hospital Trust, 09047 Cagliari, Italy
4. Department of Psychology, Educational Science and Human Movement, University of Palermo, 90141 Palermo, Italy; michele.roccella@unipa.it
5. Oasi Research Institute-IRCCS, Via Conte Ruggero 73, 94018 Troina, Italy
6. Rehabilitation and Education Center "Dismed Onlus-Centro Studi per Le Disabilita' del Mediterraneo", 98100 Messina, Italy
7. Department of Clinical and Experimental Medicine, University of Messina, 98122 Messina, Italy
* Correspondence: costanza.scaffidi@unipa.it

Abstract: Evidence suggests that adolescents respond positively to simple, early interventions, including psychosocial support and educational interventions, even when offered in non-clinical settings. Cinematherapy can help manage life challenges, develop new skills, increase awareness, and offer new ways of thinking about specific problems. This pilot trial was conducted in Italy, aiming to investigate the effects of a six-week filmmaking course on the psychological well-being of adolescents (N = 52) with emotional/behavioural problems and neurodevelopmental disorders. At the end of the project, most participants showed improvements mostly in social skills, such as social cognition ($p = 0.049$), communication ($p = 0.009$), and motivation ($p = 0.03$), detected using the SRS Social Responsiveness Scale. In addition, social awareness ($p = 0.001$) increased in all patients. Statistically significant differences resulted in four sub-scales of Youth Self-Report Scale: withdrawn/depressed ($p = 0.007$), social problems ($p = 0.003$), thought problems ($p < 0.001$), and rule-breaking behaviour ($p = 0.03$); these results showed a decrease in emotional and behavioural problems. This study is an innovative therapeutic and educational approach based on the filmmaking art. This research can offer an empirical basis for the effectiveness of alternative therapeutic tools in child and adolescent psychiatric disorders. At the same time, it can be replicated in broader contexts (e.g., school and communities) to promote children's psychological well-being.

Keywords: mental health care; adolescence; internalizing/externalizing problems; social skills; neurodevelopmental disorders; filmmaking intervention

1. Introduction

Over the past 30 years, a large increase in the number of children and adolescents suffering from anxiety and major depressive disorders or behavioural and conduct disorders has been described. Worldwide, 8.8% of the paediatric population has been diagnosed with several mental illnesses, accounting for a heavy disease burden [1]. Currently, it has become a real psychiatric emergency, exacerbated by the pandemic period, that leads many children to go through moments of sadness and emotional distress. The effects of the three years of the COVID-19 pandemic and its health security measures have had a strong emotional impact on people's lives worldwide [2]. Among the most important effects are the psychological and social ones, which are insidious, as they condition the mental health of children and adolescents, with the risk of continuing into their future. Many of them have experienced episodes or states of depression and anxiety due, for example, to school closures and the consequent social isolation and physical restrictions [3]. Currently, between 30 and 40 per cent of the school-age population suffer from a psychiatric condition [4,5].

This represents a challenge for the mental health care system, with a growing need for new therapeutic and preventive interventions, such as those based on music, theatre, and film therapy. It is urgent to focus not only on diagnostic and therapeutic procedures but also on creating opportunities for personal growth and empowering positive experiences with people dealing with the same obstacles. Evidence suggests that adolescents respond positively to early interventions, including psychosocial support and educational interventions, when offered in non-clinical settings [6].

Psychosocial interventions include art and creative therapies. A small body of literature supports using art therapy to empower youth [6]. Regarding young people, participation in the arts is thought to increase confidence and self-esteem [7]. It has also been argued extensively in the literature that models of youth participation benefit mental health over the longer term [8]. As reported by previous studies [9], the inclusion of arts in mental health programs can assist people in developing and maintaining a positive identity and creating a sense of meaning and purpose in their lives. As a matter of fact, an improvement in self-esteem and social awareness was detected in our work.

Although video-based intervention and filmmaking have been previously studied in adult psychotherapy [10], their efficacy with children and adolescents still needs to be explored. In fact, in the current literature, very few studies on the recovery of social skills for children with autism spectrum disorder or intellectual disabilities are available [11,12]. Studies documenting the usefulness of filmmaking programs specifically designed for children and adolescents with neurodevelopmental and emotional disorders are very rare. Some film-based interventions have been proposed to adolescents as educational tools, but their efficacy in mental health education remains largely under-explored [13].

Differently from other figurative arts, cinema allows for different psychological benefits, such as the identification with the character's feelings and emotions, the cathartic effect (learning through the character's experiences), and the improvement in social abilities through sharing emotions and experiences with other participants. There is clinical evidence that through the use of movies and follow-up sessions, pre-adolescent children whose parents were going through a divorce improved their capacity to identify and express their feelings and developed coping skills [14,15]. A monthly cinema therapy group session, proposed to a group of girls, allowed them to identify and work through anger and conflicts and to mark their feelings about their families and social relationships. Starting from this evidence, we argue that the cooperative work required for making a film is a collective experience which may have a stronger impact on both emotions and thoughts than the vision of a film made from other people.

Creativity should be an essential element of the education process of people with disabilities and mental disorders [12]. Indeed, working on a film project could be an opportunity to create stories and characters and identify with them while maintaining distance. In this way, individuals are exposed to their psycho-physical difficulties through the stories of the characters on the screen who are coping with the same issues as the patients [16]. Such an approach is also a strong stimulus to consider their problems from a different perspective. Consequently, this can help people to ponder their own life, promoting self-exploration and improving their ability to externalize problems [17].

This study shows how a film-based intervention, with typical structural and practical phases of the filmmaking process, can actively involve children and adolescents with mental health problems. This study has several objectives.

The first objective was therapeutic and psycho-educational. It intended to represent an educational and growth experience for children and adolescents with neurodevelopmental/psychiatric disorders to make them capable of putting their skills to the test by experimenting with the various roles that cinema caters to (screenplay, direction, set design, costumes, acting, video shooting, editing). At the same time, it wanted to stimulate them to live out highly creative and cooperative work experiences. In this way, the higher-order cognitive functions (executive functions) and the energetic, motivational, and empathic aspects (warm executive functions) have been strongly stimulated and trained. The constant presence of child neuropsychiatrists and psychologists, who supported the film director, ensured the achievement of these objectives.

The second objective was to offer a theoretical and practical introduction to the key principles of filmmaking. The participants attended a series of structured lessons on the skills necessary to use the cinematographic language (from brainstorming and storyboarding to camera use or video editing) with the purpose of creating a professional audiovisual product. All participants and professionals were members of the technical and artistic cast, working under the guidance of a qualified movie director and cinema teacher. The students also received a training certificate.

Finally, the current study explores whether, and to what extent, involvement in a filmmaking program could promote the psychological well-being of children and adolescents with emotive/behavioural problems. The hypothesis is that this highly creative and cooperative group experience could both enhance participants' self-esteem and reduce the severity of their emotional/behavioural problems.

Therefore, the research project included a quantitative assessment through standardized measures of the participants' emotional, social, and behavioural profiles. In addition, the benefits of the filmmaking course have been estimated on the extent of changes in the study measures (self-esteem and emotional/behavioural problems) through a before–after comparison. Furthermore, to support the outcomes of the filmmaking intervention, the evaluation of improvements observed by the caregivers was implemented.

2. Materials and Methods

2.1. Participants

The study involved 52 participants aged between 9 and 17 years: 24 girls (mean age 114 M_{girls} = 16, SD_{girls} = 2.4) and 28 boys (age M_{boys} = 14.8, SD_{boys} = 2.6), all with a diagnosis of neurodevelopmental/psychiatric conditions. The project was developed in two consecutive courses of 6 weeks each. A first group of participants (N = 18) was selected among patients from an outpatient service at the Child and Adolescent Neuropsychiatry Unit, "A. Cao" Hospital—"G. Brotzu" Hospital Trust, Cagliari. A second group (n = 34) was chosen at Rehabilitation and Education Center "Dismed Onlus-Centro Studi per Le Disabilita' del Mediterraneo", Messina, Italy.

Inclusion criteria were: (i) clinical diagnosis of neurodevelopmental/psychiatric conditions, (ii) aged under 17 years old.

Information regarding personal data (i.e., gender and date of birth), personal history (i.e., previous diagnosis), and family history (psychiatric conditions) was collected.

The several diagnoses in the total sample were, in descending order: anxiety disorder (n = 19), ADHD (n = 15), depressive disorder (n = 14), dyslexia (n = 13), adjustment disorder or PTSD (n = 12), autism spectrum disorder (n = 11), OCD (n = 7), bipolar disorder (n = 6), psychotic disorder (n = 5), Tourette syndrome (n = 5). Most of the enrolled adolescents received more than one diagnosis. The exclusion criteria were Total IQ (TIQ) < 70, assessed using the Wechsler scale (WISC-IV).

2.2. Aims of the Study

This study explores if a therapeutic approach based on a six-week filmmaking course would help adolescents with emotional/behavioural problems and neurodevelopmental disorders. We hypothesized that an intensive training course aimed to actualize an artistic and creative product, such as a film, could lead to improving emotional and social abilities of a group of adolescents. We questioned if the peer interaction and the cooperative work on a film set could represent an effective tool for promoting adolescents' psychological well-being, as reported in most of the scientific literature [13,18].

2.3. Procedure and Phases

Different professionals (psychologists, child psychiatrists, educators) supervised all the project phases to provide appropriate support during the entire project.

An experienced movie director [19] coordinated the whole process, with the help of a professional actor who supported the participants as an acting coach [20].

First, the invitation to participate in the project was proposed to parents through the two clinical/rehabilitation centres. The interested parents were invited for a meeting during which they obtained all details and scope of the project and provided written consent for their child's participation. Subsequently, children participated in a meeting to receive information about the filmmaking project and to obtain their assent for voluntary involvement.

Then, participants started a daily course of 5–6 h per day, lasting in total three weeks. During the first two days, all project members attended theory-based lessons in filmmaking history and techniques. This phase also focused on building trust relationships among the participants.

From the third day onward, the three main stages of the film production process were structured. First of all, a pre-production workshop took place. In this phase, the participants, divided into groups, ideated and wrote many screenplays. Participants were assigned different filmmaking roles according to their interests and attitudes: scriptwriting, direction, photography, sound, costume design, make-up artistry, production organization, and digital editing. Some subjects also held more than one role. During the pre-production workshop, the participants were also engaged in storyboarding, spaces were selected, and equipment for sets was provided. A day-by-day film production timeline was also created. Additionally, following the creative (i.e., choice of the topic, narratives, roles, etc.) and technical phases (i.e., training on camera functioning), the filmmaking process took place in natural locations or public areas (sports ground, squares, etc.) that were chosen by the participants. Participants were expected to produce a few short films (lasting about 15 min), but they outperformed expectations and ultimately produced 13 short films in total (6 in the first edition and 7 in the second edition of the course). The script themes were largely inspired by the main adolescents' issues and concerns, such as unintentional injuries, violence, mental health, suicide, self-cutting, alcohol and drug use, gender dysphoria, sense of unease, etc. In addition, some scripts were inspired by social and political issues, such as the Russia–Ukraine war and the fear of the apocalypse. Only a few themes contain hopeful messages that aim to promote the power of friendship and love. However, every script and film told a good story with an exciting plot that promoted reflection on sensitive topics.

Finally, during the last two days of the programme, the video-editing crew worked with the movie director for the post-production phase: firstly, they drafted a rough cut of the film; then, they began to review and edit the footage making additions such as visual effects, background music, and sound design.

2.4. Questionnaires

Both the participants and their caregivers were asked to complete the following self-administered questionnaires at the beginning (T_0) and at the end (T_1) of the course (Supplementary Materials):

Rosenberg Self Esteem Scale (RSE [21,22]); Youth Self-Report scale (YSR; [23,24], Italian adaption by Frigerio A. et al., 2004 [25]); Social Responsiveness Scale (SRS; [26], Italian adaption Zuddas et al., 2010 [27]); and Revised Conners' Parent Rating Scale (CPRS-R; Conners, 1997, [28] Italian adaption Nobile, Alberti & Zuddas, 2007 [29]).

Firstly, children and adolescents completed the Rosenberg Self Esteem Scale, which is a 10-item questionnaire that assesses global self-esteem. All items have a 4-point Likert scale (ranging from "strongly disagree" to "strongly agree", half reversed). Higher scores indicate a higher sense of self-esteem and scores below 15 suggest low self-esteem. The Italian questionnaire has shown good internal validity (Cronbach's α = 0.84) and test–retest reliability (r = 0.76; Prezza et al., 1994 [22]).

Secondly, they filled out the Youth Self-Report Scale, which measures the severity of emotional and behavioural problems based on a sense of self-estimated evaluation. The YSR is recognized as having good psychometric characteristics, with α values ranging from 0.71 to 0.95. The questionnaire (112 items) is an instrument of the ASEBA (Achenbach System of Empirically Based Assessment; Achenbach, 1993 [23]) and includes 8 sub-scales or syndromes: anxious/depressed, withdrawn/depressed, somatic complaints, social problems, thought problems, attention problems, rule-breaking behaviour, and aggressive behaviour. Patients select responses (not true/somewhat or sometimes true/very true or often true), and syndrome scores are then calculated by summing the response of each problem item (e.g., "I am too shy or timid" and "I threaten to hurt people"). Higher scores indicate more severe levels of the measured syndromes.

Finally, all primary family caregivers were asked to complete Social Responsiveness Scale (SRS) and the Revised Conners' Parent Rating Scale (CPRS-R) at points T_0 and T_1.

The Social Responsiveness Scale (SRS) measures the severity of social impairments in children affected by autism spectrum disorder or children from the general population. This questionnaire has excellent psychometric characteristics, and it has also been proven to be a useful tool for verifying changes in the severity of social impairment following intervention [30].

The 65-item questionnaire includes five subscales: social awareness, social cognition, social communication, social motivation, and autistic mannerisms. Caregivers respond by estimating to what extent the item describes a child's observed behaviour on a 4-point Likert scale (from "not true" to "almost always true", "Seems much more nervous in social situations than when alone"). Higher scores indicate higher severity of social deficits in that area.

The Revised Conners' Parent Rating Scale (CPRS-R; Conners, 1997, [28] Italian adaption Nobile, Alberti & Zuddas, 2007 [29]) is a questionnaire measuring parental perception of a child's behavioural problems. The short form (27 items) comprises four subscales: oppositional behaviour, cognitive problems, hyperactivity, and ADHD index. The respondent rates on a 4-point scale how often the child engages in the described behaviour (from "not true at all/never, seldom" to "very much true/very often, very frequent"; for example, "Inattentive, easily distracted"). Higher scores indicate more severe behavioural problems than lower ones. This short form of the CPRS-R proved to be a valid tool and sensitive as a treatment outcome measure [31].

3. Results

Statistical procedures were performed using IBM SPSS 19.0 data analysis software. All participants recruited at T_0 completed the filmmaking course with no dropouts, so the measurements (n = 52) at the two assessment points (T_0 vs. T_1) from both children and caregivers were available for the statistical analysis.

Firstly, descriptive statistics for dependent variables were calculated (see Table 1). The assumption of normality for all measures was verified by the Kolmogorov–Smirnov, with Lilliefors correction and Shapiro–Wilk tests: all $p < 0.05$. Therefore, Wilcoxon signed-rank tests were performed to estimate pairwise differences between the measures. These tests were employed as a non-parametric alternative to the paired t-test, as it does not rely on the assumption of normality. Specifically, they were utilized to identify significant differences ($p < 0.05$) between the YSR, SRS, and CPRS-R measures (T scores) at two different time points (T_0 vs. T_1). Results are reported in Table 2.

Primarily, an increase in self-esteem scores (RSE) can be observed (see Table 1), even though the differences between phases do not reach statistical significance. Nevertheless, the number of participants at T_0 with low vs. normal/high self-esteem was 16 (30.8%)

and 36 (69.2%), respectively; at T_1, the percentage of participants with low self-esteem was halved (8 participants, 15.4%), and 44 participants (84.6%) reported normal/high self-esteem levels. Then, the number/percentages of participants with high vs. low RSE were tested for the independence of distributions at T_0 and T_1 using the chi-square test (χ^2). However, the test showed no significant association between self-esteem levels and phases: χ^2 (1) = 1.56, p = 0.21.

Moreover, all the subscales measured by the Youth Self-Report scale were decreased from T_0 to T_1. A significant decrease in YSR scores from T_0 to T_1 resulted in four sub-scales: withdrawn/depressed (p = 0.005), social problems (p = 0.007), thought problems (p < 0.001), and rule-breaking behaviour (p = 0.04) (see Table 2).

Moreover, in the Social Responsiveness Scale (see Table 2), all parameters decreased significantly between T_0 and T_1, with the only exception being autistic mannerisms. Most importantly, the parameters that reached the widest statistically significant improvement were the social awareness subscale (p = 0.001) and social motivation subscale (p = 0.03). Social awareness increased in all patients.

Finally, while a decrease in CPRS-R scores was observed (subscales and ADHD index), the differences (T_0 vs. T_1) did not reach statistical significance. This finding was highly predictable since the programme was too short to change core aspects of a disorder, such as hyperactivity or oppositional behaviour.

Table 1. Descriptive statistics of scores at single items for every scale used. Youth Self-Report scale (YSR), Rosenberg Self Esteem Scale (RSE), Social Responsiveness Scale (SRS), and Revised Conners' Parent Rating Scale (CPRS-R). T_0 = scores before treatment; T_1 = scores after treatment; M = Means values; DS = Standard Deviation; M = Mean; DS = Standard Deviation; Mdn = Median; Min = lowest score; Max = Highest score.

		N = 52 at T_0					N = 52 at T_1				
		M_0	DS_0	Min_0	Max_0	Mdn_0	M_1	DS_1	Min_1	Max_1	Mdn_1
YSR	Anxious/depressed	64.00	11.892	50	89	61.00	61.63	12.638	50	89	57.50
	Withdrawn/Depressed	63.87	12.361	50	91	62.00	59.83	13.704	50	100	52.00
	Somatic Complaints	57.33	9.699	50	90	52.00	57.79	11.141	50	93	52.00
	Social problems	61.77	9.893	50	87	59.00	58.38	10.642	50	88	54.00
	Thought problems	59.25	8.277	50	78	58.00	56.00	8.287	50	78	51.00
	Attention problems	58.92	11.596	50	96	54.00	57.58	10.541	50	87	52.00
	Rule-breaking behaviour	55.81	8.889	50	81	51.00	54.38	8.117	50	81	50.00
	Aggressive behaviour	56.67	8.340	50	78	52.00	55.00	6.097	50	72	53.00
RSE	Rosenberg Self-Esteem	16.23	7.183	3	30	17.50	17.87	5.347	3	30	17.00
SRS Dimensions	Social awareness	45.15	27.967	0	90	47.00	40.27	23.185	3	72	49.00
	Social cognition	46.92	27.112	4	90	51.00	45.38	25.461	4	83	51.00
	Social communication	53.94	25.430	8	90	57.00	51.75	24.204	3	85	57.00
	Social motivation	54.75	31.153	5	90	63.00	50.85	29.579	1	90	56.00
	Autistic mannerisms	50.75	28.253	1	90	60.00	48.75	28.165	0	86	55.00
	Total score	66.19	13.393	45	90	65.00	63.12	14.438	42	88	63.50
CPRS-R	Oppositional	59.44	17.875	36	88	49.50	57.92	14.650	38	88	54.50
	Cognitive problems	57.25	14.835	41	87	55.00	55.87	17.029	15	88	49.50
	Hyperactivity	57.38	16.408	35	88	52.00	57.10	17.628	35	90	49.00
	ADHD Index	57.40	15.872	32	93	53.00	56.50	17.968	32	99	48.50

Table 2. Differences ($p < 0.05$) between the YSR, SRS, and CPRS-R measures (T scores) at two different time points (T_0 vs. T_1). Youth Self-Report scale (YSR), Rosenberg Self Esteem Scale (RSE), Social Responsiveness Scale (SRS), and Revised Conners' Parent Rating Scale (CPRS-R). T_0 = scores before treatment; T_1 = scores after treatment.

		Z	Two-Tailed Significance Test
YSR	Anxious/depressed—T_1-T_0	−1.841 [a]	0.066
	Withdrawn/Depressed—T_1-T_0	−2.779 [a]	0.005
	Somatic Complaints—T_1-T_0	−0.083 [a]	0.934
	Social problems—T_1-T_0	−2.693 [a]	0.007
	Thought problems—T_1-T_0	−3.382 [a]	0.001
	Attention problems—T_1-T_0	−1.235 [a]	0.217
	Rule-breaking behaviour—T_1-T_0	−2.035 [a]	0.042
	Aggressive behaviour—T_1-T_0	−1.353 [a]	0.176
RSE	Rosenberg Self-Esteem—T_1-T_0	−1.536 [b]	0.125
SRS	Social awareness—T_1-T_0	−3.475 [a]	0.001
	Social cognition—T_1-T_0	−1.967 [a]	0.049
	Social communication—T_1-T_0	−2.599 [a]	0.009
	Social motivation—T_1-T_0	−2.175 [a]	0.030
	Autistic mannerisms—T_1-T_0	−1.764 [a]	0.078
	Total score—T_1-T_0	−2.496 [a]	0.013
CPRS-R	Oppositional—T_1-T_0	−0.806 [a]	0.420
	Cognitive problems—T_1-T_0	−0.756 [a]	0.450
	Hyperactivity—T_1-T_0	−0.584 [a]	0.559
	ADHD Index—T_1-T_0	−1.842 [a]	0.065

[a] Based on positive ratings. [b] Based on negative ratings.

4. Narrative and Qualitative Reports

In addition to the numerical data that we have collected and analysed via statistical methods, we included a qualitative research approach, collecting descriptions of thoughts and emotions from participants through observation and interviews.

The focus is on exploring subjective experiences, with the aim to better clarify the impact of the intervention on the participants and to uncover insights and meanings of the experience.

The filmmaking programme represented a growth opportunity not only for the young participants, but also for all the professionals that contributed to the realization of the project. The power of this experience and the impact it can have on individuals is evident in the following reports. All of them shared a common experience of learning new skills, feeling like professionals, and becoming part of a group.

4.1. The Point of View of the Filmmaking Master

The filmmaking master was highly enthusiastic about the experience of mentoring the students in this pilot study. He commented positively on such issues as the changes he saw in the students, the positive impact on the participants, and how impressed he was with their participation. Figure 1 shows a behind-the-scenes photo shot on the film set.

As the filmmaker noted:

"For many years I have been carrying out intensive filmmaking courses, including academic ones, in various parts of the world. I have had students of all kinds, preparation, culture, age, language, and professions, but this has genuinely been my most surprising, gratifying and pleasant experience. Implementing a cinema project with such young kids was a challenge. Knowing then that these students had a difficult background and had psychiatric disorders left me uncertain about the possibility of helping them in my role as a director. But, surprisingly, I could see them following the first lessons with interest, travelling together on the bus for site inspections, casting, auditions and becoming more and more passionate. Then I saw them write their stories enthusiastically, get in front of and behind the cameras, stand at the microphones, and take the clapperboard. I saw them smile, communicate, and participate as a real team in an often tiring job full of responsibility and moments of stress. They came out stronger, aware of their abilities and proud to participate in something unique and unrepeatable. This was the real result that gratified me and made me proud. But even the strictly cinematographic results have been beyond all expectations. The stories of these short films, so intense and derived from an authentic and painful experience, have impressive communicative power. I called these young boys and girl "little giants" because of what they were capable of doing. But I would also call them little "seismographs" due to their incredible sensitivity in recording even the slightest painful movements of the world around them".

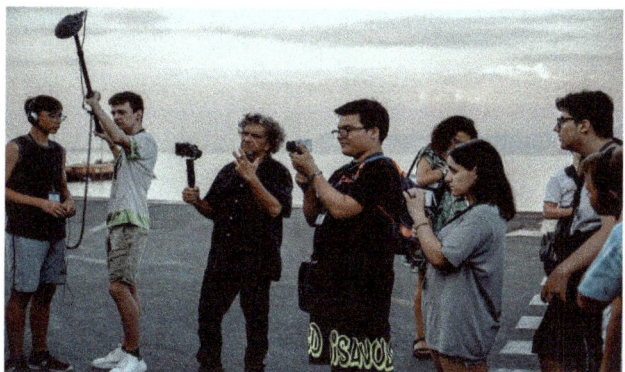

Figure 1. A behind-the-scenes photo shot on the film set.

4.2. The Narration from the Students

The participants of the filmmaking course were also elated to be part of the programme. The course provided a space for these young individuals to explore their creativity and discover their strengths, ultimately leading to a sense of empowerment. Through their words, we see how the magic of filmmaking can transcend barriers and inspire young minds to pursue their dreams.

Federico, a 13-year-old with a diagnosis of OCD and tic disorder says:

"It is impossible to describe in a few words the magic emotions that I experienced during the course. All of us learned new abilities. We felt like professionals, and we had the responsibility to use complex equipment. But above all, we felt like a big family. Unfortunately, it's all over, but everything we have done is still within us, in a special place in our heart. After this course I've decided that when I grow up, I'll work in the movie industry".

Alessio, a 12-year-old with dyslexia and autism spectrum disorder commented on the filmmaking experience. Even if the text is ungrammatical and full of errors, the meaning is clearly understandable:

"We don't know if this was a sign of destiny or if we are made to do things that giants do, but no one can express the emotions of this project. (In the sense that it is difficult to describe them). This project was beautiful (Arianna's thread). From this experience, I

understood that each of us has skills. Participating in a movie set with all the other kids was an incredible adventure. I hope more similar things are done. Anyone who has yet to experience it cannot understand." (Figure 2. Alessio's chat screenshot)

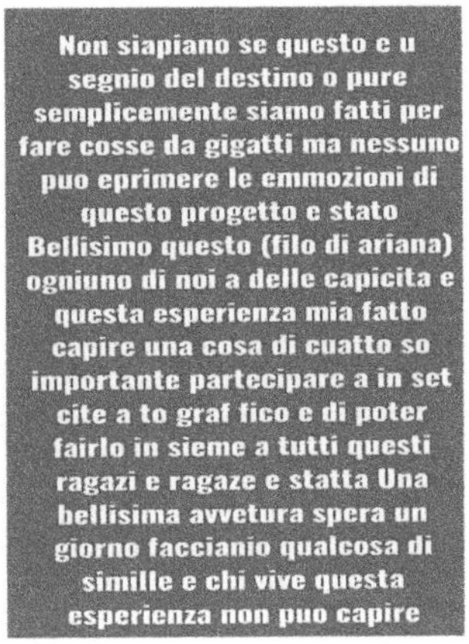

> Non siapiano se questo e u segnio del destino o pure semplicemente siamo fatti per fare cosse da gigatti ma nessuno puo eprimere le emmozioni di questo progetto e stato Bellisimo questo (filo di ariana) ogniuno di noi a delle capicita e questa esperienza mia fatto capire una cosa di cuatto so importante partecipare a in set cite a to graf fico e di poter fairlo in sieme a tutti questi ragazi e ragaze e statta Una bellisima avvetura spera un giorno faccianio qualcosa di simille e chi vive questa esperienza non puo capire

Figure 2. Alessio's chat screenshot.

5. Discussion

This pilot study aimed to explore the benefits of filmmaking therapy for individuals diagnosed with psychiatric or neurodevelopmental disorders in a consecutive sample of children and adolescents. This research is motivated by finding alternative and innovative ways to help children and adolescents with neuropsychiatric disorders in managing life challenges.

In this work, we measured the benefits of a filmmaking course by applying standardized scales widely used in the clinical assessment of developmental age. A systematic outcome measure was carried out pre- and post-programme in the context of a specialized mental health care team.

One of the strengths of this study is that it proves the effectiveness of filmmaking projects on children and adolescents affected by various psychiatric disorders, unlike previous studies that had enrolled patients affected by specific disorders such as ASD [11]. The study shows how an inclusive group offers to participants the opportunity to share their different skills and in a highly cooperative environment. It may improve creativity and self-expression, giving the participants a platform to share their perspectives with others. In fact, through storytelling, participants could learn how to convey emotions, communicate ideas, and engage their audience. Moreover, this requires effective communication between team members, and they learn how to explain their ideas clearly and persuasively and how to listen and constructively respond to others.

A second strength of the project Is that It allows the participants to create the stories and, therefore, to express their inner thoughts. The participants had the opportunity to translate their ideas and feelings into cinematic language, one of the most powerful and complete means of expression. They could learn to empathize with their characters and explain their message in a way that resonates with their audience.

The increase in the number of participants with high self-esteem we have noticed suggests that some of them changed the opinion they have of themselves. Improving the self-esteem or confidence of children and adolescents with psychiatric diseases is one of the main goals of educational interventions, with the purpose to avoid common behaviours, such as avoiding social situations and new and challenging experiences. In accordance with this result, the reduction in withdrawn/depression problems, measured by the Youth Self-Report scale, suggests a positive effect on the internalizing symptoms found in many psychiatric disorders.

Another important result was the decrease in social problems. Filmmaking requires collaboration and teamwork, as different people with different skills and perspectives come together to create a final product. Moreover, the "Social awareness" and the "Social motivation subscale", measured by the Social Responsiveness Scale, increased in all participants. Given that some of the patients were diagnosed as having ASD and that the SRS also offered a reasonable interpretation of characteristics regarding the improvement of reciprocal social interaction [22], we can expect a positive outcome of the course on social abilities, even in participants affected with ASD. Our data suggest that, as shown in previous studies focused exclusively on children with ASD [11], film production promotes the development of social skills in participants with diverse psychiatric diseases. In this way, participants learn to communicate effectively, listen actively, and provide constructive feedback. These skills are critical in any social setting and could help them develop empathy, respect, and cooperation. In addition, this could stimulate people to appreciate different perspectives and opinions, which is an essential component of social-emotional intelligence.

Our data also suggest that filmmaking could be a powerful tool for children and adolescents, providing creative expression, communication, collaboration, social awareness, and problem-solving opportunities. In fact, the thought problems and rule-breaking behaviours significantly decreased after the course.

Filmmaking is a complex and challenging creative endeavour that requires the use of a variety of cognitive skills and executive functions (EF) (motor response inhibition, working memory, sustained attention, response variability, and cognitive switching), which are mental control processes needed to carry out goal-directed behaviours and are fundamental to successful daily functioning across the lifespan [32]. Efs refer to a family of top-down mental processes needed to concentrate and pay attention when acting automatically or relying on instinct or intuition would be ill-advised, insufficient, or impossible [33–35]. Therefore, Efs are particularly important in children because they support the complex behaviours necessary for successful social interactions [36]. Deficient executive functioning has been implicated in social skills problems for many clinical populations of children. Moreover, EF impairment is commonly observed in many neurodevelopmental disorders, particularly autism spectrum disorder and attention-deficit/hyperactivity disorder. It has been estimated that 41% to 78% of individuals with ASD exhibit executive dysfunctions [37], and around 89% of children with ADHD were classified as impaired on at least one executive function component [38].

Lack of executive functioning was also detected in externalizing disorders (oppositional defiant disorders and conduct disorders) and some mood disorders (major depression, bipolar disorder). However, there are some variations in effect sizes. Apart from the classical "cold" EF, other mechanisms, including the so-called "hot" EF, i.e., motivational dysfunction, delay aversion, sensitivity to reward and punishment, and emotional processing, could be involved.

Creating a film involves many stages, from writing the script to planning the shots, filming, and editing. These stages require using a range of cognitive skills, including all the critical components of executive functioning.

Planning and organization are fundamental, from writing the script to scheduling the shoot and arranging locations and equipment. Filmmakers need to remember many details, such as camera angles, lighting, and sound while filming. It requires working memory, which is remembering information while using it to complete a task. Additionally, filming requires sustained attention to detail and the ability to switch focus between different aspects of the production. On the other hand, during the production schedule, it could be common to deal with unexpected changes, such as finding creative solutions to technical issues. It could help to improve the executive function of problem solving, which is the ability to identify and solve problems creatively and efficiently. Moreover, making decisions throughout the production process, such as selecting the location, choosing camera angles, and deciding on the best takes to use in the final edit, could enhance the decision-making steps.

During their work, participants had to be flexible and adapt to the changes in the group and the environment, maintain concentration by reducing external interference and distractions, and tolerate denials, frustrations, and routine changes.

In conclusion, participants could learn how to analyse situations, identify potential problems, and develop creative solutions. Consequently, this suggests that filmmaking, in the same way as other psychosocial interventions, could positively affect some executive functions. In the case of ADHD subjects, this can lead to the reduction in hyperactivity and inattention. This was not recorded in our work, due to the short time of the project and to the lack of psychometric assessments specifically for cognitive functions. We could hypothesize that more prolonged work might improve these outcomes.

Last but not least, thanks to this experience, which requires technology and media tools, participants could learn how to use cameras, edit software, and use other tools to create a final digital product. Some of the participants were inspired by the project to work in the cinema field in the future. This is another important result for adolescents having difficulty in designing their personal, social, and educational development.

The study had some potential limitations, represented by the small size of the sample and the absence of a control group, that limit the generalizability of the findings. In addition, it was conducted with limited time and resources, which can reduce the ability to collect detailed data. However, on the other hand, pre- and post-test comparisons were tested, and different statistically significant results were found. The group encompassed subjects with different and multiple diagnoses, and most participants affected by neurodevelopmental disorders show co-occurring psychiatric symptoms. However, the group was rather homogeneous since the participants shared neuropsychological and affective profiles and developmental trajectories. Additional research is needed in order to explore the effect of this kind of intervention on separate groups. Considering that the sample was not so wide, this was a denotative result, and with a larger sample, more significant results would emerge. More extensive studies will be necessary to test and refine research methods, procedures, and instruments. Larger patient samples and a systematic collection of standardized outcome measures are also needed. As more research is conducted in this area, we will better understand the benefits and limitations of this project as a therapeutic intervention.

6. Conclusions

This is a pilot study, but the preliminary results demonstrate that a filmmaking programme can result in measurable changes in emotional, behavioural, and social domains in children and adolescents with psychiatric or neurodevelopmental disorders. The projects that involve movies or videos could help develop new skills, increase awareness, and offer new ways of thinking about specific problems in various patient populations. Projects like this may also encourage children and adolescents with psychiatric disorders to develop skills in their personal and academic lives, explore their passions, and engage with the world around them.

Findings from this research project can offer an empirical basis for the effectiveness of a structured filmmaking method to be replicated in broader contexts (e.g., school and communities) in promoting children's psychological well-being.

In conclusion, the filmmaking programme proved to be a valid and complete psychosocial intervention to promote mental well-being in general and to strengthen specific weaknesses in young patients suffering from a psychiatric disorder.

Supplementary Materials: The following supporting information can be downloaded at: https://www.mdpi.com/article/10.3390/healthcare11121695/s1. Supplementary File S1: All scales we used for testing our sample are reported in this supplementary section. 1. Rosenberg Self Esteem Scale (RSE); 2. Youth Self-Report scale (YSR); 3. Social Responsiveness Scale (SRS); 4. Revised Conners' Parent Rating Scale (CPRS-R).

Author Contributions: Conceptualization, A.G., M.G. and L.B.; methodology, M.I. and L.B.; software, M.I., C.C. and L.V.; validation, L.V. and M.R. (Michele Roccella); formal analysis, M.I. and

L.B.; investigation, M.B., L.F. and M.R. (Micaela Rizzi); resources, C.S.A. and F.L.; data curation, C.C. and L.V.; writing—original draft preparation, M.B. and L.F.; writing—review and editing, C.C., A.G. and M.I.; visualization, C.S.A.; supervision, A.G. and M.G.; project administration, M.R. (Michele Roccella). All authors have read and agreed to the published version of the manuscript.

Funding: This research received no external funding. Participation in the filmmaking program was voluntary, without a reward system or financial or educational incentives.

Institutional Review Board Statement: The study was conducted in accordance with the Declaration of Helsinki and approved by the Ethics Committee of the Psychological Research and Intervention Center (CeRIP), University of Messina, code number n. 0032071 [UOR: SI001165-Classif. III/11].

Informed Consent Statement: Written informed consent was obtained from all subjects involved in the study. All caregivers received a full explanation of the study methods and purposes.

Data Availability Statement: The data presented in this study are available on request from the corresponding author. The data are not publicly available for privacy reasons due to the presence of sensitive information about the participants.

Acknowledgments: Special thanks go to Alessandro Zuddas, a great man and scientist who prematurely died, leaving a great void between scientific communities worldwide. He firmly believed in the usefulness of this course purpose to adolescents. His enthusiasm, knowledge, and passion have been an inspiration. We thank the AIFA APS association (Italian Association of ADHD Families), the Asperger Group ONLUS, (CuoreMenteLab), and the Buona Spa Società Benefit for support in organizational management.

Conflicts of Interest: The authors declare no conflict of interest. The funders had no role in the design of the study; in the collection, analyses, or interpretation of data; in the writing of the manuscript; or in the decision to publish the results.

References

1. Piao, J.; Huang, Y.; Han, C.; Li, Y.; Xu, Y.; Liu, Y.; He, X. Alarming changes in the global burden of mental disorders in children and adolescents from 1990 to 2019: A systematic analysis for the Global Burden of Disease study. *Eur. Child Adolesc. Psychiatry* **2022**, *31*, 1827–1845. [CrossRef]
2. Meherali, S.; Punjani, N.; Louie-Poon, S.; Abdul Rahim, K.; Das, J.K.; Salam, R.A.; Lassi, Z.S. Mental Health of Children and Adolescents Amidst COVID-19 and Past Pandemics: A Rapid Systematic Review. *Int. J. Environ. Res. Public Health* **2021**, *18*, 3432. [CrossRef]
3. Viner, R.; Russell, S.; Saulle, R.; Croker, H.; Stansfield, C.; Packer, J.; Nicholls, D.; Goddings, A.-L.; Bonell, C.; Hudson, L.; et al. School Closures During Social Lockdown and Mental Health, Health Behaviors, and Well-being Among Children and Adolescents During the First COVID-19 Wave: A Systematic Review. *JAMA Pediatr.* **2022**, *176*, 400–409. [CrossRef]
4. Patel, V.; Flisher, A.J.; Hetrick, S.; McGorry, P. Mental health of young people: A global public-health challenge. *Lancet* **2007**, *369*, 1302–1313. [CrossRef]
5. Panchal, U.; de Pablo, G.S.; Franco, M.; Moreno, C.; Parellada, M.; Arango, C.; Fusar-Poli, P. The impact of COVID-19 lockdown on child and adolescent mental health: Systematic review. *Eur. Child Adolesc. Psychiatry* **2021**, *1*, 1–27. [CrossRef]
6. Wallace-DiGarbo, A.; Hill, D.C. Art as Agency: Exploring Empowerment of At-Risk Youth. *Art Ther.* **2006**, *23*, 119–125. [CrossRef]
7. Boyd, C. Development and Evaluation of a Pilot Filmmaking Project for Rural Youth with a Serious Mental Illness | Candice Boyd—Academia.edu, 2010. Available online: https://www.academia.edu/1214133/Development_and_evaluation_of_a_pilot_filmmaking_project_for_rural_youth_with_a_serious_mental_illness (accessed on 27 March 2023).
8. Oliver, K.G.; Collin, P.; Burns, J.; Nicholas, J. Building resilience in young people through meaningful participation. *Aust. e-J. Adv. Ment. Health* **2006**, *5*, 34–40. [CrossRef]
9. Bradshaw, W. Finding a Place in the World: The Experience of Recovery from Severe Mental Illness—William Bradshaw, Marilyn Peterson Armour, David Roseborough, 2007. 2007. Available online: https://journals.sagepub.com/doi/abs/10.1177/1473325007074164 (accessed on 27 March 2023).
10. Johnson, J.L.; Alderson, K.G. Therapeutic filmmaking: An exploratory pilot study. *Arts Psychother.* **2008**, *35*, 11–19. [CrossRef]
11. Lepage, P.; Courey, S. Filmmaking: A Video-Based Intervention for Developing Social Skills in Children With Autism Spectrum Disorder. *Interdiscip. J. Teach. Learn.* **2011**, *1*, 88–103.
12. Smieszek, M. Cinematherapy as a Part of the Education and Therapy of People with Intellectual Disabilities, Mental Disorders and as a Tool for Personal Development. 2019. Available online: https://www.researchgate.net/publication/331832032_Cinematherapy_as_a_Part_of_the_Education_and_Therapy_of_People_with_Intellectual_Disabilities_Mental_Disorders_and_as_a_Tool_for_Personal_Development (accessed on 27 March 2023).
13. Goodwin, J.; Saab, M.M.; Dillon, C.B.; Kilty, C.; McCarthy, A.; O'Brien, M.; Philpott, L.F. The use of film-based interventions in adolescent mental health education: A systematic review. *J. Psychiatr. Res.* **2021**, *137*, 158–172. [CrossRef]

14. Marsick, E. Cinematherapy with preadolescents experiencing parental divorce: A collective case study. *Arts Psychother.* **2010**, *37*, 311–318. [CrossRef]
15. Bierman, J.S.; Krieger, A.R.; Leifer, M. Group Cinematherapy as a Treatment Modality for Adolescent Girls. *Resid. Treat. Child. Youth* **2003**, *21*, 1–15. [CrossRef]
16. Sacilotto, E.; Salvato, G.; Villa, F.; Salvi, F.; Bottini, G. Through the Looking Glass: A Scoping Review of Cinema and Video Therapy. *Front. Psychol.* **2022**, *12*, 6103. [CrossRef] [PubMed]
17. Dermer, S.B.; Hutchings, J.B. Utilizing Movies in Family Therapy: Applications for Individuals, Couples, and Families. 2000. Available online: https://www.researchgate.net/publication/261645349_Utilizing_Movies_in_Family_Therapy_Applications_for_Individuals_Couples_and_Families (accessed on 27 March 2023).
18. Christiansen, A. Social and Emotional Skills Training for Children: The Fast Track Friendship Group Manual. *J. Dev. Behav. Pediatr.* **2019**, *40*, 668. [CrossRef]
19. Available online: https://filmitalia.org/en/filmography/0/13194/ (accessed on 13 March 2023).
20. Available online: https://www.mymovies.it/persone/carmelo-bacchetta/278057/ (accessed on 13 March 2023).
21. Rosenberg, M. Rosenberg self-esteem scale. *J. Relig. Health* **1965**, *1*, 59–66.
22. Prezza, M.; Trombaccia, F.R.; Armento, L. La Scala Dell'Autostima di Rosenberg: Traduzione e Validazione Italiana. *Boll. Psicol. Appl.* **1997**, *223*, 35–44.
23. Achenbach, T.M.; Dumenci, L.; Rescorla, L.A. *Ratings of Relations between DSM-IV Diagnostic Categories and Items of the CBCL/6-18, TRF, and YSR*; University of Vermont: Burlington, VT, USA, 2001; pp. 1–9.
24. Ivanova, M.Y.; Achenbach, T.M.; Rescorla, L.A.; Guo, J.; Althoff, R.R.; Kan, K.J.; Almqvist, F.; Begovac, I.; Broberg, A.G.; Chahed, M.; et al. Testing syndromes of psychopathology in parent and youth ratings across societies. *J. Clin. Child Adolesc. Psychol.* **2019**, *48*, 596–609. [CrossRef]
25. Frigerio, A.; Cattaneo, C.; Cataldo, M.; Schiatti, A.; Molteni, M.; Battaglia, M. Behavioral and emotional problems among Italian children and adolescents aged 4 to 18 years as reported by parents and teachers. *Eur. J. Psychol. Assess.* **2004**, *20*, 124–133. [CrossRef]
26. Constantino, J.N.; Gruber, C.P. *Social Responsiveness Scale: SRS-2*; Western Psychological Services: Torrance, CA, USA, 2012.
27. Zuddas, A.; Di Martino, A.; Delitala, L.; Anchisi, L.; Melis, G. Ital-ian Norms and Italian Technical Manual of JN Constantino, CP Gruber. In *Social Responsivenss Scale â'SRS*; Giunti, OS: Firenze, Italy, 2010; pp. 1–67.
28. Conners, C.K.; Sitarenios, G.; Parker, J.D.; Epstein, J.N. Conners' parent rating scale--revised. *J. Abnorm. Child Psychol.* **1997**. [CrossRef]
29. Nobile, M.; Alberti, B.; Zuddas, A. *CRS-R. Conners' Rating Scales. Revised. Manuale*; Giunti Editore: Florence, Italy, 2007.
30. Bölte, S.; Poustka, F.; Constantino, J.N. Assessing autistic traits: Cross-cultural validation of the social responsiveness scale (SRS). *Autism Res.* **2008**, *1*, 354–363. [CrossRef]
31. Gianarris, W.J.; Golden, C.J.; Greene, L. The conners' parent rating scales: A critical review of the literature. *Clin. Psychol. Rev.* **2001**, *21*, 1061–1093. [CrossRef] [PubMed]
32. Dajani, D.R.; Llabre, M.M.; Nebel, M.B.; Mostofsky, S.H.; Uddin, L.Q. Heterogeneity of executive functions among comorbid neurodevelopmental disorders. *Sci. Rep.* **2016**, *6*, 36566. [CrossRef] [PubMed]
33. Burgess, P.W.; Simons, J.S. Theories of frontal lobe executive function: Clinical applications. In *Effectiveness of Rehabilitation for Cognitive Deficits*; Oxford University Press: Oxford, UK, 2005. [CrossRef]
34. Espy, K.A.; McDiarmid, M.M.; Cwik, M.F.; Stalets, M.M.; Hamby, A.; Senn, T.E. The Contribution of Executive Functions to Emergent Mathematic Skills in Preschool Children. *Dev. Neuropsychol.* **2004**, *26*, 465–486. [CrossRef]
35. Miller, E.K.; Cohen, J.D. An Integrative Theory of Prefrontal Cortex Function. *Annu. Rev. Neurosci.* **2001**, *24*, 167–202. [CrossRef] [PubMed]
36. Hunter, S.J.; Sparrow, E.P. Executive Function and Dysfunction: Identification, Assessment and Treatment Edited Executive Function and Dysfunction Identification, Assessment and Treatment. 2012. Available online: www.cambridge.org (accessed on 27 March 2023).
37. Alsaedi, R.H.; Carrington, S.; Watters, J.J. Behavioral and Neuropsychological Evaluation of Executive Functions in Children with Autism Spectrum Disorder in the Gulf Region. *Brain Sci.* **2020**, *10*, 120. [CrossRef]
38. Kofler, M.J.; Irwin, L.N.; Soto, E.F.; Groves, N.B.; Harmon, S.L.; Sarver, D.E. Executive Functioning Heterogeneity in Pediatric ADHD. *J. Abnorm. Child Psychol.* **2018**, *47*, 273–286. [CrossRef] [PubMed]

Disclaimer/Publisher's Note: The statements, opinions and data contained in all publications are solely those of the individual author(s) and contributor(s) and not of MDPI and/or the editor(s). MDPI and/or the editor(s) disclaim responsibility for any injury to people or property resulting from any ideas, methods, instructions or products referred to in the content.

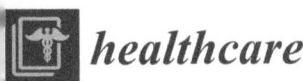

Systematic Review

Prospect Theory: A Bibliometric and Systematic Review in the Categories of Psychology in Web of Science

Júlia Gisbert-Pérez [1], Manuel Martí-Vilar [1,*] and Francisco González-Sala [2]

[1] Departamento de Psicología Básica, Universitat de València, Avgda. Blasco Ibañez 21, 46010 Valencia, Spain
[2] Departamento de Psicología Evolutiva y de la Educación, Universitat de València, Avgda. Blasco Ibañez 21, 46010 Valencia, Spain
* Correspondence: manuel.marti-vilar@uv.es

Abstract: Prospect Theory (PT) is an alternative, dynamic explanation of the phenomenon of risky decision making. This research presents an overview of PT's history in health fields, including advancements, limitations, and bibliometric data. A systematic and bibliometric review of the scientific literature included in the psychological categories of Web of Science (WoS) was performed following the PRISMA 2020 statement for systematic reviews. A total of 37 studies (10 non-empirical and 27 empirical) were included in the sample. Bibliometric results showed thematic variability and heterogeneity regarding the production, researchers, and methodologies that are used to study PT. The systematic results highlight three main fields of PT research: preventive and screening behaviors, promotion of healthy habits, and COVID-related decision making. Personal and contextual factors which alter the usual pattern specified by PT are also described. To conclude, PT currently has an interdisciplinary character suitable for health promotion, with recent studies broadening its applicability.

Keywords: prospect theory; applied psychology; health; decision making; behavior; prevention

1. Introduction

Decision making under risk has been a subject of social research for several centuries. This extensive scientific interest has allowed the development of a large theoretical and experimental body on decision making under risky conditions [1], leading to new models that have attempted to solve problems such as the excessive emphasis on normativity. This paper highlights the contribution of Prospect Theory (PT).

PT was created by Kahneman and Tversky [2,3]. It developed as an alternative explanation of risky decision-making processes to Expected Utility Theory [4]. PT contemplates the presence of heuristics and limitations in human cognition, which result in biases and deviations from what is considered normative. However, these deviations are considered systematic and could be studied to improve decision making [5].

PT is based on two fundamentals. The first points out that, in deciding between the different choice options, we depend on a frame of reference and not so much on the absolute value of the options, which violates the economic conception of rationality. The second foundation of the theory is loss aversion bias. Loss aversion refers to a greater sensitivity to potential losses than to potential gains of equal magnitude [5].

To justify these assumptions, controlled experiments were developed in which participants had to choose between different alternatives (usually two) with different probabilities of achieving certain outcomes [2,6]. The obtained results showed that the decision process comprised two phases, the editing phase and the evaluation phase. First, a reference point was set and the possible outcomes were framed as benefits or losses. The process ends with a personal assessment of the usefulness of the options [2,7]. Among the basic findings and principles of Kahneman and Tversky's theory [2,3], the S-shaped value function, the four-fold pattern of risk preferences, the "probability weighting function", the uncertainty effect, and "the reflection effect" are worth mentioning.

PT is a descriptive theory of human behavior which does not explain how people should theoretically make their decisions, but how they actually do [8]. It has been applied, not without difficulties, to different contexts, such as economics [5,9] and politics [10–12]. Likewise, its assumptions have been analyzed in more specific conditions, such as energy efficiency investment [13], terrorism [14], political participation [15], or climate policies [16].

One of Kahneman and Tversky's key insights was that the way risky decisions are framed influences what is selected, and it does so in a way captured by the assumption of an S-shaped value function defined on changes from the status quo [2,17]. Health decisions inherently involve risky choices [18]. Thus, consistent with what PT predicts, subsequent work demonstrated that the way in which health information is framed (to focus on potential gains (e.g., benefits of healthy behavior) versus losses (e.g., harms of unhealthy behavior)) systematically influences decisions and choices [17,19]. In addition, the COVID pandemic also involved risky decision making at the societal level. Consistent also with PT, gain- or loss-framing of health information influenced decision making, and risk-free behaviors may be promoted [20].

In addition to the framing effect, alterations in the expected pattern of loss aversion have also been studied. Regarding PT in the psychological field, its application in substance addictions stands out for its inherent risky decision making. [21]. According to PT, low levels of loss aversion increase the likelihood of engaging in addictive behaviors. Drug users have been found to show lower loss aversion than non-users [21]. All of this can be taken into account by healthcare personnel to understand the resistance and ambivalence in the decision-making processes in consumer patients.

Given its long-standing interest and applicability, the aim of this study is to conduct a bibliometric and systematic review of the PT literature in health settings within the psychology categories of Web of Science (WoS), in order to provide an overview of the usefulness, applicability and limitations of the theory within this scientific discipline. This will allow the creation of a new resource pool from which replications of previous studies, scientifically argued critiques, or even new experiments or theories can emerge, leading to more critical and informed scientific developments. It may also help psychology and health professionals to understand human cognitive issues and promote good health.

2. Materials and Methods

A systematic and bibliometric review of the scientific literature of Prospect Theory [2,3] in the main WoS database was conducted. A protocol was registered in PROSPERO, with identification code CRD42022348325. The search was conducted in September 2022 following PRISMA 2020 statement for systematic reviews [22]. SPSS 22 statistical package, R package Bibliometrix [23] and WoS analysis were used for the bibliometric review.

2.1. Information Sources and Search Strategy

A search was performed in the Web of Science database (Core Collection) with the search term "prospect theory" and "health". Other databases were not consulted due to the number of studies identified and the objective of exploring the WoS psychology categories.

2.2. Eligibility Criteria and Selection Process

In the systematic search, the inclusion criteria were (a) containing the term "prospect theory" and "health" in topic, (b) being a scientific article, (c) being included in one of the psychological WoS categories: "behavioral sciences", "neurosciences", "psychology", "psychology applied", "psychology biological", "psychology clinical", "psychology educational", "psychology experimental", "psychology mathematical", "psychology multidisciplinary", "developmental psychology", "psychology psychoanalysis", or "psychology social", and (d) being written in English or Spanish.

The exclusion criteria consisted o" (a)'addressing other topics (n = 80), (b) articles on other theories (n = 20), and (c) articles that were book chapters (n = 7). The selection and screening process is shown in Figure 1.

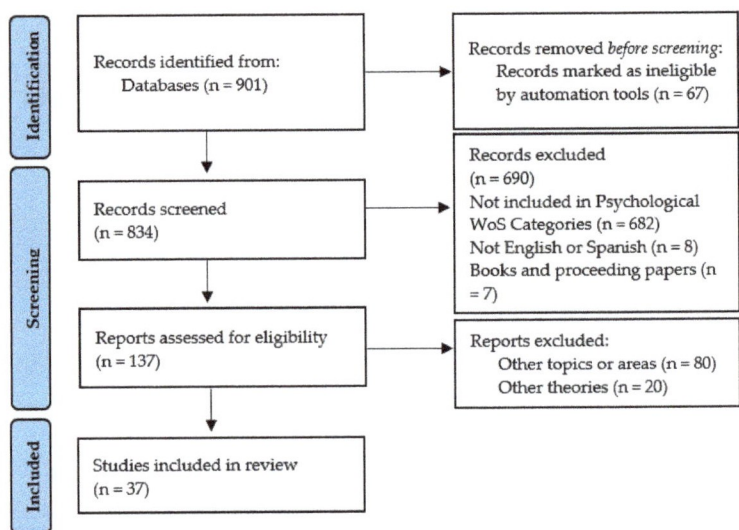

Figure 1. Flowchart of the selection and screening process of the systematic review articles according to the PRISMA method.

The selection process was performed by two investigators independently and then combined to reach a consensus. A third investigator supervised the results to confirm the quality of their work.

2.3. Data Extraction

After the selection and analysis process, the final sample contained 37 articles.

For the bibliometric review, the following variables were considered: year of publication, number of authors, distribution by country and continent, university affiliations, areas of research in psychology according to WoS, scientific journals, and key concepts. To perform the keyword co-occurrence networks), not all the terms were included, eliminating isolated nodes. For the systematic review, the following variables were considered: authors, year of publication, type of study, and main objective. For the empirical studies, we also extracted information on the sample, the methodology, the existence of a control group, and the main results and limitations. The bibliometric data extraction process was carried out using the WoS indicators, while data extraction for the systematic review was performed in the same way as the study selection process.

3. Results

3.1. Results of Bibliometric Review

Regarding TP production in the health field, the Figure 2 presents an irregular and increasing distribution with the highest production peak in 2021. In this year, several of the publications focused on the study and promotion of health behaviors in the COVID pandemic. The interest in applying PT to the field of health seems to have started in 1997, 18 years after the original study [2], indicating that the initial interests of this theory were focused on other fields. The last decade (2012–2022) accumulates 57% of the publications, highlighting the growing interest.

The sample includes 112 authors. Mainly, the contribution of P. Salovey (Yale University) to the field of health in PT (4 publications) stands out, followed by G. J. De Bruijn

(University of Amsterdam) and A. J. Rothman (University of Minnesota System) (3 publications). The rest of the authors contribute in 2 (12% of authors) or 1 publication (86%).

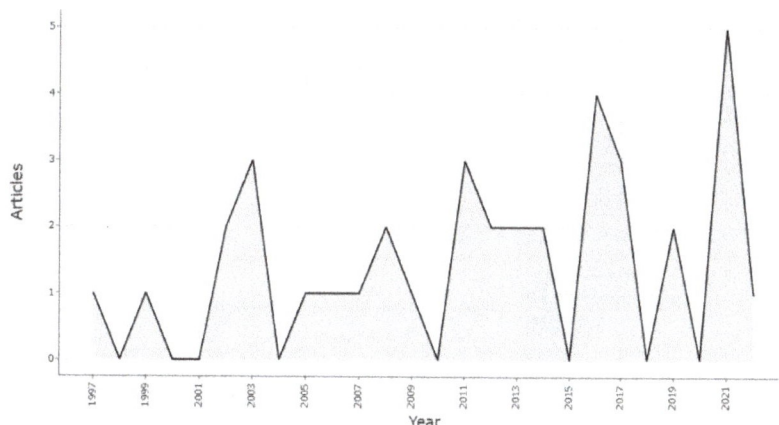

Figure 2. Annual scientific production.

Figure 3 shows the distribution of scientific production by country, considering both internal (CMI) and international (CCM) collaborations. The sample included 12 countries in the Americas, Europe, Asia, and Oceania, and a total of 142 related publications. The USA had 81 linked publications (57%), followed by the Netherlands (16; 11%) and Canada, China, and Germany (7; 5%). Accordingly, the top five universities with the highest affiliations are Yale University (4), Maastricht University (3), University of Amsterdam (3), University of Minnesota System (3), and University of Minnesota Twin Cities (3).

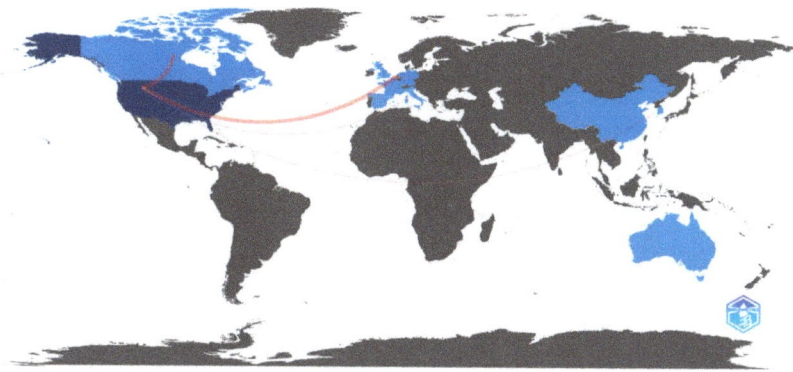

Figure 3. Country scientific production.

With 5 or fewer linked publications are Singapore, the UK, Australia, and France (4), Italy (3), South Korea (2), and Spain (1). Regarding international collaborations, the USA stands out with Canada and the Netherlands with two collaborations, followed by Germany–Spain–Netherlands, USA–Italy, and USA–South Korea with one collaboration.

Regarding the WoS psychology categories, the areas that appeared to be most linked to PT and health are Multidisciplinary Psychology (13 publications), Clinical Psychology (10), Psychology and Social Psychology (8), Applied Psychology (3), Experimental Psychology and Behavioral Sciences (2), and Developmental Psychology and Neurosciences (1). Among the categories that did not belong to Psychology, Economics and Public Environmental

Occupational Health (2) and Gerontology, Hospitality Leisure Sport Tourism, Management, Nutrition Dietetics, Oncology, Psychiatry, Social Sciences, and Biomedical and Sport Sciences (1) stood out (Table A1).

A total of 27 scientific journals present articles related to PT and health. The scientific journals with the highest number of articles on PT in the area of health are the *British Journal of Health Psychology, Health Psychology,* and *Journal of Applied Social Psychology* (3, respectively). *Journal of Behavioral Medicine, Journal of Economic Psychology, Psychology Health and Social,* and *Personality Psychology Compass* have two publications each. The remaining 20 have only one publication.

By analyzing the keyword co-occurrence networks, a general picture of the predominant terms in the study of PT and health was obtained. Figure 4 shows that "prospect-theory" was the term with the highest intermediation, i.e., presenting the highest number of links to other keywords. The other terms with the least intermediation were "intentions", "loss-framed messages", "behavior", "perceptions", "information", and "attitudes." The size of each block indicates the frequency of occurrence as an intermediate word. The figure shows three groups of keywords (blue, red, and green) and a closer link (by the thickness of the link) between "prospect-theory-behavior" and "behavior-intentions".

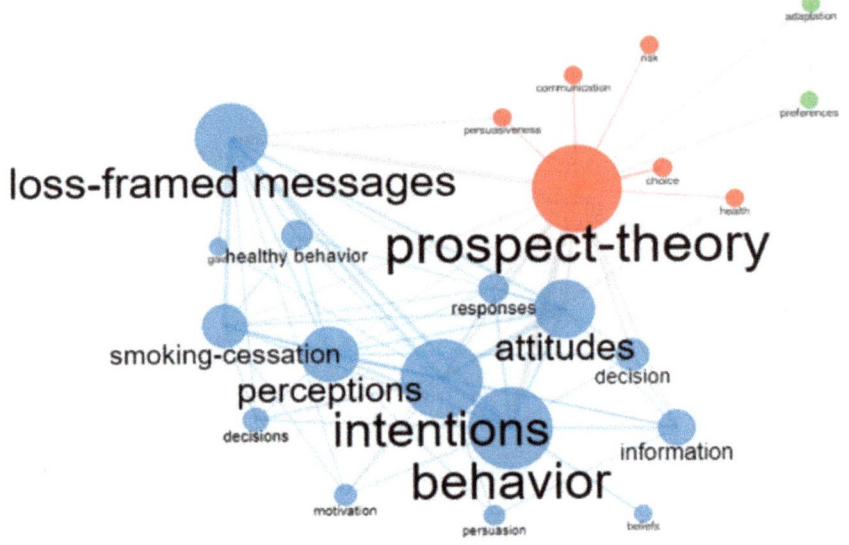

Figure 4. Co-occurrence network.

3.2. Results of Systematic Review

Tables A1 and A2 in Appendix A (non-empirical studies and empirical studies, respectively) show a synthesis of the data from the studies in the sample. Ten non-empirical studies (published between 1997 and 2021) and twenty-seven empirical studies (published between 1999 and 2022) were found.

3.2.1. Prospective Theory and Health Care Field

According to DeStasio [18], there are three main contributions of PT to the health domain. First, PT indicates that people will act differently depending on whether a situation is gain- or loss-framed compared to some reference point. Second, the reference point may have a particular impact on preventive health behaviors that are unpleasant themselves (e.g., vaccinations or invasive screening tests), where the risk of the immediate negative outcome (e.g., pain) is felt higher than the risk of the potential long-term outcome. Third, PT predicts that reframing health outcomes with respect to certainty would change decisions about health behaviors (as there is often an overweighting certainty).

PT assumes that people respond predictably to potential gains and losses. They are risk-seeking when confronted with information about losses, but risk-averse when confronted with information about gains [19]. Thus, in the health field, gain-frames may be more beneficial to promote preventive behaviors, as well as loss-frames to favor detection behaviors [24]. One possible explanation is that prevention behaviors are perceived as low risk, while detection behaviors are perceived as high risk [19,25,26].

There have been many examples of successful use of PT in modeling decision making in health care settings. For example, it has been used to model health behaviors such as disease treatment [26], disease prevention [27–31], and encouraging altruistic behaviors such as egg donation [32]. On the one hand, Fridman et al. [26] investigated the relationship between physicians' gain-loss recommendations and prostate cancer patients' treatment choices. Results showed that physicians' use of loss-related words correlated with recommendations for cancer treatment, and loss words were associated with patients' choice of treatment. On the other hand, similar results to those hypothesized by PT were obtained in disease prevention studies, but variables have been found to influence the framing effect such as cultural differences [28] and credibility of the result [30]. However, having family members with the disease to prevent did not influence decision making [31].

Another focus of PT study has been life attitudes in healthy and sick patients and reference point [33–37]. Current health status determines one's reference point. The reference point for an advanced cancer patient with a short life expectancy will be closer to death compared to an older adult with many years of expected survival. Thus, ill patients would prefer prolonging their life over quality of life, as was found in the results [33,34,36]. Likewise, sick patients rated a mild and a severe disease situation very differently, but healthy patients rated the two scenarios as much more similar [35]. In addition, having an overly pessimistic view of old age (e.g., not correctly predicting one's own ability to adapt to the health problems of old age) may produce a self-fulfilling prophecy, showing reduced sensitivity to loss and impacting their health behaviors (e.g., underinvesting in future health) [37].

Given PT usefulness, public health (PH) agencies could perhaps benefit from utilizing PT in a way that would optimize the effectiveness of PH messaging to increase overall local and global adherence [24]. On the one hand, expectations and disappointment regarding health may influence happiness. A practical implication would be that doctors exaggerate the risk of bad health outcomes in the future, and emphasize that patients could not have prevented bad current outcomes [38]. On the other hand, the differences in reference point in healthy and sick people can be applied to the promotion of care or insurance plans, considering the preferences of both groups [33]. Lastly, depending on the intention to prevent or treat, gain-loss frameworks can be applied to achieve attitudinal and behavioral changes [24].

Despite all the potentialities of PT, it also has weaknesses. For instance, Van't Riet's review [39] includes studies of framing in the health care setting with contradictory results [39,40]. Therefore, it is necessary to carry out precise analyses of the subtle differences in the messages that may influence the receptors' reactions.

It should be noted that in decision making, it is important to consider variables beyond framing and risk. Among the studies reviewed, personality aspects such as psychopathy, ambivalence (e.g., persistence of attitudes, resistance to change), impulsivity, anxiety, or health involvement stand out [41–43]. Overall, personality characteristics of the respondents played a more important role as predictors of risk choices mainly in the negative frame [42,43]. Likewise, with individuals with high ambivalence, a greater persuasion appears with a negative framing (and vice versa), due to a possible negativity bias [41].

3.2.2. Prospect Theory on Promoting Healthy Habits

PT has also been used to promote health-related attitudes and behaviors, which may reduce the occurrence of diseases. In the study of the framing effects on health issues, gain frames generally had an advantage over loss frames in promoting preventive behaviors (e.g., physical activity) [44,45]. Gallagher and Updegraff [44] concluded that "how a health message is framed is an important consideration in designing messages that promote preventive behaviors". In this regard, a gain message was associated with better semantic and affective evaluations of the message, but also a prime/frame and frame/source valence match was found more persuasive [45]. Hence, semantic consistencies must be taken into account, as they moderate the influence of message framing.

Therefore, it makes sense that, in the case of health-affirming behaviors such as physical activity (PA), messages framed around gains (i.e., benefits) rather than losses (i.e., costs) are often more effective [19,45,46]. PT has been applied through framed messages to promote PA [47], as well as the use of fitness apps [48]. The results of these studies showed an advantage of gain-framed messages in promoting sport intentions and attitudes, self-efficacy and sport practice itself [46,48]. Likewise, the effects of the framed PA messages were studied across all age and sex groups, demonstrating that older men may especially benefit from PA messages due to a possible age-related positivity effect [47].

In this context, although the gain frame in PA promotion is often more effective, it is important to consider the motivations associated with PA behavior and how the frame fits with these motivations [44]. All of this implies that the effect of framed messages is not simply based on the function of detection or prevention, but that personal motivations and interpretations must be considered. In addition, a possible interaction between source credibility and frame should be considered, as the gain frame together with a credible source (e.g., a physician) indicated higher exercise intentions and behaviors [49].

PT has also been applied to the promotion of healthy eating. On the one hand, PT predicted that the perceived positive value (i.e., benefit) associated with accumulating gains grows in an asymptotic, rather than linear, function [2]. This function applied to healthy intake suggests that less health gain may be associated with eating more pieces of fruit, and consequently, after having eaten a piece of fruit, individuals may see less value in eating more. This hypothesis was somewhat supported; health benefits that people assign to consuming increasing amounts of fruit appear to increase, but only if consumption of a variety of fruits throughout the day is considered [50]. On the other hand, the effect of autonomy on framing effects and fruit and vegetable consumption has been studied. Churchill and Pavey [51] observed that gain-framed messages only boosted fruit and vegetable consumption among those with high levels of autonomy; therefore, autonomy moderated the framing effect.

This gain-framing effect on preventive behaviors was also present in the use of sunscreen. Individuals who read gain-framed messages compared to the loss-framed ones were more likely to ask, repeatedly apply, and use sunscreen at the beach [52]. At the neural level, these results are consistent with greater activation of the medial prefrontal cortex (MPFC) to gain-framed messages. Higher MPFC activation reliably predicts subsequent behavior [53].

Moreover, in this sense, de Bruijn [54] explored the message framing effects to promote dental health using mouth rinse for 2 weeks. Their results coincided with the promotion of preventive actions, the gain-framed information to emphasize the preventive use of mouthwash being more appropriate. No framing effects were found in the detection conditions.

Frame effect on tobacco smoking cessation has also been studied [55]. Through messages framed in gain and loss and images illustrating positive and negative consequences, it was found that the intention to quit smoking was greater when negative images (e.g., unhealthy mouths) appeared, as well as when pictures of healthy mouths illustrated the presence of preventive action. On a practical level (e.g., health campaigns), the use of fear appealing communications with vivid negative images is one way to reduce tobacco use.

3.2.3. PT, COVID Pandemic, and Social Behaviors

Understanding framing effects in PH messaging is important for improving adherence, and it is particularly important when considering messaging where loss of life can be avoided, such as during the COVID-19 pandemic [24]. PT has been used to study risky decision making and the promotion of behaviors to reduce virus transmission, such as physical distancing or vaccination. People's behavioral response to a health crisis depends on how they perceive threat and their level of risk tolerance. Through PT, public health messages can be framed to influence adherence to health recommendations, taking into account other factors that may affect adherence.

Doerfler et al. [56] focused on risky decision making during the pandemic and its relationship with Dark Triad traits. Their results coincided with those presented by Tversky and Kahneman [57]. In a gain scenario (lives saved), individuals were more likely to opt for the certain option, thereby displaying a bias toward risk-aversion. In a loss scenario (lives lost), individuals were more likely to take greater risks.

During the COVID pandemic, maintaining an adequate physical safety distance was necessary to prevent the spread of the virus, especially indoors. Neumer et al.'s [58] online and field experiment with manipulated gain- or loss-framed messages showed that loss-framed messages were more effective than gain-framed ones promoting physical distancing. The loss-frame advantage suggests that uncertainty about the true effectiveness of distancing to avoid contracting COVID-19 is high and that people are more willing to accept this uncertainty when faced with a potential loss than gain.

Another behavior studied since PT has been vaccination during the pandemic. Vaccination is an important tool to end pandemics, but the majority of the public must be willing to be vaccinated to reach herd immunity. Using health message framing, Reinhardt and Rossman [43] conducted an online experiment with framed messages with younger and older samples. Loss frames lead to significantly more positive vaccination attitudes in younger adults than gain frames, which affects their vaccination intentions. However, the effects of gain- and loss-framed messages on vaccination attitudes and intentions in older adults did not differ significantly. This difference was explained by an age-related positivity effect in the older sample, since they ignored the negatively framed information in the loss frame condition and focused on the positive ones.

Finally, some moderators studied in relation to the framing of health message interventions during pandemics have been respondents' age, targeted beneficiaries (self or community), uncertainty (as mentioned above), loss-framing reactance, and personality traits as psychopathy, as mentioned above [24,43,56]. In relation to health, the age of respondents may imply differences in framing effects for variables such as positivity in older people [43]. Furthermore, greater persuasion has been found when messages are directed at the respondents themselves as opposed to the general community. Reactance is directly associated with attitudes and behaviors and is expressed in negative cognitions and emotions; therefore, it may result in more negative attitudes towards the promoted behavior [56]. Lastly, psychopathy emerged as the significant predictor of risk taking during the COVID-19 crisis.

4. Discussion

PT is a theory that attempts to explain dynamic changes in decision making, including aspects ignored by rational choice theories and highlighting the importance of situation and value in decision making [59]. In this study, a systematic review and bibliometric analysis of the literature on PT and health-related fields included in the WoS psychology categories was performed. The results of the bibliometric analysis have shown a growing international interest in the application of PT in health issues. The USA, followed by the Netherlands and Canada, have contributed the largest amount of literature on PT in health care settings. The analysis of the co-occurrence networks showed that the most frequent terms were prospect theory, intentions, behavior, and loss-framed messages, indicating the main interests of the application of PT in health.

Regarding the results of the systematic review, heterogeneity has been found in the topics, methodology, and even in some results. The application of PT in health has mostly focused on the framing effects to promote health behaviors and the importance of people's reference point. On the one hand, it has generally proven useful to use a gain frame to promote preventive health behaviors, whereas a loss frame seems to be more useful for treatment or detection behaviors. Therefore, when decision making involves low risk, gain-framed messages may be more effective, as well as loss framed messages in high-risk decisions. On the other hand, current health status is a key factor in decision making, as it determines the personal reference point. Current health status can influence the choice of future treatments or preferences about longevity or quality of life.

Other areas in relation to health that have been studied in PT have been the promotion of healthy habits. PT has been shown to be useful in promoting healthy habits, using gain-framing primarily. These behaviors, in turn, can be preventive, thus promoting wellness. Furthermore, the COVID pandemic situation has allowed numerous applications of PT in an intrinsically risky and uncertain context, especially in the promotion of preventive behaviors (e.g., social distancing, vaccination).

In summary, from a PT perspective, it is possible to encourage certain health-related behaviors depending on the framing, decision risk, and variables that may influence decision making. It is important to note that some results have been shown to be contradictory, thus requiring an analysis of the choices to be balanced, as well as consideration of variables that may influence decision making (e.g., personality traits, certainty of sources, cultural differences, age). All this can be taken into account when developing preventive or screening programs, as well as to promote healthy behaviors, considering the particularities of the targeted social sector (e.g., healthy or sick people).

In conclusion, this systematic and bibliometric review provides interdisciplinary evidence of the functionality of PT for the study of decision making under risk, highlighting both PT basis and factors that modify the expected decision patterns. Although these factors can be considered to hinder the applicability of PT, knowing its limitations can be very beneficial in extending the theory to new fronts. Understanding cognitive aspects such as decision making is essential in fields such as psychology and health, as it allows planning better assessments and interventions to promote well-being.

4.1. Limitations

The present study has several limitations. First, including only articles in the sample limits the complete knowledge of the study topic. Second, due to the size of the sample and the interest in the psychological categories of the WoS, other databases were not consulted. This meant that only studies categorized within the areas of psychology in WoS were included, thus providing a bibliometric and systematic approach limited to this area, which explains why studies such as the original [2] are not included in the sample. The interest in the psychological fields and PT lies in the importance of the cognitive part in decision making and its importance as a health science. Third, aspects such as the sampling method or the method of information extraction have not been considered because little information was provided in the articles in the sample.

4.2. Future Directions

First, a study of similar characteristics is proposed in other fields to broaden the study of PT. Second, it is proposed to conduct empirical studies that apply PT to specific fields or problems related to cognitive aspects or decision making within psychology and health, such as behavioral addictions. Third, it would be interesting to continue with the study of variables that alter the patterns expected by PT in order to extend the scientific knowledge. In this way, a more complete scientific framework would be obtained and the scope of the theory itself would be broadened. Fourth, it would be very useful to create a training program for health care and health professionals to promote preventive health behaviors and treatment. In this line, it would be interesting to test the applicability of PT with minors, in order to promote healthy habits in early ages.

Author Contributions: Conceptualization, J.G.-P.; methodology, M.M.-V. and J.G.-P.; software, M.M.-V., F.G.-S. and J.G.-P.; formal analysis, J.G.-P.; data curation, J.G.-P.; writing—original draft preparation, M.M.-V. and J.G.-P.; writing—review and editing, M.M.-V. and F.G.-S.; visualization, M.M.-V. and F.G.-S.; supervision, M.M.-V. and F.G.-S.; project administration, M.M.-V. All authors have read and agreed to the published version of the manuscript.

Funding: This research received no external funding.

Institutional Review Board Statement: Not applicable.

Informed Consent Statement: Not applicable.

Data Availability Statement: The raw data supporting the conclusions of this article will be made available by the authors, without undue reservation.

Conflicts of Interest: The authors declare that there is no conflict of interest.

Appendix A

Table A1. Non-empirical articles included in the systematic review.

Year	Author	Main Aim	Methodology
2021	Edwards [24]	Literature from behavioral economic, heuristic, and behavioral analysis in relation to explaining how cognitive biases in public health messaging, and how best to improve the effectiveness of PH messages	Review
2021	Kocas [32]	To apply PT and the anchoring heuristic to demonstrate how donors' initial exposure to information during recruitment, as well as the way in which risk is framed throughout, may influence their perception and decision making	Theoretical
2019	DeStasio et al. [18]	To describe how health psychology and neuroeconomics can be mutually informative in the study of preventative health behaviors	Theoretical
2016	Van't Riet et al. [39]	To examine the validity of the risk-framing hypothesis anew by providing a review of the health message-framing literature	Review
2016	Detweiler-Bedell & Detweiler-Bedell [25]	To explore the application of message framing, regulatory focus, construal level and psychological minds to goal setting and self-regulation, and they illustrate the powerful role of subjectivism in determining the effectiveness of health communication.	Theoretical
2012	Gallagher & Updegraff [44]	To distinguish the outcomes used to assess the persuasive impact of framed messages (attitudes, intentions, or behavior)	Review
2011	Mace & Le Lec [37]	To show that this fatalistic behavior can be explained through prospect theory by modeling this overly pessimistic view of old age as a failure to predict the change in the reference point due to hedonic adaptation	Theoretical
2008	Schwartz et al. [27]	To develop two approaches to reducing disutility by directing the decision maker's attention to either (actual) past or (expected) future losses that result in shifted reference points, on the basis of PT	Theoretical
2007	Siu [45]	To examine effective message design in the promotion of exercise through PT and other theories	Theoretical
1997	Rothman & Salovey [19]	To consider how health recommendations are framed, focusing on the differences in how message framing is operationalized in formal decision problems and experiments in applied domains To examine the impact of message framing on health-relevant decision To explore if the persuasiveness of a framed recommendation relies on the extent to which the message is accepted or deflected by its recipient	Review

PT: Prospect Theory.

Table A2. Systematic data of empirical studies.

Year	Author	Aims	Sample	Methodology	Control Group	Results	Limitations
2022	Neumer et al. [58]	To use a health message intervention to motivate customers to engage in distancing behavior	$N_1 = 206$ (M = 32.99, SD = 13.87, age range 14–78), $N_2 = 268$ (M = 43.68, SD = 17.14, age range 15–86)	Online and field experiment 2 × 2 (gain-loss framed messages and targeting different beneficiaries)	No-intervention baseline	The intervention was more effective when targeting customers than citizens (Exp. 1–2). Loss-framed messages were more effective than gain-framed ones (Exp. 2). Perceptions of risk/worry statistically mediated the effect of messages targeting self-benefits on distancing intentions and behavior	(1) Loss-frame manipulation represents the worst-case consequence (2) Self-developed shortened items (3) Not assess demographics for the Exp. 2
2021	Reinhardt & Rossman [43]	To investigate the effects of framing on younger and older adults' reactance arousal, attitudes toward the coronavirus vaccination, vaccination intention, and recognition performance	$N = 281$ (M = 50.1, SD = 23.5)	Online experiment 2 × 2 (gain-loss frame and participants' age)	Control variables	Loss framing positively influenced vaccination attitudes and led to stronger vaccination intentions among younger adults, but decreased recognition accuracy. No framing effects in older adults	(1) Cross-sectional data (2) Higher predisposition to vaccination in older adults (vulnerability for infectious diseases) (3) Possible socially desirable responding (4) Text-only stimuli
2021	Doerfler et al. [56]	To investigate the effects of message framing and personality in relation to risky decision-making during the COVID-19 crisis	$N = 294$ (M = 39.01, SD = 13.75, age range: 18–78)	Asian Disease Problem (modified) and Dirty Dozen Scale (personality)	No	Both gain- and loss-framing influenced risk choice in response to COVID-19, with more risk-averse in the loss condition. Psychopathy emerged as a significant predictor of risk-taking	(1) 40-year-old instrument (2) Brief measure of the Dark Triad traits (3) Sample limited to US-located participants
2021	Fridman [26]	To explore the association between words related to gains or losses and patients' choices following physician-patient consultations	$N = 208$	Analysis of transcribed consultations and pre-post treatment decisions	Control variable	Physicians who recommended immediate cancer treatment for cancer used fewer words related to losses and significantly fewer words related to death from cancer. Physicians' use of loss-related words correlated with recommendations for cancer treatment, and loss words were associated with patients' choice of treatment	(1) Automated text analysis (2) Focus on "gains" and "losses", just related to cancer survival or cancer death (3) Only male patients
2019	De Bruijn [54]	To explore the effects of message framing to promote dental hygiene	$N = 549$ (M = 47.4, SD = 16.1, age range 18–87)	2-weeks online experimental study 2 × 2 (behavioral function (detection or prevention) and message frame (gain or loss))	No Baseline	Participants were more likely to select a mouth rinse product that had a preventive function when that prevention function message emphasized gain-framed information. Message frame did not impact choice in the detection function condition	(1) Self-reported post-intervention measurement (2) 20% of participants were excluded (3) Priming task to induce either a general non-behavior specific risk-seeking or averse mindset
2017	Lim & Noh [48]	To examine the effect of message framing on users' intentions to adopt fitness applications	$N = 100$ (M = 22.3, age range 18–31)	Laboratory experiment employing a designed fitness app (gain- and loss-framed)	No	Advantage of gain-framed messages over loss-framed messages in increasing user's intentions to use the app. Gain-framed messages on users' intentions to use the fitness app was mediated through exercise self-efficacy and outcome expectations of exercise	(1) No long-term tracking of the behavioral change (2) One period of data collection (3) Text-based message intervention (4) Exercise limited to simple sit-ups

165

Table A2. Cont.

Year	Author	Aims	Sample	Methodology	Control Group	Results	Limitations
2017	Vezich et al. [53]	To extend predict real-world behaviors (sunscreen use) from neural activity by making direct links to select theories relevant to persuasion	N = 37 women (M = 20.43, SD = 2.44)	Questionnaires, fMRI and 40 text-based ads promoting sunscreen use	No Control ads	Greater MPFC activity to gain- vs. loss-framed messages, and this activity was associated with behavior Stronger relationship for those who were not previously sunscreen users results reinforce that persuasion occurs in part via self-value integration	(1) Not representative sample (2) Response rate could not be calculated
2016	Malhotra et al. [33]	To compare attitudes of community-dwelling older adults and patients with advanced cancer for length and quality of life and assess whether these attitudes change with age	N = 1067 CDOAs N = 320 stage IV cancer patients	Quality-quantity (QQ) questionnaire	Control for differences in sociodemographic characteristics	Lower proportion of CDOAs (26%) than patients (42%) were relatively more inclined towards length over quality of life. With increasing age, the difference in relative inclination between CDOAs and patients increased	(3) Possible differences in patients (4) Decisions possibly influenced by recommendations
2016	Burns & Rottman [50]	To examine how evaluations of healthiness change as participants consider eating increasing quantities of fruit and to explore how additional contextual features	N = 55 (M = 21.98) N = 72 (M = 20.6)	A 5 (quantity: 1, 2, 3, 4, 5) × 2 (variety: same, variety) × 5 (fruit type: apple, pear, orange, banana, peach) within-subjects design	No	Health benefits that people assign to eating increasing quantities of fruit seem to increase, but only if eating a variety of fruits throughout the day is considered	(1) Lack of ecological validity (2) Individual differences may interact with the manipulations employed
2016	Lucas et al. [28]	To examine the effect of gain versus loss-framed messaging as well as culturally targeted personal prevention messaging on African Americans' receptivity to colorectal cancer (CRC) screening	N = 132 African-American sample	Online education module about CRC, and exposition to a gain-framed or loss-framed message about CRC screening (2 × 2 × 2)	Yes	Cultural difference in the effect of message framing on illness screening White Americans were more receptive to CRC screening when exposed to a loss-framed message and African Americans were more receptive when exposed to a gain-framed message	(1) Statistically significant differences were not always observed for the reported health messaging differences (2) Small sample size and specific sociodemographic sample (3) CRC screening behavior was not presently assessed
2014	Van't Riet et al. [40]	To examine the validity of the risk-framing hypothesis	N_1 = 282 (M = 23.3, SD = 4.55, age range = 18–53) N_2 = 542 (M = 31.8, SD = 9.96, age range = 18–75) N_3 = 672 (M = 44.7, SD = 14.6, age range = 15–82) N_4 = 679 (M = 44.4, SD = 13.9, age range = 18–79) N_5 = 80 (M = 21.6, SD = 4.25, age range = 18–49) N_6 = 125 (M = 22.9, SD = 5.94, age range = 18–58)	Six empirical studies on the interaction between perceived risk and message Framing (two different countries and employed framed messages targeting skin cancer prevention and detection, physical activity, breast self-examination and vaccination behavior)	No	No evidence in support of the risk-framing hypothesis	(1) Behavioral intention as primary outcome (weak evidence that framing affects behavioral outcomes differently than attitudinal/intentional outcomes) (2) Some samples are women only

Table A2. Cont.

Year	Author	Aims	Sample	Methodology	Control Group	Results	Limitations
2014	Li et al. [47]	To compare message-framing effects on physical activity (PA) across age and gender groups	N = 111 younger adults (M = 2.31, SD = 3.04, age range = 18–35) N = 100 older adults (M = 71.66, SD = 7.48, age range = >60)	Questionnaires (IPAQ pre-post, Instrumental Activities of Daily Living and Subjective evaluation of the messages), accelerometer during 14 days.	No Manipulation check (demographics)	Significant age-by-gender by-framing interactions predicting self-report and accelerometer-assessed PA. Older men may benefit particularly from gain-framed PA promotion messages	(1) Self-report items (2) Limited generalizability (3) Not representative groups in terms of the demographic and health-related variables (4) More physical than social benefits
2013	Mathur et al. [29]	To investigate the effectiveness of health message framing (gain/loss) depending on the nature of advocacy (prevention/detection) and respondents' implicit theories (entity/incremental)	N_1 = 68 N_2 = 93 N_3 = 251	Exp 1. Two-part experiment randomly assigned to a gain or loss frame condition Exp 2. 2 × 2 (implicit theory × frame) between-subjects experiment Exp 3. 2 × 2 × 2 (implicit theory × frame × advocacy) between-subjects design	No	For detection advocacies, incremental theorists are more persuaded by loss-frames. For prevention advocacies, incremental theorists are more persuaded by gain-frames. For both advocacies (detection and prevention), entity theorists are not differentially influenced by frame. Entity theorists are message advocacy sensitive, regardless of the message frame.	
2013	Churchill & Pavey [51]	To explore whether autonomy moderated the effectiveness of gain-framed vs. loss-framed messages encouraging fruit and vegetable consumption	N = 177 (M = 21.46, SD = 5.89, age range = 18–57)	Prospective design involving two waves of data collection Questionnaires (demographics, baseline fruit and vegetable consumption, autonomy, framed messages, BMI)	No	Autonomy moderated the effect of message framing. Gain-framed messages only prompted fruit and vegetable consumption amongst those with high levels of autonomy	(1) Self-report measure
2012	Foster et al. [38]	To test the empirical implications of competing theories about how expectations of outcomes affect utility	N = 13,479 (M = 46.05, SD = 16.70)	6-year survey (demographics, SF-36 and health relevant behaviors scale)	No Baseline	Expecting good health in the future increases happiness now	(1) No direct effect of expected outcomes (2) Not clearly if it is sufficiently controlled for current health (3) Individuals relate their health to their prior expectations or to their actual health in the past

Table A2. Cont.

Year	Author	Aims	Sample	Methodology	Control Group	Results	Limitations
2011	Verlhiac et al. [55]	To examine if preventive-behavior framing and outcomes of action framing moderate behavioral intention to stop smoking when health messages are illustrated by pictures	N = 11 (M = 2.1, SD = 0.65)	2 (Preventive Action: presence vs. absence) × 2 (Outcome Behavior: gain vs. loss) × 2 (Outcome Pictures: healthy mouths vs. unhealthy mouths) between-subjects factorial design and questionnaires (State anxiety, behavioral intention)	Yes	Behavioral intention was higher when pictures of unhealthy mouths were presented, regardless of framing, and when pictures of healthy mouths illustrated the presence of preventive action	(1) External validity issues
2011	Gallagher & Updegraff [44]	To examine the effect of fit between the frame and the type of outcome emphasized in a message on subsequent physical activity	N = 192 sedentary adults (M = 19.0, SD = 1.91, age range 16–35)	2 × 2 (frame and extrinsic or intrinsic outcomes) and questionnaires (18-item Need for Cognition (NC) Scale, Exercise Attitudes, Follow-up Exercise, Past Exercise)	No	The predicted interaction between frame, outcome and NC was found such that a 'fit' message promoted somewhat, but not significantly, greater exercise for those with high NC, but a 'non-fit' message promoted significantly greater exercise for those with low NC	
2009	Winter et al. [34]	To examine through PT if sicker people evaluate quality of life in future health status more positively, compared to healthier people	N = 230 elderly people (M = 76.8, SD = 5.5, age range 69–95)	YDL questionnaire, ADL and IADL (current physical functioning) and demographics	Yes	Interaction between current health status and health scenario supported the relative acceptability of poor-health prospects to sicker individuals	
2008	Latimer et al. [46]	Messages to motivate the practice of physical activity emphasizing the benefits (gains) and the costs of inactivity (losses)	N = 332 sedentary people	Sending framed messages and a mixture of the two, and study of cognitive variables and self-reported physical activity in interviews on three occasions	Yes	Gain and mixed frame messages resulted in higher intentions and greater self-efficacy than the loss frame messages (week 2) Gain messages implied increased physical activity (week 9)	
2006	Lacey et al. [35]	To look at how patients and non-patients rate descriptions of health conditions that differ in severity	N = 159 lung disease patients (M = 67.5, SD = 11.3, age range 23–90) N = 196 healthy participants (M = 39.9, SD = 13.1, age range 18–83)	Survey materials with lung conditions with different levels of severity and QoL questionnaire	Context and no context condition	Perspective of the raters (i.e., their own current health relative to the health conditions they rated) influences the way they distinguish between different health states that vary in severity	(1) Measurement limitations (2) Sample homogeneity (3) Participant-related factors

(1) Relatively healthy sample
(2) Cross-sectional study
(3) Possible race effect

Table A2. Cont.

Year	Author	Aims	Sample	Methodology	Control Group	Results	Limitations
2005	Lauriola et al. [42]	To examine how personality factors affected both risk-taking in decision-making tasks and in real-world health behaviors	N = 240 (M = 46.99, SD = 19.01, age range 20–80)	Framing experiments 3 × 2 (framing condition × valence) about blood cholesterol level or vitamin consumption level Questionnaires (EPQ-R, BIS-BAS, Barratt Scale, the Multidimensional Health Questionnaire, and Coronary Heart Disease items	No	More risk-taking in the negative risky choice framing valence condition and more negative health status evaluation in the negative attribute-framing valence condition. Impulsiveness, Anxiety, Health Involvement and Health Negative Affect correlated with message effectiveness in the goal-framing task and with the observed risk attitude in the risky choice task	
2003	Apanovitch et al. [30]	To compare the effectiveness of 4 videotaped educational programs designed to motivate HIV testing among low-income, ethnic minority women	N = 480 (M = 32, SD = 8.76, age range 18–50)	Structured interviews pre-post, framed videotaped program, self-reported information (HIV and risk factors)	No	Participants' perceptions of the certainty of the outcome of an HIV test moderated the effects of framing on self-reported testing behavior 6 months after video exposure. In the certain outcome, those who saw a gain-framed video reported a higher rate of testing than those who saw a loss-framed message.	(1) Self-reported information (2) Increased perception of risk and uncertainty diminished the effects of message framing (3) No control condition
2003	Jones et al. [49]	To study the influence of the source credibility and message framing in the promotion of physical exercise in university students	N = 192 (M = 19.81, SD = 4.05)	Positively or negatively skewed messages and questionnaires to assess the impact on intentions and physical exercise	No	It is helpful to provide exercise-related information highlighting the benefits to motivate clients to exercise	(1) Homogeneous sample (2) Non-objective techniques (3) Lack of impact of persuasive communication on attitudes towards exercise
2003	Winter et al. [36]	To test PT as a model of preferences for prolonging life under various hypothetical health states	N = 384 older people in shared housing (M = 80.6, SD = 7.0)	QoL (Quality of life) questionnaire	No	Participants with health problems preferred a longer life with poorer health conditions than did healthy participants.	(1) General problems due to the type of sample
2002	Broemer [41]	To test the hypothesis that the degree of experienced ambivalence toward health behaviors moderates the impact of differently framed messages	Exp. 1. N = 80 (M = 24.4, SD = 3.89) Exp. 2. N = 120 (M = 25.2, SD = 3.15) Exp. 3. N = 80 (M = 17.6, SD = 2.65)	Health attitudes survey with two framed conditions and questionnaires (perceived personal risk, perceived relevance of health issue, ambivalence, evaluation of the message, attitudes, cognitive elaboration)	No	Highly ambivalent individuals are more persuaded by negatively framed messages whereas individuals low in ambivalence are more persuaded by positively framed messages	(1) Only male participants (exp.1) (2) Not provide direct evidence that ambivalence determines how much subjective weight is given to different health-related outcomes (3) Role of salient behavioral norms might affect reactions to persuasive appeals

Table A2. Cont.

Year	Author	Aims	Sample	Methodology	Control Group	Results	Limitations
2002	Finney & Iannotti [31]	To evaluate an intervention derived from prospect theory that was designed to increase women's adherence to recommendation for annual mammography screening	N = 929 (age range 40–69)	1 of 3 reminder letters (positive frame, negative frame, or standard hospital prompt	No	The hypothesis that women with a positive history would be more responsive to negatively framed messages, whereas women with a negative history would be more responsive to positively framed letters was not confirmed	(1) Small sample size (2) Is it possible that someone hadn't receive the message (3) Previous experience with mammography messages
1999	Detweiler-Bedell et al. [52]	Use PT to predict that messages highlighting potential "gains" should promote prevention behaviors such as sunscreen use best	N = 217 (M = 38.7, age range 18–79)	Experiment to compare the effectiveness of 4 differently framed messages (2 highlighting gains, 2 highlighting losses) to obtain and use sunscreen Questionnaires (attitudes and intentions)	No	People who read either of the 2 gain-framed brochures, compared with those who read either of the 2 loss-framed brochures, were significantly more likely to (a) request sunscreen, (b) intend to repeatedly apply sunscreen while at the beach, and (c) intend to use sunscreen with a sun protection factor of 15 or higher	(1) Brief intervention (2) Restricted nature of primary behavioral measure: requests for sunscreen with an SPF of 15 (3) Not collect long-term data

N: sample size, M: mean; SD: standard deviation.

References

1. Edwards, W. The theory of decision making. *Psychol. Bull.* **1954**, *5*, 380–417. [CrossRef] [PubMed]
2. Kahneman, D.; Tversky, A. Prospect Theory: An Analysis of Decision under Risk. *Econometría* **1979**, *47*, 263–292. [CrossRef]
3. Tversky, A.; Kahneman, D. Rational choice and the framing of decisions. In *Rational Choice: The Contrast between Economics and Psychology*; Hogarth, R.M., Reder, M.W., Eds.; University of Chicago Press: Chicago, IL, USA, 1987; pp. 67–94.
4. Von Neumann, J.; Morgenstern, O. *Theory of Games and Economic Behavior*; Princeton University Press: Princeton, NJ, USA, 1944.
5. Molins, F.; Serrano, M.A. Bases neurales de la aversión a las pérdidas en contextos económicos: Revisión sistemática según las directrices PRISMA. *Rev. De Neurol.* **2019**, *68*, 47–58. [CrossRef]
6. Holmes, R.; Bromiley, P.; Devers, C.; Holcomb, T.; McGuire, J. Management Theory Applications of Prospect Theory: Accomplishments, Challenges, and Opportunities. *J. Manag.* **2011**, *37*, 1069–1107. [CrossRef]
7. Mayer, R. To win and lose—Linguistic aspects of Prospect-Theory. *Lang. Cogn. Process.* **1992**, *7*, 23–65. [CrossRef]
8. Lim, S.L.; Bruce, A. Prospect theory and body mass: Characterizing psychological parameters for weight-related risk attitudes and weight-gain aversion. *Front. Psychol.* **2015**, *6*, 330. [CrossRef]
9. Barberis, N.C. Thirty years of prospect theory in economics: A review and assessment. *Natl. Bur. Econ. Res.* **2012**, *27*, 18621.
10. Clarke, S. A Prospect Theory Approach to Understanding Conservatism. *Philosophia* **2017**, *45*, 551–568. [CrossRef]
11. Vieider, F.M.; Vis, B. Prospect Theory and Political Decision Making. *Oxf. Res. Encycl. Politics* **2019**, *3*, 334–343.
12. Vis, B. Prospect Theory and Political Decision Making. *Political Stud. Rev.* **2011**, *9*, 334–343. [CrossRef]
13. Heutel, G. Prospect Theory and Energy Efficiency. *J. Environ. Econ. Manag.* **2019**, *96*, 236–254. [CrossRef]
14. Du Bois, C. A Prospect Theory Perspective on Terrorism. *Int. J. Bus. Soc. Res.* **2017**, *7*, 1–8. [CrossRef]
15. Herrmann, O.; Jong-A-Pin, R.; Schoonbeek, L. A prospect-theory model of voter turnout. *CESifo Work. Pap.* **2019**, *168*, 362–373.
16. Osberghaus, D. Prospect theory, mitigation and adaptation to climate change. *J. Risk Res.* **2017**, *20*, 909–930. [CrossRef]
17. Nan, X.; Daily, K.; Qin, Y. Relative persuasiveness of gain-vs. loss-framed messages: A review of theoretical perspectives and developing an integrative framework. *Rev. Commun.* **2018**, *18*, 370–390. [CrossRef]
18. DeStasio, K.L.; Clithero, J.A.; Berkman, E.T. Neuroeconomics, health psychology, and the interdisciplinary study of preventative health behavior. *Soc. Pers. Psychol. Compass* **2019**, *13*, e12500. [CrossRef]
19. Rothman, A.J.; Salovey, P. Shaping perceptions to motivate healthy behavior: The role of message framing. *Psychol. Bull.* **1997**, *121*, 3–19. [CrossRef]
20. Hameleers, M. Prospect Theory in Times of a Pandemic: The Effects of Gain versus Loss Framing on Risky Choices and Emotional Responses during the 2020 Coronavirus Outbreak—Evidence from the US and the Netherlands. *Mass Communitacion Soc.* **2021**, *24*, 479–499. [CrossRef]
21. Cabedo-Peris, J.; González-Sala, F.; Merino-Soto, C.; Pablo, J.Á.C.; Toledano-Toledano, F. Decision Making in Addictive Behaviors Based on Prospect Theory: A Systematic Review. *Healthcare* **2022**, *10*, 1659. [CrossRef]
22. Page, M.J.; McKenzie, J.E.; Bossuyt, P.M.; Boutron, I.; Hoffmann, T.C.; Mulrow, C.D.; Shamseer, L.; Tetzlaff, J.M.; Akl, E.A.; Brennan, S.E.; et al. The PRISMA 2020 statement: An updated guideline for reporting systematic reviews. *BMJ* **2021**, *372*, n71. [CrossRef]
23. Aria, M.; Cuccurullo, C. bibliometrix: An R-tool for comprehensive science mapping analysis. *J. Informetr.* **2017**, *11*, 959–975. [CrossRef]
24. Edwards, D.J. Ensuring Effective Public Health Communication: Insights and Modeling Efforts From Theories of Behavioral Economics, Heuristics, and Behavioral Analysis for Decision Making Under Risk. *Front. Psychol.* **2021**, *12*, 715159. [CrossRef] [PubMed]
25. Detweiler-Bedell, B.; Detweiler-Bedell, J.B. Emerging trends in health communication: The powerful role of subjectivism in moderating the effectiveness of persuasive health appeals. *Soc. Personal. Psychol. Compass* **2016**, *10*, 484–502. [CrossRef]
26. Fridman, I.; Fagerlin, A.; Scherr, K.A.; Scherer, L.D.; Huffstetler, H.; Ubel, P.A. Gain–loss framing and patients' decisions: A linguistic examination of information framing in physician–patient conversations. *J. Behav. Med.* **2021**, *44*, 38–52. [CrossRef]
27. Schwartz, A.; Goldberg, J.; Hazen, G. Prospect theory, reference points, and health decisions. *Judgm. Decis. Mak.* **2008**, *3*, 174–180.
28. Lucas, T.; Hayman, L.W., Jr.; Blessman, J.E.; Asabigi, K.; Novak, J.M. Gain versus loss-framed messaging and colorectal cancer screening among African Americans: A preliminary examination of perceived racism and culturally targeted dual messaging. *Br. J. Health Psychol.* **2016**, *21*, 249–267. [CrossRef] [PubMed]
29. Mathur, P.; Jain, S.P.; Hsieh, M.-H.; Lindsey, C.D.; Maheswaran, D. The influence of implicit theories and message frame on the persuasiveness of disease prevention and detection advocacies. *Organ. Behav. Hum. Decis. Process.* **2013**, *122*, 141–151. [CrossRef]
30. Apanovitch, A.M.; McCarthy, D.; Salovey, P. Using message framing to motivate HIV testing among low-income, ethnic minority women. Health psychology: Official journal of the Division of Health Psychology. *Am. Psychol. Assoc.* **2003**, *22*, 60–67.
31. Finney, L.J.; Iannotti, R.J. Message framing and mammography screening: A theory-driven intervention. *Behav. Med.* **2002**, *28*, 5–14. [CrossRef]
32. Kocas, H.D.; Pavlenko, T.; Yom, E.; Rubin, L.R. The long-term medical risks of egg donation: Contributions through psychology. *Transl. Issues Psychol. Sci.* **2021**, *7*, 80–88. [CrossRef]
33. Malhotra, C.; Xiang, L.; Ozdemir, S.; Kanesvaran, R.; Chan, N.; Finkelstein, E.A. A comparison of attitudes toward length and quality of life between community-dwelling older adults and patients with advanced cancer. *Psycho-Oncology* **2017**, *26*, 1611–1617. [CrossRef] [PubMed]

34. Winter, L.; Moss, M.S.; Hoffman, C. Affective forecasting and advance care planning: Anticipating quality of life in future health statuses. *J. Health Psychol.* **2009**, *14*, 447–456. [CrossRef] [PubMed]
35. Lacey, H.P.; Fagerlin, A.; Loewenstein, G.; Smith, D.M.; Riis, J.; Ubel, P.A. It must be awful for them: Perspectives and task context affects ratings for health conditions. *Judgm. Decis. Mak.* **2006**, *1*, 146–152.
36. Winter, L.; Lawton, M.P.; Ruckdeschel, K. Preferences for Prolonging Life: A Prospect Theory Approach. *Int. J. Aging Hum. Dev.* **2003**, *56*, 155–170. [CrossRef] [PubMed]
37. Macé, S.; Le Lec, F. On fatalistic long-term health behavior. *J. Econ. Psychol.* **2011**, *32*, 434–439. [CrossRef]
38. Foster, G.; Frijters, P.; Johnston, D.W. The triumph of hope over disappointment: A note on the utility value of good health expectations. *J. Econ. Psychol.* **2012**, *33*, 206–214. [CrossRef]
39. Van 't Riet, J.; Cox, A.D.; Cox, D.; Zimet, G.D. Does Perceived Risk Influence the Effects of Message Framing? Revisiting the Link between Prospect Theory and Message Framing. *Health Psychol. Rev.* **2016**, *10*, 447–459. [CrossRef]
40. Van 't Riet, J.; Cox, A.D.; Cox, D.; Zimet, G.D.; De Bruijn, G.J.; Van den Putte, B.; De Vries, H.; Werrij, M.Q.; Ruiter, R.A. Does perceived risk influence the effects of message framing? A new investigation of a widely held notion. *Psychol. Health* **2014**, *29*, 933–949. [CrossRef]
41. Broemer, P. Relative effectiveness of differently framed health messages: The influence of ambivalence. *Eur. J. Soc. Psychol.* **2002**, *32*, 685–703. [CrossRef]
42. Lauriola, M.; Russo, P.M.; Ludici, F.; Violani, C.; Levin, I.P. The role of personality in positively and negatively framed risky health decisions. *Personal. Individ. Differ.* **2005**, *38*, 45–59. [CrossRef]
43. Reinhardt, A.; Rossmann, C. Age-related framing effects: Why vaccination against COVID-19 should be promoted differently in younger and older adults. *J. Exp. Psychol. Appl.* **2021**, *27*, 669–678. [CrossRef] [PubMed]
44. Gallagher, K.M.; Updegraff, J.A. When 'fit' leads to fit, and when 'fit' leads to fat: How message framing and intrinsic vs. extrinsic exercise outcomes interact in promoting physical activity. *Psychol. Health* **2011**, *26*, 819–834. [CrossRef] [PubMed]
45. Siu, W.L. Prime, frame, and source factors: Semantic valence in message judgment. *J. Appl. Soc. Psychol.* **2007**, *37*, 2364–2375. [CrossRef]
46. Latimer, A.E.; Rench, T.A.; Rivers, S.E.; Katulak, N.A.; Materese, S.A.; Cadmus, L.; Hicks, A.; Keany Hodorowski, J.; Salovey, P. Promoting participation in physical activity using framed messages: An application of prospect theory. *Br. J. Health Psychol.* **2008**, *13*, 659–681. [CrossRef]
47. Li, K.K.; Cheng, S.T.; Fung, H.H. Effects of message framing on self-report and accelerometer-assessed physical activity across age and gender groups. *J. Sport Exerc. Psychol.* **2014**, *36*, 40–51. [CrossRef]
48. Lim, J.S.; Noh, G.-Y. Effects of gain-versus loss-framed performance feedback on the use of fitness apps: Mediating role of exercise self-efficacy and outcome expectations of exercise. *Comput. Hum. Behav.* **2007**, *77*, 249–257. [CrossRef]
49. Jones, L.W.; Sinclair, R.C.; Courneya, K.S. The effects of source credibility and message framing on exercise intentions, behaviors, and attitudes: An integration of the elaboration likelihood model and prospect theory. *J. Appl. Psychol.* **2006**, *33*, 179–196. [CrossRef]
50. Burns, R.J.; Rothman, A.J. Evaluations of the health benefits of eating more fruit depend on the amount of fruit previously eaten, variety, and timing. *Appetite* **2006**, *105*, 423–429. [CrossRef]
51. Churchill, S.; Pavey, L. Promoting fruit and vegetable consumption: The role of message framing and autonomy. *Br. J. Health Psychol.* **2013**, *18*, 610–622. [CrossRef]
52. Detweiler, J.B.; Bedell, B.T.; Salovey, P.; Pronin, E.; Rothman, A.J. Message framing and sunscreen use: Gain-framed messages motivate beach-goers. Health psychology. *Off. J. Div. Health Psychol.* **1999**, *18*, 189–196. [CrossRef]
53. Vezich, I.S.; Katzman, P.L.; Ames, D.L.; Falk, E.B.; Lieberman, M.D. Modulating the neural bases of persuasion: Why/how, gain/loss, and users/non-users. *Soc. Cogn. Affect. Neurosci.* **2017**, *12*, 283–297. [CrossRef] [PubMed]
54. De Bruijn, G. To frame or not to frame? Effects of message framing and risk priming on mouth rinse use and intention in an adult population-based sample. *J. Behav. Med.* **2019**, *42*, 300–314. [CrossRef]
55. Verlhiac, J.-F.; Chappé, J.; Meyer, T. Do Threatening Messages Change Intentions to Give Up Tobacco Smoking? The Role of Argument Framing and Pictures of a Healthy Mouth Versus an Unhealthy Mouth. *J. Appl. Soc. Psychol.* **2011**, *41*, 2104–2122. [CrossRef]
56. Doerfler, S.M.; Tajmirriyahi, M.; Dhaliwal, A.; Bradetich, A.J.; Ickes, W.; Levine, D.S. The Dark Triad trait of psychopathy and message framing predict risky decision-making during the COVID-19 pandemic. *Int. J. Psychol.* **2021**, *56*, 623–631. [CrossRef] [PubMed]
57. Tversky, A.; Kahneman, D. The Framing of Decisions and the Psychology of Choice. *Science* **1981**, *211*, 453–458. [CrossRef] [PubMed]
58. Neumer, A.; Schweizer, T.; Bogdanić, V.; Boecker, L.; Loschelder, D.D. How health message framing and targets affect distancing during the COVID-19 pandemic. *Health Psychol.* **2022**, *41*, 630–641. [CrossRef] [PubMed]
59. McDermott, R. Prospect theory in political science: Gains and losses from the first decade. *Political Psychol.* **2004**, *25*, 289–312. [CrossRef]

MDPI
St. Alban-Anlage 66
4052 Basel
Switzerland
www.mdpi.com

Healthcare Editorial Office
E-mail: healthcare@mdpi.com
www.mdpi.com/journal/healthcare

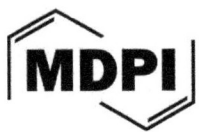

Disclaimer/Publisher's Note: The statements, opinions and data contained in all publications are solely those of the individual author(s) and contributor(s) and not of MDPI and/or the editor(s). MDPI and/or the editor(s) disclaim responsibility for any injury to people or property resulting from any ideas, methods, instructions or products referred to in the content.

www.ingramcontent.com/pod-product-compliance
Lightning Source LLC
LaVergne TN
LVHW070656100526
838202LV00013B/978